D1694348

SPRINGER
LABORATORY

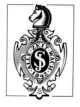

A. Rolfs   I. Schuller   U. Finckh   I. Weber-Rolfs

PCR: Clinical Diagnostics and Research

With 95 Figures

Springer-Verlag
Berlin Heidelberg New York London Paris
Tokyo Hong Kong Barcelona Budapest

Dr. med. ARNDT ROLFS
IRMELA SCHULLER
ULRICH FINCKH
INES WEBER-ROLFS

Freie Universität Berlin
Universitätsklinikum Steglitz
Abteilung für Neurologie
Hindenburgdamm 30
D-1000 Berlin 45

ISBN 3-540-55440-8 Springer-Verlag Berlin Heidelberg New York
ISBN 0-387-55440-8 Springer-Verlag New York Berlin Heidelberg

This work is subject to copyright. All rights are reserved, whether the whole or part of the material is concerned, specifically the rights of translation, reprinting, reuse of illustrations, recitation, broadcasting, reproduction on microfilm or in any other way, and storage in data banks. Duplication of this publication or parts thereof is permitted only under the provisions of the German Copyright Law of September 9, 1965, in its current version, and permission for use must always be obtained from Springer-Verlag. Violations are liable for prosecution under the German Copyright Law.

© Springer-Verlag Berlin Heidelberg 1992
Printed in Germany

The use of general descriptive names, registered names, trademarks, etc. in this publication does not imply, even in the absence of a specific statement, that such names are exempt from the relevant protective laws and regulations and therefore free for general use.

Product liability: The publishers cannot guarantee the accuracy of any information about dosage and application contained in this book. In every individual case the user must check such information by consulting the relevant literature.

Typesetting: Camera ready by author
25/3145-5 4 3 2   — Printed on acid-free paper

Foreword

In 1985, Kary Mullis was driving late at night through the flowering buckeye to the ancient California redwood forest, cogitating upon new ways to sequence DNA. Instead he came upon a way to double the number of specific DNA modules, and to repeat the process essentially indefinitely.[1] He thought of using two oligonucleotide sequences, oppositely oriented, and a DNA polymerase enzyme, to double the number of DNA targets. Each product would thene become the target for the next reaction, effectively yielding a product which doubled in quantity with each repeated cycle. Like the chain reaction leading to nuclear fission, with each cycle event each initial reactant (neutron or DNA molecule) yields two similar products, each of which can serve as the initial reactant. The invention of this exponentially increasing amplification system quickly became known as the polymerase chain reaction (PCR).

The tremendous sensitivity of PCR ultimately resides in the necessity for *each* of *two* specific oligonucleotide annealing reactions to occur at the same time in the proper orientation. The DNA annealing reaction is a very specific reaction. Single genes have been detected by hybridization of a DNA probe to chromosome preparations together with sensitive fluorescence microscopy. This is the equivalent to detecting a gene present in a single copy per cell genome. It is the combination of *two* such specific annealing reactions which makes possible the amplification needed to detect a single molecule with a specific DNA sequence in over 100,000 cell genomes. Although often a third "probe" nucleotide is used to determine the result of a PCR, it only provides a small proportion of the amplification and hence the sensitivity.

The PCR procedure *itself* has undergone a near exponential increase in interest. In 1985 and 1986, there was one article on the topic listed in the Medline (USA) database increasing each subsequent year to 4, 7, 337, 2046, and reaching 4436 articles in 1991. The ultimate in sensitivity, together with increasing ease of performance, have placed PCR in a central position in molecular biological research.[2] PCR promises to achieve similar status in clinical diagnosis.

The major advance in PCR practice was the development of a polymerase stable at the near-boiling temperatures employed in the PCR. The other major advance was the development of automated thermal cyclers. since these advances, other issues such as defining the proper primer sequences, and optimizing temperatures and times for denaturation, annealing and extension, have risen to the fore. The recently popularized "hot start" protocol may qualify as a third major advance.

For clinical diagnostic use PCR requires considerations of performance ease and reproducibility not a priority in research applications. PCR, especially when used to detect RNA genomes of immunodeficiency virus (HIV), is likely the most laborious procedure in the clinical diagnostic laboratory. Because it is a technically difficult and labor intensive procedure, it is not yet in armamentarium of the average clinical laboratory. Commercial efforts are underway to make the assay less labor intensive, and less prone to contamination. Homogenous detection systems, which require no seperation of the PCR products, would be ideal for this application. New opportunities for clinical diagnosis abound and commercial tests are just beginning to appear.

The authors have written a handbook of PCR techniques for those who would like to perform these in the research or clinical laboratory. Clinical diagnostic applications are emphasized. They have broken down the procedure into its component elements, carefully discussing the theoretical and practical details of each element. They have presented and explained the "rules of thumb" which guide the application of PCR theory to PCR practice. On the practical side, there are 14 detailed manuscripts in the Addendum which show specific cases of how PCR are put to clinical diagnostic use. The volume is replete with examples and specific recommendations derived from the experience of the authors.

The principles of PCR are presented in Chapter 1, with particular emphasis on the function of the initial denaturation and first extension steps and how these can be modified for optimum reaction. Specific optimization strategies are presented for both analytical and preparative PCR in Chapter 2.

The different applications of PCR are summarized in Chapter 3, and each of these applications are expanded upon in subsequent chapters. The authors present many "pearls", such as the observation that the single point mutation may be detected even if the concentration of the mismatched target is as much as 100 times higher than that of the target with the perfectly matched sequence. An exasperating phenomenon in the clinical application of PCR has been occasional sporadic failure of the procedure for no apparent reason. Chapter 4 details many of the causes and cures for such failures. Not only are inhibitory substances which interfere with the procedure detailed, but several specific procedures to eliminate them are presented.

No handbook on PCR is complete without consideration of the problem of contamination. Even such an insensitive procedure as the Southern blot has been prone to contamination of reagents. When a procedure, such as PCR, is sensitive enough to detect downwards to a single molecule, the possibility for contamination is extreme. Since the liquid in which the reaction takes place acts like aerosol, the sources of contaminants can include extraneous sample on a worker's fingers or pipets. Much more insidious and dangerous is the contamination of fingers, hair, doorknobs, or reagents with *PCR products*, since these products may be present in enormous concentrations. Procedures to avooid contamination are considered in detail in Chapter 5.

The preparation of samples is carefully considered in Chapter 6 and 7, which introduce three different procedures for isolating DNA from peripheral blood leukocytes as well as procedures for isolating DNA from mouthwashes and sputum, cells and tissue. The isolation of RNA from cells and tissue is detailed in Chapter 8, with procedures for avoiding endogenous and exogenous RNase contamination delineated in extreme detail. Three different methods to isolate RNA are presented.

Chapter 9 covers amplification of RNA targets, such as messenger RNA or viral RNA. RNA is amplified using so-called reverse transcription/PCR, or "RT-PCR", in which a reverse transcription step is the first step transcribing the RNA target to DNA for subsequent amplification. The usual reverse transcriptase enzymes have rigid pH optima and they are not very efficient enzymes. Thermostable enzymes with reverse transcriptase activity are introduced as possible alternatives.

The methods to assess the result of the PCR are covered in Chapter 10. In addition to the usual technique of gel electrophoresis, variations on this technique are presented, including several non radioactive detection methods. Chapter 11 covers methods of detection which use restriction endonucleases.

Although theoretically PCR is both extremely sensitive and extremely specific, practical considerations, such as the natural variation in nucleic acid sequences of infectious organisms or the many possible mutations possible in a single gene, often interferes with the procedure's success. Chapter 12 details an example of multiplex PCR detecting mycobacteria, in which more than one primer pair is incorporated into the same reaction.

Single base mutations are often the basis of genetic diseases. The detection of single base changes using PCR is detailed in Chapter 13, which presents different methods. Some of these depend on subtle differences in efficiency of elongation or on the exact primer-target mismatches on the 3' end of the primer.

PCR may also be used to sequence DNA. Unlike most other analytical uses for PCR, for this purpose the fidelity of the amplification is of paramount importance. Chapter 14 presents a system to sequence both single stands of a product using manual or automated sequencing methods.

Although PCR is generally a technique which requires knowledge of the target sequence, it can also be used to find "flanking sequences" adjacent to the known one. If a peptide sequence is known, the limited information imputed about the DNA sequence may be used to fish out the entire gene. The technique of "inverse PCR" is presented in Chapter 15, as are four additional related procedures.

Since PCR amplifies exponentially, the quantity of product varies markedly with very small differences in procedure efficiency. This characteristic makes PCR essentially nonquantitive. Nevertheless, there are very clever co-amplification or so called "competitive" amplification techniques which can result in a highly quantitive PCR or "QPCR". These techniques involve co-amplification of two targets - a known amount of nucleotide with a sequence minimally different from the target sequence, and an unknown amount of target sequence. The products are carefully quantitated. In Chapter 16 the authors provide theoretical background for competitive amplification, noting amplification efficiencies of various sized fragments as well as discussing possible solutions to the problem of product quantitation, such as differential liquid phase hybridization.

Two uses for PCR mainly of interest to the research laboratory are the creation of specific mutations, and cloning DNA in micro-organisms. These are discussed in Chapter 17 and 18.

One goal of molecular biologists has been the development of an *in situ* PCR - that is a PCR which could be performed on cell preparations or tissue sections. Since a simple non-radioactively labeled probe suffices to detect a single copy gene on a chromosomal preparation, why does one need *in situ* PCR? Either to detect a single copy gene in less favorable preparations such as tissue sections, or to detect less than a single copy gene such as a single HIV infected cell oout of 10,000. Two general techniques have been developed for this. The first partially cross-links cell membrane constituents in cytological preparation, making the cell membrane permeable to PCR reagents but not to the PCR products, the latter of which stay inside the cell and are then detected. The second utilizes a procedure to inhibit diffusion of products and is intended for use on tissue sections. They are discussed in Chapter 19.

One unsettled aspect of PCR methodology is how to determine the optimal primers for any given protocol. The lore is replete with guidelines, computer programs, and rules of thumb for producing well behaved primers that sensitively and specifically amplify but fail to produce non-specific product. In Chapter 20 the authors detail points of theoretical importance as well as practical importance in choosing optimal primers and purifying them appropriately.

The other major ingredient in the polymerase chain reaction is the DNA polymerase. If Taq polymerase is good, why isn't another more heat stable polymerase even better? It might be. These findings, and others regarding enzymes are detailed in Chapter 21.

For those readers contemplating the purchase of a thermal cycler, or optimal use of the one they already own, Chapter 22 details the different features of thermal cyclers and their consequences in PCR performance.

Finally, there are alternative amplification or chain reaction systems which may be better than the PCR in certain circumstances. Four are detailed in Chapter 23 including the robust ligase chain reaction.

A compendium of manuscripts are presented in the addendum which offer extensive information on specific techniques in three areas: the characterization of oncogenes, the detection of infectious agents, and basic methodology. These manuscripts cover topics which are likely to be of interest to many readers and describe procedures which, with modification only of primers and target, may be used directly in the reader's laboratories. Among the topics covered in this manner are the use of PCR for the detection of single base mutations, and direct sequencing of PCR products. Infectious agents for which PCR assays are presented include *Borrelia burgdorferi* - the bacteria causing Lyme disease; cytomegalovirus - a virus causing major complications in the immunosuppressed, and sequences related to the HIV virus. Specific methodological procedures presented include PCR based site directed mutagenesis, and the production of PCR synthesized probes for non-radioactive in situ hybridization.

This handbook is the complete source for PCR strategies, from introductory to advanced, for those who want to apply PCR to research or clinical diagnostic problems. There are concise compilations of proven methods, together with alternatives and rules of thumb, all designed to result in PCRs that will work in the reader's laboratory. This volume should be an invaluable reference for both the molecular biology and clinical diagnostic laboratories.

David Myerson
Fred Hutchinson Cancer Research Center, Pathology Section, SC-111, 1124 Columbia Street, Seattle, USA

---

[1] Mullis, KB: The unusual origin of the polymerase chain reaction. Scientific American 262;4:56-65,1990
[2] Science. Molecule of the Year

Preface

To write a book today dealing with the method of polymerase chain reaction seems a nearly superfluous undertaking when one takes a look at the flood of publications that have appeared since the first description in 1985 by K Mullis. However, in spite of the unusual enthusiasm surrounding this technique and the at times enormous sums spent for its further development, PCR is still performed by only a few centres routinely as a clinical service. Why is it that this method has not gained more acceptance in routine diagnostics in the last 7 years? Besides the problems and obstacles that have resulted from restrictions on licensing agreements, technical problems above all have prevented the PCR from becoming a clinical laboratory bench procedure. It has therefore been our goal - esp. in view of said numerous publications - to summarize PCR internal problems and describe the methods and measures that might be helpful to solve them. We have tried to make clear that numerous details must be taken account of for an optimal performance of PCR, esp. in the areas of patient sample requirements, rapid sample preparation techniques and elimination of inhibitors of PCR that are ubiquitous in biological samples.

Many thoughts and suggestions regarding PCR problems have emerged in the last two years in the framework of PCR practice laboratory courses that were run in Berlin by our working group. Here, we have repeatedly been confronted with basic questions that were not blocked by the expert's view and partly remain unsolved even today. Many original data on the methodology and improvement of individual detail problems in the PCR field have entered the book which would not have been worthwhile publishing separately, but which will certainly be able to give many new suggestions in the framework of a book. Numerous co-workers from our own working group have worked, with much effort and ardor, on the realization of this project. Of the many, only a few can be specially mentioned: thus, George Trendelenburg designed numerous figures and illustrations with much devotion to detail, Björn Heidrich contributed to the development of the data banks and DNA sequencing data, Joachim Beige made available hard-earned know-how regarding the preparation of DNA from difficult biological samples, Frank Tiecke contributed his experiences regarding the application of paraffin-embedded tissues, Andreas Ney the first results for the technique of DAF, and Thomas Plath his findings regarding new thermocyclers. All other co-workers of the laboratory, Heike Kallisch, Eva Lanka, Kay Lipka, Jan Lokies, Viviana Simon, Dagmar Steinhoff, Barbara Trampenau, Mathias Vallée, Freimut Wilborn, and our nice guest Hartwig Schwaibold, can here only be thanked for their support. The linguistic revision of this volume and its layout were, for the most part, undertaken by Maria Finckh and Kendall Martin (Corvallis, Oregon), Claus-Peter Eichhorst, Rainer Schaub, Christine Kebel, Justin Price, John O'Leary (Ireland), Beate Mildenberger and many others, kindly and always ready to help. By all means, mention must also be made of Mary Knoop, who influenced much - albeit indirectly - regarding the development of PCR technology in our laboratory.

We would also like to thank, above all, the scientists who, through their contributions to the addendum, have presented those subjects that the authors could not include in their contributions. The individual authors' experiences have, to a higher or lesser extent, also found their way into the 23 chapters of the book. However, it should not be left unmentioned that, above all, Ulrich Finckh devoted himself to fundamental problems of the PCR (e.g., chapters 1 and 2), Ines Weber-Rolfs, to the automation of the sequencing of PCR fragments, and Irmela Schuller to the basic problems of RNA methodology and reverse transcriptase PCR. Finally, we would like to thank Peter Marx, Director of the Department of Neurology at the Klinikum Steglitz, Free University of Berlin, for his patient support for the project, as well as Hanna Hensler-Fritton, Heike Berger and Thomas Narr from Springer Verlag/Berlin-Heidelberg for their permanent help, constant readiness to give information and infinite patience.

Berlin, August 1992   Arndt Rolfs (for the authors)

Table of contents

1. PCR: principles and reaction components — 1
    1.1. PCR: A cyclic, exponential, in vitro amplification process — 1
    1.2. Temperature and time profile of thermal cycling — 4
        1.2.1. Initial denaturation — 4
        1.2.2. Primer annealing — 4
        1.2.3. Primer extension — 6
        1.2.4. Denaturation step — 6
        1.2.5. Cycle number — 7
        1.2.6. Final extension — 7
    1.3. Taq DNA polymerase and reaction buffer — 7
    1.4. Deoxynucleotide triphosphates (dNTPs) — 9
    1.5. Primers — 9
        1.5.1. Primer-related PCR artifacts — 10
        1.5.2. Melting temperature (T_m) and optimized annealing temperature — 11
        1.5.3. Primer concentration — 12
    1.6. Oil overlay and reaction volume — 13
    1.7. DNA sample — 13
        1.7.1. Purity of samples — 13
        1.7.2. Homogeneity of samples — 14
        1.7.3. DNA content of samples — 14
    1.8. Size and structure of amplification products — 14
    1.9. PCR set-up strategies — 16

        Method: Mastermix PCR — 18

2. Optimization strategies — 22
    2.1. Analytical PCR — 22
        2.1.1. Specificity — 22
        2.1.2. Product analysis (agarose gel) and trouble-shooting — 25
        2.1.3. Sensitivity — 25
    2.2. Preparative PCR — 26
        2.2.1. Reamplification — 26
        2.2.2. Incorporation of label using Taq polymerase — 27

        Method 1: Reamplification of PCR products — 29
        Method 2: PCR synthesis of double- and single-stranded probes — 30

3. General applications of PCR
    3.1. Asymmetric PCR   34
    3.2. Allele-specific amplification (ASA)   34
    3.3. Nested PCR   35
    3.4. Multiplex PCR   36
    3.5. Differential PCR   36
    3.6. Competitive PCR   37
    3.7. Amplification of unknown sequences   37
    3.8. Application of PCR for genetic examinations, DNA amplification fingerprinting   38
    3.9. Amplification with consensus primers   40
    3.10. Expression PCR   40
    3.11. Detection of infectious agents or rare sequences   41

4. Substances affecting PCR: Inhibition or enhancement   51
    4.1. Inhibition introduced by native material   51
        4.1.1. Blood   52
        4.1.2. Fixed paraffin-embedded tissue   52
    4.2. Inhibition introduced by reagents during DNA isolation:
    Detergents, Proteinase K and Phenol   53
        4.2.1. Detergents   53
        4.2.2. Proteinase K   54
        4.2.3. Phenol   54
        4.2.4. Salts and buffer systems   54
    4.3. Additives influencing the efficiency of PCR   55
        4.3.1. Dimethyl sulfoxide (DMSO)   55
        4.3.2. Glycerol   55
        4.3.3. Formamide   56
        4.3.4. Polyehtylene glycol (PEG)   56
        4.3.5. TWEEN   57
    4.4. Evaluation of the effect of individual additives   58

        Method: Improving the efficiency of PCR amplification of HIV-1-
            provirus DNA from patient samples using a panel of additives   58

5. PCR: Contamination and falsely interpreted results   61
    5.1. Control experiments   61
    5.2. Sources of contaminations   63
        5.2.1. Pre-PCR contaminations   63
        5.2.2. Post-PCR contaminations   63
    5.3. Prevention and elimination of contamination   64
        5.3.1. Laboratory architecture   64
        5.3.2. Autoclave   64
        5.3.3. Working place and equipment   64
        5.3.4. Influence of contamination risks on experimental design   65

5.3.5. Decontamination procedures	65
5.3.6. Chemical modification of PCR products to prevent carryover	66

6. Biological material amenable to PCR — 68
    6.1. Sample preparation and storage — 68
        6.1.1. Peripheral blood leucocytes — 68

            Method 1: Selective lysis of red blood cells — 69
            Method 2: Buffy coat — 70
            Method 3: Isolation of mononuclear cells using FICOLL-PAQUE™ — 71

        6.1.2. Pharyngeal and mouthwashes — 73
        6.1.3. Sputum, bronchoalveolar fluids — 73

            Method 4: Preparation of mycobacterial DNA from sputum — 74

        6.1.4. Cerebrospinal fluid — 76
        6.1.5. Urine — 76
        6.1.6. Plasma, serum and other samples without host cellular DNA — 76
        6.1.7. Biopsies and solid tissue samples — 76
        6.1.8. Formalin-fixed, paraffin-embedded tissue — 76

7. Isolation of DNA from cells and tissue for PCR — 79
    7.1. Alkaline lysis — 79

            Method 1: Isolation of DNA using alkaline lysis — 80

    7.2. Guanidinium rhodanid method (GuSCN) — 81
    7.3. Proteinase K digestion for the isolation of DNA — 81

            Method 2: Proteinase K/phenol-chloroform extraction — 81
            Method 3: PCR-adapted proteinase K method for leucocytes or whole blood — 84
            Method 4: DNA isolation from paraffin-embedded tissue — 85
            Method 5: Detection of viral DNA from serum — 87

    7.4. Automated DNA extraction — 88

8. Isolation of RNA from cells and tissue for PCR — 90
    8.1. General preparations — 90
    8.2. Inhibition of endogenous RNases — 90
    8.3. Methods for the isolation of RNA suitable for RT-PCR — 91

        Method 1: Acid guanidinium thiocyanate-phenol-chloroform extraction   92
        Method 2: Microadaption of the guanidinium-thiocyanate/CsCl
                    ultracentrifugation method   95
        Method 3: Quick RNA isolation   96

9. Reverse transcription/PCR (RT-PCR)   99

    9.1. Setting up an RT-PCR   100
    9.2. Selective RT-PCR   102

        Method 1: RNase-free DNase treatment of RNA samples   103
        Method 2: Reverse transcriptase using MoMLV-RT   108

10. Methods for identification of amplified PCR products   112

    10.1. Agarose gel electrophoresis   112
        10.1.1. Electrophoresis equipment   112
        10.1.2. Gel loading buffer (GLB)   113
        10.1.3. UV-illumination and photography of stained gels   113
        10.1.4. Molecular weight markers and semiquantitative gel analysis   113

        Method 1: Agarose gel casting   115
        Method 2: Post-PCR sample loading   116

    10.2. DNA blot transfer and nonradioactive hybridization /detection   117
        10.2.1. Capillary transfer (Southern blot)   117

        Method 3: Southern blot from agarose gels   117

        10.2.2. Dot blot and slot blot procedures   119

        Method 4: Dot blot protocol   120

        10.2.3. Hybridization with digoxigenin-11-dUTP labeled DNA probes   120

        Method 5: Membrane hybridization procedure   121

    10.3. Detection systems of digoxigenin labeled hybrids   122

        Method 6: Chromogen detection (NBT/BCIP)   123
        Method 7: Chemiluminescence detection (AMPPD™)   124

    10.4. Polyacrylamide gel (PAGE) electrophoresis   125
        10.4.1. Separation of radioactive labeled amplification products and autoradiography   126

        Method 8: Vertical denaturing polyacrylamide gel   127

10.4.2. Detection of non-radioactive amplification products in PAGE using silver stain	131
Method 9: Silver stain of denaturing PAGE	133
11. Restriction fragment analysis	**136**
11.1. Restriction endonucleases	137
11.2. Endonuclecase selection	138
11.3. Optimal digestion conditions	139
Method: Restriction digest of PCR products	140
12. Multiplex PCR	**143**
Method: Detection of three different mycobacterial genom regions in a single PCR tube	145
13. Detection of single base changes using PCR	**149**
13.1. Allele-specific amplification (ASA, PASA, ASP, ARMS)	149
13.2. Allele-specific oligonucleotide hybridisation (ASO)	153
Method 1: Oligonucleotide hybridization using TMACl buffer	154
13.3. Chemical mismatch cleavage method	155
Method 2: Chemical cleavage of mismatches in PCR products	156
13.4. Denaturing gradient gel electrophoresis (DGGE)	159
Method 3: Denaturing gradient gel elctrophoresis	160
13.5. PCR single-strand conformation polymorphism (PCR-SSCP)	163
Method 4: Sngle-strand conformation polymorphism (SSCP)	165
14. Non-radioactive, direct, solid-phase sequencing of genomic DNA obtained from PCR	**168**
14.1. Generation of single-stranded DNA fragments	169
14.2. Sequencing of biotinylated PCR products	172
Method 1: Manual sequencing procedure	172
Method 2: Automatic sequencing procedure	180
15. Application of PCR to analyze unknown sequences	**184**

15.1. Inverse PCR ... 184

  Method 1: Inverse PCR ... 186

15.2. Alternative methods to inverse PCR ... 189
 15.2.1. "Alu-PCR" ... 189
 15.2.2. Targeted gene walking PCR ... 190
 15.2.3. "Panhandle PCR" ... 191
 15.2.4. Rapid amplification of cDNA ends (RACE-PCR) ... 193

  Method 2: Rapid amplification of 3´cDNA ends (3´-RACE) ... 196
  Method 3: Rapid amplification of 5´cDNA ends (5´-RACE) ... 197

16. Quantification of PCR-products ... 201

17. Cloning methods using PCR ... 208

  Method: Cloning and purification of a partial gag-sequence of HIV-1 using PCR ... 209

18. Site-directed mutagenesis using the PCR ... 216

19. In-situ polymerase chain reaction ... 219

20. Oligonucleotides in the field of PCR ... 221
20.1. Guidelines for designing PCR primers ... 221
20.2. Synthesis of primers ... 224
20.3. Purification of oligonucleotides ... 226

  Method 1: Purification of oligonucleotides by gel electrophoresis ... 227

  Method 2: Purification of oligonucleotides by reverse-phase HPLC ... 229

  Method 3: Quick purification of oligonucleotides using anion-exchange columns (OligoPak™) ... 232

20.3. Chemical modification of primers ... 233

  Method 4: Labelling of oligonucleotides by T4polynucleotide kinase ... 234

Method 5: Chemical labelling of oligonucleotides using photoactive biotin   236
Method 6: 3´-end biotin labelling by terminal deoxynucleotidyl transferase   237
Method 7: Modifications of the 3´terminus with a primary aliphatic amine   238
Method 8: 5´-end labelling by an amino linker during synthesis   240
Method 9: 5´-end labelling by introduction of a sticky-and restriction site in the PCR with subsequent incorporation by Klenow polymerase   242

21. Review of different heat-stable DNA polymerases   244
21.1. Taq DNA polymerase   244
21.2. Vent polymerase (Thermococcus litoralis)   248
21.3. Thermus thermophilus DNA polymerase   250
21.4. Pfu DNA polymerase (Pyrococcus furiosus)   250

Method: Amplification of a 365bp HIV-1-fragment using Pfu polymerase and influence of DMSO on amplification efficiency   251

21.5. Bst polymerase   252
21.6. Fidelity of different heat-stable DNA polymerases   253

22. Physical features of thermocyclers and of their influence on the efficiency of PCR amplification   259

23. Alternative methods to PCR   263
23.1. Ligase chain reaction (LCR)   263
23.2. Transcription-based amplification system (TAS)   265
23.3. Self-sustained sequence replication (3SR)   267
23.4. Q-beta replicase   268

Addendum:

Methodological examples for the application of the Polymerase chain reaction

A) Characterization of oncogenes

Detection of mutations at codon 61 of the c-Ha-ras gene in small precancerous liver lesions of the C3H mouse   A1
R Bauer-Hofmann, A Buchmann, F Klimek, M Schwarz

Isolation and direct sequencing of PCR-cDNA fragments from tissue biopsies — A4
H Klocker, F Kaspar, J Eberle, G Bartsch

Differential PCR: Loss of the ß1-interferon gene in chronic myelogenous leukemia (CML) and acute lymphoblastic leukemia (ALL) — A11
A Neubauer, C Schmidt, B Neubauer, W Siegert, D Huhn, E Liu

B) Detection of infectious agents

Long-term persistence of Borrelia burgdorferi in neuroborreliosis detected by polymerase chain reaction — A15
S Bamborschke, A Kaufhold, A Podbielski, B Melzer, A Porr, B Rehse-Küpper

Two-stage polymerase chain reaction for the identification of Borrelia burgdorferi in the tertiary stage of neuroborreliosis — A18
H Bocklage, R Lange, H Karch, J Heesemann, HW Kölmel

Screening for CMV infection following bone marrow transplantation using the PCR technique — A22
H Einsele, M Steidle, M Müller, G Ehninger, JG Saal, CA Müller

Detection of spumaviral sequences by polymerase chain reaction — A26
W Muranyi, R M Flügel

The use of PCR for epidemiological studies of HNANB viruses in arthropod vectors — A32
R Seelig, CF Weiser, HW Zentraf, C Bottner, HP Seelig, M Renz

C) Basic methodology and research applications

In vitro amplification and digoxigenin labelling of single-stranded and double-stranded DNA probes for diagnostic in situ hybridisation — A37
U Finckh, P A Lingenfelter, K W Henne, C Schmidt, W Siegert, D Myerson

Differentiation of arylsulfatase A deficiencies associated with metachromatic leukodystrophy and arylsulfatase A pseudodeficiency — A44
V Gieselmann

Molecular genetics of neuromuscular diseases - the role of PCR in diagnostics and research — A48
B Kadenbach, P Seibel

The application of polymerase chain reaction for studying the phylogeny of bacteria — A56
G Köhler, W Ludwig, KH Schleifer

Site-directed mutagenesis facilitated by PCR — A60
O Landt, U Hahn

Ectopic transcription in the analysis of human genetic disease — A63
J Reiss

Appendix I: Suppliers of specialist items — *A67*
Appendix II: List of Contributors — *A70*
Appendix III: DNA sequencing chromatograms — *A73*

Index — *A76*

1. PCR Principles and Reaction Components

1.1. PCR: A cyclic, exponential, in-vitro amplification process

The polymerase chain reaction (PCR) permits the selective in vitro amplification of a particular DNA region by mimicking the phenomena of in vivo DNA replication. The following reaction components are required: single-stranded DNA template, primers (oligonucleotide sequences complementary to the ends of a defined sequence of DNA template), deoxynucleotide triphosphates (dNTPs) and a DNA polymerase enzyme. A new DNA strand complementary to the desired template can then be enzymatically synthesized under appropriate conditions (see figure 1.1). The various reaction components for PCR are readily available. Single-stranded DNA template is easily generated by heat-denaturing (melting) double stranded DNA. Synthetic oligonucleotide primers can either be synthesized in one's own laboratory or purchased. The commonly used reaction buffers in PCR contain Mg^{2+}, monovalent cations and some co-solvents. The co-solvents may help to stabilize the enzyme, influence the enzyme processivity and/or DNA melting temperature (T_m). The introduction of a heat stable DNA polymerase (Saiki 1988, Mullis 1985), brought significant improvements to PCR and automation became a typical feature of PCR methods. Most of the DNA polymerases used in PCR are heat-stable and can withstand temperatures up to 95-97°C. The polymerase chain reaction itself requires three

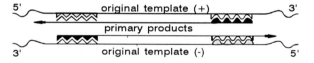

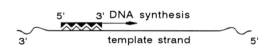

Figure 1.1: Enzymatic synthesis of a DNA strand starting at the free 3'-OH terminus of the primer. The newly synthesized strand will be complementary to the template. For symbols, see legend from fiigure 1.2.

Figure 1.2: First DNA thermoamplification cycle. DNA synthesis is started at two different priming sites on the two original template strands. Through the position of the primer annealing sites, each primary product contains again a newly synthesized primer annealing site. The newly synthesized strands from the primary products do not have a distinct length.

thermal steps: (1) denaturation of duplex DNA at 92-96°C, (2) annealing of the primers to a complementary site of the template at 45-72°C and (3) extension of the primer at the 3´OH by successive additions of dNTPs. DNA strand extension occurs at 72°C. The scheme of denaturation, annealing and extension with each step defined by a fixed period of time is called a cycle. The repetition of such cycles then leads to the amplification of DNA.

If two different primers - each selectively binding to one of the complementary strands - are extended past each other in a cycle of amplification, then each newly created DNA strand will contain a binding site for the other primer. In this fashion, each new DNA strand becomes a template for any further cycle of amplification, thus, enlarging the template pool from cycle to cycle. Repeated cycles of amplification theoretically lead to the exponential synthesis of a DNA fragment with a length defined by the 5´ termini of the primer pair employed. Exponential synthesis of a DNA fragment is expressed in the formula:

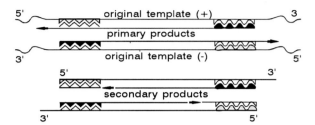

Figure 1.3: Second DNA thermoamplification cycle. After denaturation of the primary products from the first cycle, the primers anneal to the original strands and to the DNA synthesis products from the first cycle. Now, primary products and secondary products are created. The newly synthesized strands from the secondary products have a distinct length corresponding to the distance between the 5´ends of the two primers. For symbols, see legend from figure 1.2.

$$(2^n - 2n)x \qquad [1]$$

where n = number of temperature cycles,
$2n$ = primary and secondary extension products with indeterminate length,
x = number of copies of original template.

As depicted in figure 1.2, the primary extension products result from DNA synthesis on the original template during the first cycle. The secondary extension products result from DNA synthesis after denaturation of primary products and are amplified linearly during the next cycles (see figure 1.3 and table 1.1). They are of indeterminate length. In the third cycle, the first "target" fragments of a defined length are synthesized on the denatured secondary products (see figure 1.4). The length and genomic position of these fragments are defined through the primer sequences. After the first four cycles, an exponential amplification of such "target" fragments is to be expected.

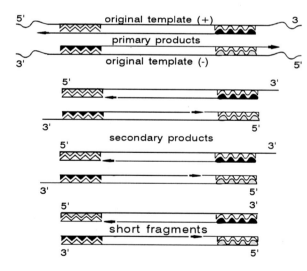

Figure 1.4: After the third cycle (only partially shown). The first short double-stranded fragments are synthesized on the denatured secondary products from the second cycle. In addition, again, primary and secondary products are synthesized. The short double-stranded fragments are amplified exponentially during the further cycles, the secondary products are amplified linearly. For symbols, see legend from figure 1.2.

In principle, each physical and chemical component

Exponential amplification of double-stranded short fragments

after cycle no (n)	copies (x) of double stranded template	double stranded amplification products 2nx		short fragments $(2^n-2n)x$	total $2^n x$
		primary products 2x	secondary products $x(2n-2)$		
0	1	0	0	0	1
1	0	2	0	0	2
2	0	2	2	0	4
3	0	2	4	2	8
4	0	2	6	8	16
5	0	2	8	22	32
6	0	2	10	52	64
7	0	2	12	114	128
8	0	2	14	240	256
9	0	2	16	494	512
10	0	2	18	1004*	1024
20	0	2	38	1048538*	1024^2
30	0	2	58	~1.1×10^9 *	1024^3
40	0	2	78	~1.1×10^{12}*	1024^4
50	0	2	98	~1.1×10^{15}*	1024^5

* assuming a 100 µl reaction volume are
- 10^3 molecules (~ 0.0017 amol)   17 aM = 17×10^{-18} M
- 10^6 molecules (~1.7 amol)   17 fM = 17×10^{-15} M
- 10^9 molecules (~1.7 fmol)   17 pM = 17×10^{-12} M
- 10^{12} molecules (~1.7 pmol)   17 nM = 17×10^{-9} M
- 10^{15} molecules (~1.7 nmol)   17 µM = 17×10^{-6} M

Table 1.1: Theoretical numbers of the various amplification products with indeterminate-length and short products. Numbers are given for x = 1 starting double-stranded template copy and assuming (1) 100% amplification efficiency, (2) that only one DNA strand per molecule of DNA polymerase is synthesized per cycle and (3) that the enzyme concentration is not reaction limiting. See 1.2.5 for further discussion.

of a PCR assay can be considered as a variable factor to be modified for a potential increase in quality. As will be shown, these factors are not independent of one another. Only for didactic reasons are they described in separate sections. These factors include:

1. Equipment, i.e., type of reaction tube, type of thermocyclers (see chapter 22).

2. Temperature and time profile of thermal cycling and cycle number.

3. DNA polymerase concentration; type of enzyme and reaction buffer including co-solvents (see also chapter 4).

4. Deoxynucleotide triphosphates (dNTPs) concentrations.

5. Primers (see also chapter 20).
6. Oil overlay and reaction volume.
7. DNA sample (amount and purity).
8. Size and structure of amplification product.
9. Set-up strategy.

1.2. Temperature and time profile of thermal cycling

The cycling parameters outlined here were found to be suitable for thermal cyclers with a **metal block** (DNA Thermal Cycler, DNA Thermal Cycler 480, *GeneAmp* PCR System 9600, Perkin-Elmer Cetus Instruments, USA; Polychain I, Polychain II, Polygen, FRG) or with **circulating water** (Thermocycler 60/1, Thermocycler 60/2, Biomed, FRG) using 500µl reaction tubes (Eppendorf Safelock™; Perkin-Elmer GeneAmp™) and a final reaction volume of 25-100µl. In all assays, Taq DNA polymerase from Perkin-Elmer was used.

1.2.1. Initial denaturation

One could attempt to remove impurities in a DNA sample, such as proteases or chloroform by heating the sample to 95°C once for approx. 10min before setting up a PCR.

Initial heating of the PCR mixture for 3 to 5 min at 95°C is enough to completely denature complex genomic DNA so that primers can anneal after cooling. The genomic DNA will never completely renature under the conditions of the following thermal cycles. The half-life of Taq DNA polymerase activity is 40 mins at 95°C (Gelfand and White 1990).

Heat damage of DNA leads to an increased nucleotide misincorporation rate during PCR (Eckert and Kunkel 1991). If high fidelity is desired, a minimum incubation time at high temperatures may be preferable.

1.2.2. Primer annealing

During PCR, the primer annealing step is the phase with the lowest prevailing temperature, provided a hot start technique (see 1.9.) is performed. Probably the most critical component for optimization of the specificity of a PCR assay is the choice of the annealing temperature.

In the very first cycles of an analytical PCR with genomic DNA as a template, primers must perform a "genomic screening" (Ruano 1991) until they find the complementary annealing sites. Among other things, the probability and specificity of primer annealing depends on temperature, time and the product of the concentrations of the single-stranded target (annealing site) and the primer. Under the right conditions, in the first cycles the target concentration doubles with each cycle and the relative decrease in primers is negligible. Thus the probability of successful primer annealing in the very first cycles is mainly determined by the target copy number and whether there is enough "genomic screening time" to find a target (provided the temperature allows specific annealing exclusively). If the temperature is too high, no annealing occurs at all, but if the temperature is too low, nonspecific annealing might increase dramatically. All primers that anneal at any site at their 3' terminus, irrespective of whether they anneal specifically or not, are elongated at the 3' end, even at the annealing temperature (synthesis rate of Taq DNA polymerase is 24 nucleotides/sec at 55°C and 1.5 nucleotides/sec at 37°C). In addition, at low temperatures, primers may hybridize to any genomic site with partial complementarity, not involving the 3´end, and thus, also not be available for specific screening.

For most purposes, the annealing temperature has to be optimized empirically and may sometimes depend on the method of sample DNA isolation. The T_m calculated with equation [2] in 1.5.2. is not necessarily a true estimate of the optimized annealing temperature

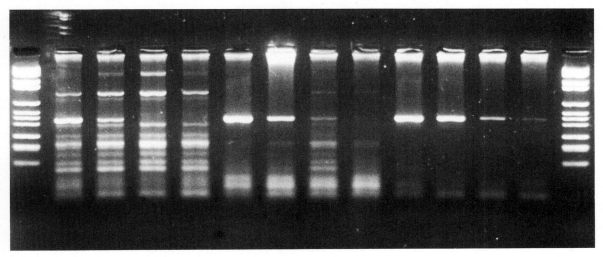

Figure 1.5: Amplification of a 435bp CMV IE-DNA fragment with three different annealing temperatures. Lanes **2-5:** 63°C; **6-9:** 66°C; **10-13:** 68°C. Each sample (lanes 2-13) contained 700ng seronegative human DNA (corresponding to approx. 10^5 diploid genomes) plus a variable amount of a linearized plasmid containing the CMV MIE DNA region with numbers as specified: $<10^4$ (lanes **2, 5, 9**), $<10^3$ (lanes **3, 6, 10**), $<10^2$ (lanes **4, 8, 12**), <10 (lanes **5, 9, 13**). Lanes **1, 14:** 250ng molecular weight marker VI (Boehringer; see chapter 10.1.4). Thermoprofile: 3min 95°C; 35 cycles with 20sec 94°C, 30sec annealing as stated, 20sec 72°C; 10min 72°C final extension; machine: DNA Thermal Cycler, Perkin-Elmer Instruments. Primers : 5'-CCAAGCGGCCTCTGATAACCAAGCC-3' (MIE-4), 5'-CAGCACCATCCTCCTC TTCCTCTGG-3' (MIE-5)(Demmler 1988). Buffer: GeneAmp™ 10xPCR Buffer (Perkin-Elmer Cetus). 9µl PCR product per lane.

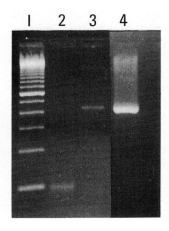

Figure 1.6: Influence on HIV provirus DNA amplification (env-region) from patient DNA by modification of the annealing time during the first 5 thermocycles in the outer fragment PCR from a nested PCR, the inner fragment PCR shown. Lanes **1:** 1µg 100bp ladder (Gibco BRL); **2:** non-DNA control, 20sec annealing; **3:** 25ng genomic DNA (approx. 3500 human genomes), 20sec annealing; **4:** 25ng genomic DNA, 2min annealing in the first 5 cycles, 20sec annealing in the following 35 cycles. Patient sample: 25ng genomic DNA phenol/chloroform extract from peripheral blood. Thermoprofiles and protocols: Outer fragment (658bp) PCR : 5min 95°C; 40 cycles with 40sec 95°C, 20sec 55°C, 60sec 72°C; final extension 10min 72°C (lanes **2** and **3**); 5 cycles 40sec 95°C, 2min 55°C, 60sec 72°C, 35 cycles 40sec 95°C, 20sec 55°C, 60sec 72°C; final extension 10min 72°C (lane **4**). 25µl reaction volume. Buffer: GeneAmp™ 10xPCR Buffer (Perkin-Elmer Cetus). 1 U Taq polymerase, 200µM dNTP, 0.6µM primers. Inner fragment (427bp) PCR: 3min 95°C; 40 cycles with 20sec 95°C, 30sec 55°C, 30sec 72°C; final extension 10min 72°C (lanes **2-4**). 100µl reaction volume. Buffer: GeneAmp™ 10xPCR Buffer (Perkin-Elmer Cetus). 2 U Taq polymerase, 200µM dNTP, 0.6µM primers. Outer primers: 5'-TAGTAGGAGGCTTGGTAGGT-3' (1246); 5'-GCTGCTGTGTTGCTACTTGT-3' (1247) [Rolfs unpubl.] Nested primers: 5'-CAGGAAACAGCTATGACC ATTGTAACGAGGATTGTGGAAC-3' (1270, sequencing primer with a 5'-terminal 18mer rM13 sequence); 5'-TAAAACGACGGCCAGTGCCAGCTGTGTTGCTACTTGTGATTG-3' (1271, sequencing primer with a 5'-terminal 20mer M13 sequence) (Rolfs unpubl.). Cycler: GeneAmp PCR System 9600 (Perkin-Elmer Instruments). 8µl PCR product per lane.

which may be up to 12°C above T_m. Note that at T_m, according to the definition, 50% of a hypothetical double-stranded oligonucleotide is melted. Thus the annealing/dissociation kinetics are shifted towards dissociation with any rise in temperature. Successful priming in PCR is not only a quantitative net result of primer annealing/dissociation kinetics, but also depends on whether or not primer extension takes place prior to primer dissociation (Wu 1991). Using Taq polymerase, the DNA synthesis rate increases with higher temperatures to an optimum at between 72 and 75°C. Thus for commonly used primers, the optimum temperature for the primer dissociation/extension balance will be higher than T_m. This and the fact that T_m increases with primer extension, might be the reason for the high optimum annealing temperatures for PCR. In other words; given sufficient excess of primers, a PCR may be run at higher annealing temperatures attain higher specificity and probably higher sensitivity (see figure 1.5).

Annealing time is usually between 20 and 40 sec. Only in cases where the ratio of target copy number to heterologous DNA is very low, as for example retroviral DNA in peripheral blood, longer annealing times (e.g., 2 min) in the first cycles might be advantageous to the genomic screening process (see figure 1.6).

Sometimes the evaluation of the optimum annealing temperature is the most time-consuming part of an optimization strategy. Higher than expected annealing temperatures may be necessary to minimize priming events due to secondary strcutures of both specific and nonspecific amplification artifacts. The highest annealing temperature giving optimum results should be used, provided that there is enough excess of primers for the later cycles.

1.2.3. Primer extension

In our experience, elongation at 72°C for 20 sec for fragments shorter than 500bp and 40 sec for fragments up to 1.2kb always gives satisfactory results. If secondary structures of amplification products are suspected to be present, longer elongation times should be tried (Gelfand, pers. communication), or an auto extension file used where the extension step lasts longer in the succeeding cylces.

Sometimes, it might be useful to integrate the elongation phase into a longer ramp time between a short annealing step and a short 72°C step to promote the elongation of the earliest annealing events.
If annealing is suitable at 68-72°C, a two-temperature PCR may be performed, with an overall incubation time of 20-40 seconds at the lower temperature.

1.2.4. Denaturation step

Denaturation at 95°C for 20-30 sec is usually sufficient. But it is essential to adapt the denaturation time to the tubes and PCR machines which are being used. In later cycles, lower denaturation temperatures may be better for preserving enzyme activity. The relatively short amplified fragments are more easily melted than complex DNA. If the denaturation temperature is too low, the incompletely melted DNA "snaps" back immediately when slightly cooled, thus giving no access to primers.

At the end of a PCR, the denaturation step should not be the last step. When they are cooled down rapidly, the resulting single-stranded fragments eventually form secondary structures instead of reannealing to the complementary fragments, which would lead to misinterpretations after product electrophoresis. Also, heteroduplexes might arise when a mixture of single-stranded PCR fragments is cooled down rapidly. Depending on the underlying specific sequence polymorphisms and prevailing artifacts, with partial sequence homologies, heteroduplexes might also disturb electrophoretic product analysis. For information on analysis of secondary structures of single-stranded DNA (= single-strand conformation) and hetero-duplexes, see chapter 13.

1.2.5. Cycle number

In an analytical PCR, the cycle number should not exceed 40. We have found that an amplification product originating from less than 10 molecules in an in an optimal reaction can generally detected in an ethidium-bromide-stained agarose gel after less than 40 PCR cycles. The most appropriate cycle counts are 25 to 35. Often, with increasing cycle numbers, unwanted amplification artifacts proliferate but not the desired product. The phenomena which arise with larger cycle numbers depend on (1) stringency and (2) which one of the components reaches reaction-limiting concentrations. One might expect that the amplification rate should change from exponential to linear ("plateau" effect) once the concentration of the amplification products exceeds the Taq concantration. Usually, in a PCR, 0.5 to 2.5 units of Taq polymerase are appropriate, corresponding to 25 to 125fmol of AmpliTaq™ enzyme (Perkin-Elmer Cetus) (Gelfand 1989, Lawyer 1989).

It is interesting to note that sometimes we observe product yields between 5-8pmol/100 µl (= 50-80 nM = $5-8 \times 10^{-8}$ M) for products shorter than 300 bp after 40 cycles with only 2 U Taq (= 100fmol/100µl = 10^{-9} M). This represents 50-80 fold excess of product concentration over Taq concentration. Such result suggest that one Taq molecule can extend more than one primer per cycle. This could happen if once annealed primers remain annealed until Taq "arrives" after completing previous extension(s).

If it is assumed that one molecule of a bacterial DNA polymerase does not catalyze the extension of more than one primer/cycle (Mullis 1991) during PCR, the maximum product synthesis rate/cycle should correspond to the absolute enzyme molecule number (here: 25-125fmol/cycle). For example, starting with 10^5 copies of template for amplification (assuming 100% amplification efficiency and no enzyme degradation) and 2U Taq (100fmol = 6×10^{10} molecules); 20 exponential cycles are required for synthesis of 100fmol of amplification product. Each additional linear cycle will then add 100fmol. Theoretically, based on this calculation 69 cycles would be required to produce 5pmol of amplification product. This is in contrast to the observed results.

When primers are consumed and there are still dNTPs available, amplificattion products and artifacts may start to prime themselves in subsequent cycles, often leading to longer products and smears in the gel. Such reactions might even lead to consumption of the extant specific product (Bell and DeMarini 1991). This phenomenon may be influenced by stringency in the annealing step, the cycle number, and primer and dNTP concentrations (see figure 1.8).

1.2.6. Final extension

Usually, after the last cycle, a 5-15min 72°C hold time is performed to promote completion of partial extension products and complete the annealing of single-stranded complementary products. After the optimization of an assay, it may be possible to omit any final extension and to allow the tubes to reach RT after a normal extension step. After PCR completion, the tubes can be stored at -20°C until needed for product analysis.

1.3. Taq DNA polymerase and reaction buffer

Only Taq DNA polymerase is mentioned in this section, because all the other components mentioned refer to this enzyme. See chapter 21 for other polymerases.
One unit of Taq DNA polymerase corresponds to 50 fmol of AmpliTaq™ enzyme (5 units/µl, Perkin-Elmer Cetus) (Gelfand 1989, Lawyer 1989).
Taq DNA polymerase lacks 3'-5' proofreading activity (Tindall and Kunkel 1988). The fidelity (i.e. nucleotide misincorporation frequency) of Taq polymerase depends upon the concentration of free Mg^{2+} and dNTPs, on whether the four dNTPs are balanced, on

pH, and on heat damage to the template DNA (see also chapter 21), among other things (Eckert and Kunkel 1991). If a DNA polymerase lacks proofreading activity, primers may be elongated in spite of a primer 3' terminus/template mismatch. In the case of Taq, the elongation will strongly depend on the type of mismatch. The following primer 3'-terminus/template mismatches significantly reduced PCR product yield after 30 cycles as indicated: C·C, G·A, A·G to <1%; A·A to <5%. All other mismatches did not decrease product yield (Kwok 1990).

The synthesis rate of Taq depends on temperature, [Mg^{2+}], detergent, template secondary structure, and [dNTP], among other things. Taq synthesis rate (nucleotides/enzyme molecule), as reviewed by Gelfand (1989) and Gelfand and White (1990), is as follows:

at 75-80°C :	150/sec
70°C :	>60/sec
55°C :	24/sec
37°C :	1.5/sec
22°C :	0.25/sec

The half-life of Taq DNA polymerase is as follows (Gelfand and White 1990)

at 92.5°C :	130min
95.0°C :	40min
97.5°C :	5-6min

The amount of polymerase is one of the more important factors to be optimized for a particular assay. For most assays, the optimum amount of enzyme will be between 0.5 and 2.5 units in a 50μl reaction volume. Increased enzyme concentrations sometimes lead to decreased specificity. But it is essential for diagnostic assays using different patient samples to use some excess of polymerase, because of the potential inhibiting activity of the sample.

The $MgCl_2$ concentration may be varied from approximately 0.5mM to 5mM to find the optimum. Mg^{2+} influences enzyme activity, increases T_m of dsDNA, and forms soluble complexes with dNTP, which is essential for dNTP incorporation. The concentration of free Mg^{2+} depends on [dNTP], [PP_i] and [EDTA]. Each of these compounds binds stoichiometrically with Mg^{2+}.

For many optimization strategies, it will be suitable to modify neither [Mg^{2+}] nor [dNTP] before all the other reaction components are optimized. If [$MgCl_2$] modification is planned, it is advisable to store $MgCl_2$ stock solutions at -20°C, due to the hygroscopic properties of $MgCl_2$, which make it impossible to weigh out the salt consistently. For optimization assays, it is possible however, to reduce [Mg^{2+}] through the addition of EDTA(see figure 1.7).

In our experience, the use of the commercially available 10 x reaction buffer (GeneAmp™ 10xPCR Buffer, Perkin-Elmer Cetus) leads to consistent and satisfactory results over a broad range of different assays. The components of the 10 x buffer are:

100 mM Tris-HCl, pH 8.3 (at room temperature)
500 mM KCl
15 mM $MgCl_2$
0.01% (w/v) gelatin

The following modified nucleotides may be used as substrates for Taq polymerase:

Nucleotide	Example of use
[α-P^{32}]dNTPs	radiolabeling of amplification product
[α-^{35}S]dATP	radiolabeling of amplification product
[α-^{35}S]dCTP	radiolabeling of amplification product
ddNTPs	chain termination sequencing reaction
dUTP	substitutes dTTP for contamination prevention after digestion by *uracil N-glycosylase(UNG)*
Biotin-11-dUTP	nonradioactive probe labeling
Biotin-16-dUTP	nonradioactive probe labeling
Biotin-21-dUTP	nonradioactive probe labeling
Digoxigenin-11-dUTP	nonradioactive probe labeling
7-deaza-dGTP	decrease of secondary structure of amplification product

Numerous substances exist which promote or inhibit the PCR process. Some of them will be reviewed in chapter 4.

Note: Some components, reported by several authors as being essential, especially detergents (for example Taylor 1991), are added to the reaction mixture with the enzyme, which is delivered in a specific storage

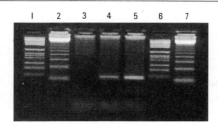

Figure 1.7: Addition of variable amounts of EDTA. Reamplification of a 139bp fragment from a CMV late gene (gp64). Initial template input: approx. 100 copies. In addition, each sample (lanes **3-5**) contained 700ng seronegative human DNA (corresponding to approx. 10^5 diploid genomes). The final EDTA concentration in lanes **3, 4, 5** respectively was 1, 0.6, 0.2 mM. The final $MgCl_2$ concentration was 1.5mM in each sample. 50µl reaction volume, 1.5 units Taq, 100µM dNTP. Buffer: GeneAmp™ 10xPCR Buffer (Perkin-Elmer Cetus). Primers: 5'-CCG CAACCTGGTGCCCATGG-3' (LA1) , 5'-CGTTTGGG TTGCGCAGCGGG-3' (LA2) (Shibata 1988). Thermoprofile: 3min 95°C; 35 cycles with 20 sec 94°C, 30sec annealing and extension at 72°C; 10min 72°C final extension; machine: DNA Thermal Cycler, Perkin-Elmer Instruments. Molecular weight markers: 1µg 123bp ladder (Gibco BRL) (lane **1**); 250ng molecular weight marker VI (Boehringer; see chapter 10.1.4) (lane **2**). 10µl PCR product per lane.

buffer. This should be considered during optimization experiments when the enzyme concentration is modified. Among other things, the storage buffer of AmpliTaq™ DNA polymerase (Perkin-Elmer Cetus) contains 50% glycerol, 0.5% Tween 20™ and 0.5% Nonidet P40™. If 1 unit enzyme (0.2µl AmpliTaq™) is added to a 50µl reaction, the final concentration of these substances will be 0.2% glycerol, 0.002% Tween 20™ and 0.002% Nonidet P40™.

1.4. Deoxynucleotide triphosphates (dNTPs)

Generally, a 10mM stock solution, equimolar with each of the four dNTPs, is suitable for multi-tube assays. For smaller experiments, 1-2mM stocks may be prepared and stored at -20°C. Imbalanced dNTP mixtures will reduce Taq fidelity. We observed, however, that signal intensity decreased significantly when using 1mM solutions that had been stored over 2 months. Thus, they should not be stored for extended periods of time. dNTP stock solutions should be neutralized to pH 7.0 with NaOH. Suitable solutions with a pH of 7.0 are commercially available as salt solutions (e.g., as 100mM Li-salts, Boehringer Mannheim).

The optimal dNTP concentration depends on
- length of amplification product
- $MgCl_2$ concentration
- primer concentration
- reaction stringency

On the other hand, dNTPs (and pyrophosphate) reduce free $[Mg^{2+}]$, thus interfering with polymerase activity and decreasing primer annealing. Taq DNA polymerase catalyzes dNTP polymerization with higher fidelity at lower dNTP concentrations (>10µM) than those which are usually suitable for the optimal sensitivity of an analytical PCR (100-200µM). But in a preparative PCR, where PCR products are reamplified to amplify single-stranded or double-stranded DNA for sequencing or to synthesize labeled probes, it may be essential to decrease dNTP concentrations (20-40µM), because of the high input number of the easily amplifiable target. We observed yields of selectively reamplified (unlabeled) double stranded product of more than 2µg/100µl with 40µM dNTPs. If dNTPs are the limiting factor of a PCR, often the problems mentioned above (see 1.2.5. cycle number) and the problems of reamplification may be contolled, even with a cycle number of 55 (Finckh 1991) to 70 (see figure 1.8).

1.5. Primers

The basic features of synthesis and purification of synthetic oligonucleotides used as PCR primers are outlined in chapter 20.

In most applications, it is the sequence and the combination of the primers that determine the overall assay success. Optimization experiments are carried out merely for "optimization".

Depending on their purpose, useful primer lengths are

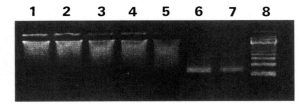

Figure 1.8: Second reamplification of a 160bp CMV IE-DNA fragment under conditions where primers and/or dNTPs are limiting. Synthesis of high molecular weight DNA due to lack of primers and/or dNTPs. Primers 0.1µM (lanes **1-7**): 5'-CCACCCGTGGTGCCAGCTCC-3' (IE1), 5'-CCCGCTCCTCCTGAGCACCC-3' (IE2) (Shibata 1988). dNTPs in lanes **1-7** in decreasing concentrations: 100µM, 80µM, 60µM, 40µM, 20µM, 10µM, 5µM. Initial template input approx. 50ng PCR product with identical sequence. In addition, each sample (lanes **1-7**) contained 700ng seronegative human DNA (corresponding to approx. 10^5 diploid genomes). Lane **8**: 1µg 123bp ladder (Gibco BRL). 50µl reaction volume, 1.5 U Taq polymerase. Buffer: GeneAmp™ 10xPCR Buffer (Perkin-Elmer Cetus). Thermoprofile: 3min 95°C initial denaturation; 45 cycles with 20sec 94°C, 20sec 66°C, 20sec 72°C; 10min 72°C final extension. Machine: DNA Thermal Cycler, Perkin-Elmer Instruments. 9µl PCR product per lane.

individual primers should not end in palindromes.
- Primers should lack secondary structure.
- Avoid imbalanced distribution of G/C- and A/T-rich domains. But oligo (dT) and poly (dC) work well.
- Primers should be specific to a single member of a gene family.

Some of the basic primer features may be checked with commercially available primer programs.

Bases which do not hybridize to the template may be added at the 5´end of a primer, e.g., for introducing restriction sites, GC-clamps or promotor sequences (see chapter 14, 17 and 23) into the amplification product. This allows higher annealing temperatures after the early cycles, because of the higher T_m of the newly amplified longer primer-target hybrid (see also chapter 3.3 and 14).

Most PCR applications are mainly controlled through the design of the primers and the choice of primer combinations, concentrations and sequence modifications. Selected applications are described in chapter 3.

14 to over 40 bases long, with a G+C content ranging from 40-75%.

Using formula [2] in 1.5.2. and a 50% G+C content of the oligonucleotide primers, the calculated T_m of primers lies between 39°C for a 14mer and 67°C for a 40mer. General guidelines for primer design are similarly summarized by Rappolee (1990):

- Primers should lie within highly conserved regions of the genome of the analyzed species.
- 3' ends of primers should use conserved amino acids, with nondegenerate codons (e.g., Trp and Met). Avoid potential third-base wobble positions at the 3' end, especially when sequence conservation is not proven.
- 3' ends of primers should avoid complementarity to prevent "primer dimer" formation and resultant waste of primers in the PCR. For the same reason,

1.5.1. Primer-related PCR artifacts

We have observed "primer dimers" that are very often longer than the theoretical primer-primer artifacts. These are additional sequences between the primers that reflect amplification artifacts due to a lack of annealing stringency rather than resulting from direct primer-primer annealing (Erlich 1991, Mullis 1991). This may be checked by gel analysis and by comparing the fragments from non-DNA and negative background DNA samples using single primers and the primer combinations.

Such short artifacts are amplified very efficiently and may significantly reduce available primers.

1.5.2. Melting temperature (T_m) and optimized annealing temperature

Pairs of primers with similar T_m should be used. The T_m indicated for primers delivered by manufacturers or from primer programs allows us to compare primer characteristics prior to their combined use. However, before starting experiments with new primers, it might be useful to calculate a T_m which reflects the reaction conditions. This is possible (as noted in Sambrook 1989, pp.11.46 and 9.51) for oligonucleotides ranging in length from 14 to 70 bases, using the following (modified) equation:

$$T_m = 81.5 + 16.6(\log_{10}[J^+]) + 0{,}41(\%G+C) - (600/l) - 0.63(\%FA) \qquad [2]$$

where
[J^+] = concentration of monovalent cations
l = length of oligonucleotide
FA = formamide

Example:
Using the GeneAmp™ PCR buffer with the final [J^+] ~60mM (KCl, $MgCl_2$, dNTP-salt), and the following human pyruvate dehydrogenase (PDH) gene sequence (Koike unpubl.) specific 20mer primers with a 55% G+C content

PDH-1: ^{5}G G T A T G G A T G A G G A C C T G G A^3
PDH-2: ^{5}C T T C C A C A G C C C T C G A C T A A^3
(Rolfs unpublished) is:

$$T_m = 81.5 - 20.3 + 22{,}6 - 30 = 53.8°C$$

Note: We prefer this calculation because it ignores the molar concentration of primer/template duplexes. The concentration of these duplexes depends on primer input and template copy number and is different for each particular analytical PCR. In addition, through the amplification process during PCR, the number of annealing sites which are produced increases and primer concentration decreases with each cycle, which probably influences the primer annealing/dissociation kinetics. Generally, suitable annealing temperatures are only roughly related to the T_m (being usually 3-12°C higher than the T_m) of a given primer, and thus have to be optimized as described above (see 1.2.2).
In the PDH-example mentioned above, the best annealing temperature is 62°C for patient samples with regard to sensitivity (0.4µM primer concentration), e.g. see figures 2.1 and 7.1.

An alternative formula for the determination of optimum annealing temperature was reported by Wu et al. (1991):

$$T_p = 22 + 1.46(L_n) \qquad [3]$$

where:
T_p = optimized annealing temperature ± 2-5°C
L_n = effective length of oligonucleotide primer:
    L_n = 2(no. of G or C) + (no. of A or T)

This formula seems to be suitable for a limited oligonucleotide length range (L_n range of 20-35). (In the 20mer examples mentioned above, L_n would be = 31 and T_p = 67.3°C.)

The so-called "Wallace temperature" [2°Cx(A+T) + 4°Cx(C+G)] refers to a 1M salt concentration in oligonucleotide hybridization assays (Thein 1986). It is more or less a matter of mathematical and practical coincidence that a suitable annealing temperature for short (up to 20mers) primers eventually corresponds to the temperature calculated with this formula (PDH-example here: 62°C).
Particularly for short primers and primers with imbalanced base composition, it is rather the sequence that determines the melting behaviour than the overall base composition. With the "nearest-neighbour" thermodynamics the DNA duplex stability may be calculated as a sum of the relative stabilities of the pairwise interacting nearest neighbouring nucleotides (Breslauer 1986). The primer program OLIGO™ calculates the T_m with respect to the nearest neighbour values of an oligonucleotide (Rychlik 1989). Rychlik et al (1990) report that the optimized primer annealing temperature (T_a^{OPT}) depends on the T_m of the primer with the lower T_m value and the T_m of the amplification product. With longer products the T_a^{OPT} increases.

1.5.3. Primer concentration

Prior to application, accurate stock solutions of primer in water should be prepared at 10μM for each primer. If this is not wanted for specific applications, for example in single-stranded DNA amplification, non-equimolar primer concentrations should be avoided. Primer concentrations should be calculated and adjusted to reflect the real molecule number rather than ng per μl or other expressions of concentration. Given an OD_{260} for the respective primer, the molar concentration can be calculated, taking into account base composition and length, with the following equation (modified from Thein and Wallace 1986):

$$\frac{OD_{260} \times \text{dilution}}{\Sigma \text{ molar extinction coefficient of dNTPs}} = xM \quad [4]$$

Molar extinction coefficient
(1cm pathlength cuvette):
  A = 15200
  T = 8400
  G = 12010
  C = 7050

The above-mentioned examples contain for
- PDH-1: 5 A, 4 T, 9 G, 2 C.
- PDH-2: 5 A, 4 T, 2 G, 9 C.

The Σ molar extinction coefficients are for
- PDH-1: 5x15200 + 4x8400 + 9x12010 + 2x7050 = 231790,
- PDH-2: 5x15200 + 4x8400 + 2x12010 + 9x7050 = 197070,
and from a 1/100 dilution of each of the two stock solutions an OD_{260} = 0.25 was measured, and so:

$$[PDH-1] \quad \frac{0.25 \times 100}{231790} = 107.9 \mu M$$

$$[PDH-2] \quad \frac{0.25 \times 100}{197070} = 126.9 \mu M$$

Because an OD_{260} = 1 of oligonucleotides corresponds to approx. 33μg/ml (Sambrook 1989, p. 11.21), the following formula can be used as a control:

$$OD_{260} \times \text{dilution} \times 33 = z \, \mu g/ml = 0.001 \, z \, g/l \quad [5]$$

Our examples here:
  0.25 x 100 x 33 = 825μg/ml = 0.825g/l

Given the mean MW of a base = 325g/mol, the molar concentration for the 20mer examples mentioned above is:

$$\frac{0.825 g/l}{20 \times 325 g/mol} = 126.9 \mu M \quad [6]$$

Note: This would result in a 15% difference in concentration between the two primers, if formulas 5 and 6 are being used instead of formula 4 for mixing primers in equimolar proportions.

Generally, for analytical PCRs, suitable primer concentrations are between 0.1 and 1 μM. In many cases, the optimum primer concentration is related to the length of the amplified fragment:

Yield of produced ds fragment	incorporated primers per strand (molar concentration)		incorporated dNTPs absolute (molar conc./* A, C, T, G), irrespective of fragment length
	200 bp fragment	800 bp fragment	
1μg/100μl	8 pmol (0.08μM)	2 pmol (0.02μM)	3.2 nmol (8μM)
3μg/100μl	24 pmol (0.24μM)	6 pmol (0.06μM)	9.6 nmol (24μM)

* 325 daltons / incorporated nucleotide and equimolar content of each A, C, T, G is assumed.

The commonly used dNTP concentration of 200µM in a 100µl reaction volume corresponds to 80nmol dNTPs. As can be seen in the table (page 12) this is approximately an 8- to 24-fold molar excess over the incorporated DNA fraction, depending on product yield and irrespective of fragment length. We usually work with constant dNTP concentrations and prefer to modify primer concentration in optimization strategies. Remember that the modification of dNTP concentration would influence the other components of PCR (see 1.4). The optimum primer amount often corresponds to that concentration, which is theoretically necessary for amplification of 2-4µg product.

For optimized assays, this means that in most cases after PCR, whether there is amplified product or not, residual nonextended primers should be visible in the gel.

expelling air in the water phase with a pipet, so that the air bubbles come up, and the correct volume may be drawn into the pipet tip. The oil on the outer surface of the tip should be wiped off with a lint-free paper towel. Positive displacement pipets may be used for this method of removing oil in order to prevent cross-contaminations. Sometimes less than 10^{-3}µl of a post-PCR sample is detectable in hybridization assays (depending on specific fragment yield). Such minute amounts might exist in aerosols (see chapters 5 and 10.1).

Depending on the robustness of a particular assay, it may be necessary to reduce the reaction volume, which allows shorter ramp and hold times and might increase specificity. We routinely perform 25µl reactions in 500µl tubes for analytical assays, which allows us to repeat product analysis at least once.

1.6. Oil overlay and reaction volume

Most thermal cyclers do not heat the lids of the reaction tubes. Therefore, an overlaying of the amplification mix with light mineral oil is necessary to prevent evaporation. Any evaporation would lead to higher reagent concentration and to a decrease in temperature (Mezei 1990). In addition, the oil helps to prevent cross-contaminations. On the other hand, too much oil slows down the thermal profile. It is necessary to standardize the amount of oil overlay in order to minimize these factors. The type of thermocycler will determine how much oil represents the best compromise. In thermal cyclers, where the lid of the reaction tube is heated continuously to >96°C, a PCR can be run without oil overlay (e.g., *GeneAmp* PCR System 9600, Perkin-Elmer Cetus Instruments # 801-0001/2/3). For most applications, 70µl oil for 100µl reactions, 40µl oil for 50µl reactions, and 30µl oil for 25µl reactions is probably sufficient (mineral oil light white, Sigma # M-5904; paraffin oil, Bayol F, Serva # 14500).

If necessary, the oil may be removed with chloroform. In most cases, it is enough to avoid including it in samples for electrophoresis. This may be done by

1.7. DNA sample

A DNA sample may be contaminated, inhibit PCR or contain no DNA. It is crucial for diagnostic assays to include controls that check all of these possibilities (see chapter 5).

1.7.1. Purity of samples

Besides DNA, there may be other substances in the sample which interfere with the PCR process. Many of these are mentioned in chapter 4. Sometimes it is the purity of a sample which limits the sensitivity of an assay. In some cases, even the freezing of a sample just once or several times seems to affect reproducibility.

For clinical samples, it is important to be aware of the presence of the potential PCR inhibitory compounds EDTA, heparin, porphyrins and related compounds and $H_xPO_4^{n-}$.

EDTA and heparin may be present in blood samples as anticoagulants. They can be removed from blood samples simultaneously with the hemoglobin from hemo-lyzed erythrocytes prior to lysis of the washed leuko-cytes.

More than 0.25mM $Mg_3(PO_4)_2$ will precipitate in aqeuous solutions at RT. This means that small amounts of PO_4^{2-} (e.g., from PBS buffers in alkaline preparations) will significantly reduce free $[Mg^{2+}]$, which might interfere with the reaction. Note that 1 x PBS (Dulbecco's, Gibco BRL) contains approx. 9.3mM $H_xPO_4^{n-}$. If 1/10 of a PCR reaction volume consists of 1 x PBS, this will result in 0.9mM $H_xPO_4^{n-}$, which would probably decrease free $[Mg^{2+}]$ compared to the original 1.5mM Mg^{2+} in a standard PCR.

1.7.2. Homogeneity of samples

Patient samples, whether genomic DNA preparations or crude cell extracts, are never homogeneous solutions. High-quality genomic DNA cannot even be handled with narrow pipet tips. Thus, it is sometimes useful to dilute an aliquot of the sample before PCR analysis, and to use a larger, diluted sample volume in the reaction mixture. One of the crucial factors of reproducibility is whether or not it is possible, to pipet a given sample identically at any date. For many samples, this is influenced by storage conditions and heating and freezing of the sample.

1.7.3. DNA content of sample

The optimum DNA content of a sample for PCR analysis depends on its purity and the underlying purpose of the assay. For genetic analysis, it is useful to analyze a sufficient standard amount of DNA (100-500ng) or cell numbers to minimize the impact of nucleotide incorporation errors. For the detection of an unknown copy number of target DNA, as for example infectious agents, the maximum amount of sample DNA or cells which do not inhibit the PCR, has to be determined empirically.

1.8. Size and structure of amplification products

PCR is very often less efficient with longer products. One possible cause might be the nature of the secondary structure of single-stranded templates. Secondary structures could have several deleterious effects:

1. A hairpin or a loop within the fragment, still giving access to a primer at its 3' terminus, either slows down the polymerase or is degraded through the 5'-3' exonuclease activity of Taq polymerase (Holland 1991). See figure 1.9.

   Erlich (1991) mentioned the efficient amplification of long fragments with a mutant Taq DNA polymerase lacking 5'-3' exonuclease activity. The commercially available Stoffel fragment, a truncated Taq (Perkin-Elmer Cetus # N808-0038), which has the same properties, might be suitable for such purposes.

2. A loop, where the 3' end of the product anneals somewhere within the product, becomes a primer structure. If such a structure is elongated once, a new primer annealing site is created on the "wrong"

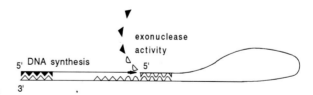

Figure 1.9: Model of a looping-back 5' terminus of an amplification product. The annealing of the partially hybridizing 5' terminus (primer) is cooperatively enhanced through neighboring sequences. Degradation of the DNA loop or retardation of the DNA synthesis might result. For symbols, see legend figure 1.2.

strand. In the next cycles, a product with distinct length (longer than the one wanted originally) may be created and exponentially amplified with only one primer(see fig. 1.10). Similar annealing events at the 3' end of such fragments to the same strand of another product with an identical sequence may occur with an increase in the concentration of the fragments. This will produce artifacts identical to those produced by the above self-priming effect. These artifacts will contain intended internal sequences, if such unwanted priming events happened originally with specific products. If the created sequences prefer their own intra-strand secondary structure (due to the complementarity of the ends), shorter products than were originally planned will come up, again containing specific sequences. This phenomenon is the basic feature of a method referred to as "panhandle PCR" (Jones 1992; see chapter 15.4 for further information). All this may be checked with southern blot analysis of gels where many "nonspecific bands" or smears hybridize to a specific probe that contains only internal sequences of the desired product.

Another approach is to check the DNA sample and a small amount of its post-PCR products with only one of the two primers in a particular PCR. If similar or identical artifacts come up as described with a pair of primers, redesigning one or both primers might be necessary.

One of the major effects of additional components in the PCR, is their influence on secondary structure stability (see chapter 4). When secondary structures are a problem, adding reagents which lower the T_m of dsDNA (e.g., formamide) and increasing primer concentration to compensate for interference with primer annealing, might improve the yield of long amplification products.

Secondary structures of template DNA may be destabilized through enzymatic incorporation of the modified nucleotide 7-deaza-dGTP so that the template might be amplified more efficiently (Innis 1988).

3. If products are very long, they might preferentially reanneal at particular domains close to one terminus, especially with higher product concentrations. Eventually this will interfere with

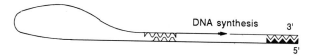

Figure 1.10: Model of a looping-back 3' terminus of an amplification product. This structure is a typical priming site for DNA synthesis. DNA synthesis will stop at the 5' terminus, forming a new primer annealing site for the 5' terminal primer. In the following cycles, the generated artefact can be amplified exponentially with the 5' terminal primer only. For symbols, see legend figure 1.2.

elongation of a primer on the other end. As in paragraph 1., the polymerase will be slowed down, or the product will be degraded. If the enzyme "jumps" to the other strand, a phenomenon similar from that described in the previous paragraph might result. The product would then be exponentially amplifiable with only one primer. But the lengths of such artifacts would be highly variable, depending on the jumping location, thus creating a smear on gel analysis. Sometimes, we have

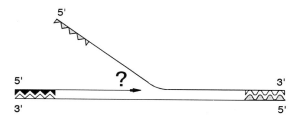

Figure 1.11: It will be hard to predict what happens under such circumstances. See text for discussion. For symbols, see legend figure1.2.

observed smears that hybridized with a probe that is internal to the amplified fragment. It is unclear whether this is a potential explanation.
4. With increasing cycle numbers, the PCR products compete with the primers for annealing sites. This creates gap- or nick-like sites which are target sites for the polymerase-independent 5'-3' exonuclease activity of Taq (Gelfand, personal communication and Holland 1991).

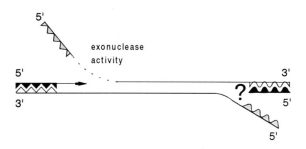

Figure 1.12: For explanation, see text. For symbols, see legend figure 1.2.

1.9. PCR set-up strategies

The conditions for any PCR set-up and the handling of PCR reagents are crucial to the overall sensitivity and to the quality of results.

It is necessary to standardize a set-up protocol in order to achieve optimal assay systems. **As long as there are contamination problems, nonspecific and implausible or false-negative results, it is impossible to establish a PCR-based assay for medical diagnostics.**

Every primer that is nonspecifically elongated at its 3' end because of unwanted annealing to partially complementary sequences is not only lost for specific priming, but also enhances further nonspecific amplifications. The competition of such nonspecific reactions might even cause false-negative results. Remember that the incorporation rate of Taq DNA polymerase is approx. 0.25 nucleotides per second at 22°C. The temperature of the reaction mixture and the time needed for the set-up of a PCR assay, especially the waiting and ramp time before a complete reaction mixture reaches initial denaturation temperature, all influence sensitivity and specificity(see fig 1.13).

Thus, an optimal set-up for a PCR should create a situation in which a thermostable DNA polymerase never comes in contact with nonspecific primer-DNA template hybrids, or other nicked or partially annealed double-stranded DNA. A 1000-fold decrease in sensitivity has been reported after leaving a reaction mixture for 5 min at room temperature, compared to more stringent handling (Mullis 1991). Several set-up strategies deal with these problems.

Usually, in a well established assay system, an aliquot of a "mastermix" is placed in a suitable reaction tube and DNA sample is added immediately before thermal cycling. This leads to an efficient and specific amplification. Each reagent and tube should be placed on ice, and the thermal cycler preheated to approx. 90°C (see Method 1).

Theoretically, the Hot Start™ PCR is closer to the optimum, in which the DNA polymerase and essential reaction components join after heating. This may be done by mixing the enzyme or other essential reaction components with a preheated reaction mixture. But with this procedure, it is difficult to maintain identical conditions for all reaction tubes. Pipets and tips are not designed for pipetting into hot media, and it becomes difficult to prevent cross-contaminations.

Generally, those procedures are preferable in which the tubes, once closed and heated, are never opened until thermal cycling is completed.

A good and safe way to perform a hot-start PCR is by physically separating the reaction components with various materials that melt at higher temperatures, such as paraffin or agarose.

A paraffin wax pellet (*AmpliWax*™ *PCR Gems*; Perkin Elmer Cetus # N808-0100) is melted and rests on top of the reaction mixture minus one essential component. With subsequent cooling, the remaining component is laid over the newly formed paraffin wax layer. In the next heating step, the liquid paraffin rises above all components and forms a vapor barrier during PCR. Compared to 2 min incubation at RT of a completed reaction mixture a Hot Start™ protocol was reported being more specific and probably more sensitive (Chou 1992). A 16-17mg paraffin pellet is suitable for 100µl reaction volumes.

A similar procedure is described in chapter 2.2., methods 1 and 2, where the template DNA for reamplification is pre-cast in agarose. A hot-start procedure with agarose may also be performed, with primers and/or dNTPs pre-cast in agarose. A melted aliquot of the agarose/reagent mixture is placed at the bottom of the reaction tubes, and the tube is then placed on ice. The gelled agarose/reagent mixture is overlayed with the remaining reaction components and will melt during the initial heating of the reaction tube.

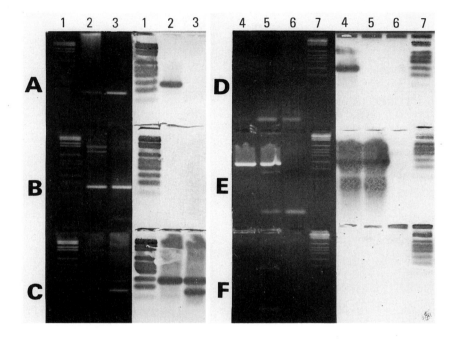

Figure 1.13: CMV 282bp late gene (gp64) DNA fragment amplification from five different patient samples (A-E) and one control DNA sample from a seronegative person (F). False-negative results (A 3, D 5) after leaving the complete reaction mixture pre-PCR at RT for 10min (lanes 3 and 5), instead of ice exclusively (lanes 2, 4, 6). A, C, E: peripheral blood leucocytes, DNA preparation with alkaline lysis, 2µl sample input. B, D, F: phenol/chloroform extracted DNA, 2µl sample input. B, F: peripheral blood leucocytes; D: cerebrospinal fluid. Lane 6: non-DNA contamination control. Lanes **1 and 7**: 250ng molecular weight marker VI (Boehringer; see chapter 10.1.4). Note the non-specific fragments visible in the gel, but not after hybridization. See chapters 6 and 7 for sample and DNA preparation methods. 3% agarose gel (left) with 10µl PCR product per lane and the southern blots (right) after hybridization with digoxigenin-11-dUTP labeled probes (CMV-LA probe, pBR328 probe) and immunological detection (as described in chapter 10) are shown. Amplification primers: 5'-CACCGACGAGGATTCCGA-3' (1192), 5'-ACCTCGGTGCTTTTTGGG-3' (1193) (Rolfs unpubl.). Protocol: 25µl reaction volume. Buffer: GeneAmp™ 10xPCR Buffer (Perkin-Elmer Cetus). Primers 0.4µM, dNTPs 200µM, 1 U Taq polymerase. Thermoprofile: 3min 95°C initial denaturation; 35 cycles with 20sec 94°C, 20sec 65°C, 20sec 72°C; 10min 72°C final extension. Machine: GeneAmp PCR System 9600 (Perkin-Elmer Instruments). Tubes: 500µl Eppendorf Safelock™. CMV-LA probe length: 139bp. The probe primers are nested to the 282 bp fragment and are identical to those described in figure 1.7 (Shibata 1988). pBR328 probe: Random-priming labeled linearized pBR328 (tube #4, labeled control-DNA from the "DNA Labeling and Detection Kit Nonradioactive") (Boehringer #1093657). The principles and methods of probe synthesis and hybridization are described in chapters 2 and 10. Hybridization: A mixture of approx. 50ng CMV-LA probe and 20ng pBR328 probe were heated to 95°C and immediately added to 5ml prewarmed hybridization solution (62°C). 12h hybridization time (for detailed method, see chapter 10).

General rules for PCR set-up:

- Be aware of contamination sources and methods for contamination prevention (for more detail see chapter 5).
- Physically separated areas for pre-PCR and post-PCR procedures, e.g., laminar flow hood, separated rooms.
- Use personal reagent sets and pipets.
- Wear gloves and change them frequently.
- Use disposable materials, bottles and tubes.
- Always place prelabeled tubes and thawed reagents on ice.
- Use different sets of pipets for reagents and DNA samples. Positive displacement pipets are preferable for DNA samples, primers and labeled reagents.
- Preheat thermal cycler.

Procedure	Comments

Method: Mastermix PCR

Protocol (10-tube assay)

Add reagents in the following order into a precooled tube:

1. H_2O 173µl

2. 10 x reaction buffer 25 µl

3. Additives ($MgCl_2$, EDTA, formamide, BSA ...)

4. dNTPs 5µl

5. Primer 1 10µl
   Primer 2 10µl

Final volume: 25µl/tube

1. e.g., sterile water; (10x25µl) - 77µl = 173µl.

2. e.g., (GeneAmp® 10xPCR Buffer, Perkin-Elmer Cetus, # 808-0006) 100 mM Tris-HCl, pH 8.3 (at RT), 500 mM KCl, 15 mM $MgCl_2$, 0.01% (w/v) gelatin.

3. For details see chapter 4.

4. Stock: 10mM; final: 200µM (Boehringer Mannheim, # 1051 440, 458, 466, 482).

5. Stock: 10µM; final: 0.4µM.

Procedure(cont.)	*Comments(cont.)*
6. Taq DNA polymerase 2μl	6. Final: 1 unit/25μl (Perkin-Elmer Cetus). Note: Mix enzyme gently and spin down briefly before use. Small volumes of native enzyme, or even a 1:5 dilution, can't be pipetted accurately, due to the high viscosity of the storage buffer and due to the enzyme solution sticking to the outside of the pipet tip. After dilution in the master mix, this becomes negligible.
7. Mix gently, spin down briefly	7. Enzymes may be destroyed at liquid-gas phase borders through excessive foaming.
8. Aliquot into precooled reaction tubes	8. 22.5μl/tube
9. Overlay with 30μl light mineral oil	9. e.g., Sigma # M-5904
10. Add 2.5μl DNA sample under oil	10. up to 2 μg DNA; depending on purity and target amount.
11. Place into a hot thermal cycler as quickly as possible.	

References

1. Bell DA, DeMarini DM. Excessive cycling converts PCR products to random-length higher molecular weight fragments. 1991, Nucleic Acids Res 19, 5079.

2. Breslauer KJ, Frank R, Blöcker H, Marky LA. Predicting DNA duplex stability from the base sequence. 1986, Proc Natl Acad Sci USA 83, 3746-3750.

3. Chou Q, Russell M, Birch DE, Raymond J, Bloch W. Prevention of pre-PCR mis-priming and primer dimerization improves low-copy-number amplifications. 1992, Nucl Acids Res 20, 1717-1723.

4. Demmler GJ, Buffone GJ, Schimbor CM, May RA. Detection of cytomegalovirus in urine from newborns by using polymerase chain reaction DNA amplification. 1988, J Infect Dis 158, 1177-1184.

5. Eckert KA, Kunkel TA. The fidelity of DNA polymerases used in the polymerase chain reactions. *In* PCR A Practical Approach; Eds.: Mcpherson MJ, Quirke P, Taylor GR, IRL Press, 1991.

6. Erlich HA, Gelfand D, Sninsky JJ. Recent advances in the polymerase chain reaction. 1991, Science 252, 1643-1651.

7. Finckh U, Lingenfelter PA, Myerson D. Producing single-stranded DNA probes with the *Taq* DNA polymerase: A high yield protocol. 1991, BioTechniques 10, 35-39.

8. Gelfand DH. Taq DNA polymerase. *In* PCR Technology Principles and Applications for DNA Amplification; Ed. Erlich H.A., Stockton Press 1989.

9. Gelfand D.H. and White T.J. Thermostable DNA polymerases. *In* PCR Protocols A Guide to Methods and Applications; Eds. Innis M.A., Gelfand D.H., Sninsky J.J., White T.J., Academic Press, 1990.

10. Holland PM, Abramson RD, Watson R, Gelfand DH. Detection of specific polymerase chain reaction product by utilizing the 5' -> 3' exonuclease activity of *Thermus aquaticus* DNA polymerase. 1991, Proc Natl Acad Sci USA 88, 7276-7280.

11. Innis MA, Mayambo KB, Gelfand DH, Brow MAD. DNA sequencing with *Thermus aquaticus* DNA polymerase and direct sequencing of polymerase chain reaction-amplified DNA. 1988, Proc Natl Acad Sci USA 85, 9436-9440.

12. Jones DH, Winistorfer C. Sequence specific generation of a DNA panhandle permits PCR amplification of unknown flanking DNA. 1992, Nucl Acids Res 20, 595-600.

13. Koike K, Urata Y, Koike M, Human Pyruvate Dehydrogenase beta-subunit-gene, complete cds. Unpublished data, EMBL accession number D90086

14. Kwok S, Kellogg DE, McKinney N, Spasic D, Goda L, Levenson C, Sninsky JJ. Effects of primer-template mismatches on the polymerase chain reaction: human immunodeficiency virus type 1 model studies. 1990, Nucl Acids Res 18, 999-1005.

15. Lawyer FC, Stoffel S, Saiki RK, Mayambo K, Drummond R, Gelfand DH. Isolation, characterization, and expression in *Escherichia coli* of the DNA polymerase gene from *Thermus aquaticus*, 1989, J Biol Chem 246, 6427-6437.

16. Mezei LM. Effect of oil overlay on PCR amplification. 1990, Amplifications A Forum for PCR Users 4, 11-13.

17. Mullis KB. The polymerase chain reaction in an anemic mode: How to avoid cold oligodeoxyribonuclear fusion. 1991, PCR Methods and Applications 1, 1-4.

18. Mullis KB, Faloona FA. Specific synthesis of DNA *in vitro* via a polymerase-catalyzed chain reaction. 1987, Methods Enzymol, 155, 335-350.

19. Rappolee DA. Optimizing the sensitivity of RT-PCR. 1990, Amplifications A Forum for PCR Users 4, 5-7.

20. Ruano G, Brash DE, Kidd KK. PCR: The first few cycles. 1991, Amplifications A Forum for PCR Users 7, 1-4.

21. Rychlik W, Spencer WJ Rhoads RE. Optimization of the annealing temperature for DNA amplification *in vitro*. 1990, Nucl Acids Res 18, 6409-6412.

22. Rychlik W, Rhoads RE. A computer program for choosing optimal oligonucleotides for filter hybridisation, sequencing and *in vitro* amplification of DNA. 1989, Nucl Acids Res 17, 8543-8551.

23. Saiki RK, Gelfand DH, Stoffel S, Scharf SJ, Higuchi R, Horn GT, Mullis KB, Erlich HA. Primer-directed enzymatic amplification of DNA with a thermostable DNA polymerase. 1988, Science 239, 487-491.

24. Saiki RK, Scharf S, Faloona F, Mullis KB, Horn GT, Erlich HA, Arnheim N. Enzymatic amplification of ß-globin genomic sequences and restriction site analysis for diagnosis of sickle cell anemia. 1985, Science 230, 1350-1354.

25. Sambrook J, Fritsch EF, Maniatis T. Molecular cloning. A laboratory manual. 2.Edition, CSH, 1989.

27. Shibata D, Martin WJ, Appleman MD, Causey DM, Leedom JM, Arnheim N. Detection of cytomegalovirus DNA in peripheral blood of patients infected with human immunodeficiency virus. 1988, J Infect Dis 158, 1185-1192.

27. Taylor GR. Polymerase chain reaction: basic principles and automation. *In* PCR A Practical Approach; Eds.: Mcpherson M.J., Quirke P., Taylor G.R., IRL Press, 1991.

28. Thein S.L., Wallace R.B. The use of synthetic oligonucleotides as specific hybridisation probes in the diagnosis of genetic disorders. *In* Human genetic diseases: a practical approach. Eds.: Davis K.E. IRL Press, Herndon, Virginia, 1986.

29. Tindall KR, Kunkel TA. Fidelity of DNA synthesis by the *Thermus aquaticus* DNA polymerase. 1988, Biochemistry 27, 6008-6013.

30. Wu DY, Ugozzoli L, Pal BK, Qian J, Wallace B. The effect of temperature and oligonucleotide primer length on the specificity and efficiency of amplification by the polymerase chain reaction. 1991, DNA and Cell Biology 10, 233-238.

2. Optimization Strategies

The criteria for PCR optimization are specificity, sensitivity, efficiency, reproducibility and fidelity. Which of these criteria has highest priority depends on the purpose of the PCR. Optimization of fidelity is of particular importance for cloning of PCR products and will be dealt with in chapter 17.

It is useful to distinguish between the two main applications:

1. Analytical PCR, often from unique samples, i.e., detection of infectious agents in patient samples, genetic analysis, tumor diagnostics, research and forensics.

2. Preparative PCR, e.g., synthesis of hybridization probes and sequencing templates.

2.1. Analytical PCR

A unique forensic or patient sample requires optimization of the PCR protocol prior to examination in an analytical PCR assay. Usually, a maximized sensitivity, specificity and reproducibility is required to avoid false-negative results. In many cases, sensitivity increases with increasing specificity. This is due to a decrease in nonspecific competing reactions which consume substrates and occupy enzyme. With increasing sensitivity, reproducibility also increases, because samples with a very low target DNA copy number are more often positive. On the other hand, it is not always possible to simultaneously optimize each criterion for both those samples containing high copy numbers or very low copy numbers of target DNA.

2.1.1. Specificity

Concept (example):

Amplification of a cytomegalovirus (CMV) specific 300bp product from patient samples.
Approximate molecular weight of 300bp product:

$$650 \times 300 = 195{,}000 \text{ g/mol}$$

With optimized conditions, it should be possible to get over 1µg product yield with a PCR from a standard positive control sample.

$$1\mu g \text{ 300bp product corresponds to 5.1 pmol.}$$

Oligonucleotide primers:

$$25\text{mers, } T_m \text{ 61.8°C (see chapter 1.5.2).}$$

For synthesis of a product-specific probe, a pair of nested primers is designed (see next section).

A DNA extract (200ng/µl) from a human fibroblast culture that contains laboratory virus strain (AD169) serves as a positive control (PC), and genomic DNA from seronegative individuals is used as a negative control (NC).

A. First Experiment: Optimizing dNTP and Primer Concentrations

Enzyme: AmpliTaq™ (Perkin-Elmer Cetus), 2U/tube.

50μl/tube, thus 1μM primer corresponds to 50pmol/tube.

Thermal cycling profile:
(suitable for Biomed or Perkin-Elmer instruments)

initial denaturation: 3min 95°C
35 cycles
   denaturation step: 20sec 95°C
   annealing step: 30sec 55°C
   elongation step: 30sec 72°C
final extension: 10min 72°C

Protocol:

Tube No.	DNA	[dNTP]	[Primers]	Taq
1.	PC 100ng	200μM	1.0μM (50pmol)	2U
2.	PC 100ng	200μM	0.5μM (25pmol)	2U
3.	PC 100ng	100μM	0.5μM (25pmol)	2U
4.	PC 100ng	100μM	0.2μM (10pmol)	2U
5.	PC 100ng	100μM	0.1μM (5pmol)	2U
6.	H$_2$O	200μM	1.0μM (50pmol)	2U
7.	NC 100ng	200μM	1.0μM (50pmol)	2U
8.	NC 100ng	100μM	0.5μM (25pmol)	2U

After the product analysis of such a primary experiment, in most cases it is possible to continue with experiments where only a single component is modified.

B. Second Experiment: Optimizing Annealing Temperature

Reduce volumes to 25μl/tube, with half of each of the reaction components. This will provide shorter ramp times and more parity of sample temperatures.

If many nonspecific bands are visible in the gel from PC and/or NC samples after the first experiment, an estimate of the best conditions from PC reactions and all NC reactions should be repeated at 58°C annealing temperature. At least one sample, consisting of a 1:1 mixture of 50ng PC and 50ng NC DNA should be included.

In many situations, exclusive amplification of the desired product is achieved after modifying the annealing temperature.

C. Third Experiment: Optimizing Cycle Number

It is now essential to include more samples where PC and NC DNA are mixed in differing ratios.

Protocol (example):

Take the best conditions from previous experiments for the following tubes.

Tube No.	PC DNA	NC DNA
1.	100ng	100ng
2.	100ng	0
3.	50ng	50ng
4.	50ng	0
5.	25ng	25ng
6.	25ng	0
7.	10ng	40ng
8.	10ng	0
9.	1ng	50ng
10.	1ng	0
11.	0 (!)	50ng
12.	0 (!)	0 (!)

Without tubes 11 and 12, neither qualitative nor quantitative estimates are possible (see chapter 5).

It is very useful to compare the results of several samples after 20, 25, 30, 35 and 40 cycles. For this experiment, the completed reaction mixtures, including the DNA samples (!) (see chapter 1.7.2 sample homogeneity), have to be aliquoted into the tubes, and

Product / Artifact	Possible Explanation	What to Do
1. Suspected specific product band, 300bp.		Prove, e.g., with southern blot.
2. Distinct bands < ca. 120bp or smears in that region.	Primer-related by-products that are preferentially amplified due to short length (primer dimers).	Check: set-up, primer concentration, annealing temperature.
3. Faint diffuse band, 100-200bp.	Single-stranded specific product.	Check primer concentrations and characteristics; southern blot.
4. Smear that stops exactly at 300bp.	Low primer concentration, specific products prime themselves.	Southern blot. Increase primers? Decrease dNTP? Decrease cycles? Increase annealing temp.?
5. Smear without distinct stop; no bands.	Nonspecific multiple priming, no target or lack of sensitivity. Note: specific priming can't be excluded with gel analysis alone. See also chapter 1.8.3.	Repeat first experiment or similarly, assess sensitivity with dilutions (see next section); southern blot.
6. Smear, starting from slot.	Degraded sample DNA.	
7. Distinct bands of any length.	Nonspecific priming, sometimes due to lack of sensitivity.	<u>Repeat reaction with one primer only</u>; check annealing temp.; Check primer concentrations, analyze product sequence and structure.
8. Distinct band(s) approx. 150-600bp.	Specific product forms a selfpriming secondary structure (see chapter 1.8).	Try to reamplify with only one primer; southern blot; try to optimize annealing temp. Check primer concentrations, analyze product sequence and structure.

Table 2.1: Product analysis (agarose gel) and trouble-shooting

the tubes taken out of the thermal cycler after their respective numbers of cycles are completed through the elongation step (at 72°C). These tubes should then be held in a water bath at 72°C for 10min, before storage(see figure 7.1).

Sometimes, problems will occur due to the lack of primer specificity. In these cases, other primers must be tested.

For assessment of specificity and sensitivity, the optimization strategy for diagnostic assays requires the inclusion of several high and faint positive patient samples.

2.1.2. Product analysis (agarose gel) and trouble-shooting (see table 2.1)

For preparation of gels, gel analysis, capillary blot and nonradioactive hybridization see chapter 10.

Irrespective of whether a single or many bands or smears are visible in the gel, a specificity control should be performed as soon as possible e.g. with hybridization on the internal nested probe after capillary transfer (southern blot) of the gel (see next section and chapter 10). Therefore, the gels from the initial experiments should be blotted for product analysis (and for establishing a hybridization assay).

We have observed hybridization of the internal probe to more than the one expected fragment. For a given assay, we have repeatedly seen hybridization of the internal probe to the same set of additional products. Points 3., 5., and 8. from table 1 contain possible explanations for such phenomena. Similar phenomena have been reported by Chou *et al.* (1992) as probably being single stranded truncation products which are hardly visible in an ethidium bromide stained gel. This truncation might be a result from sequence specific hot spots for Taq-dissociation from template (Abramson 1992, cited in Chou 1992).

2.1.3. Sensitivity

It is essential to have already optimized specificity before an assessment of sensitivity.

Results from dilutions of standard positive-control (PC) samples do not give a true reflection of the situation in diagnostic or other analytical assays, since samples vary widely from one another. But at least it is possible to analyze the number of copies of target DNA which are necessary to reproducibly yield a detectable and specific amplification product. Samples of quantified dilutions of standard positive control DNA (mixed with negative control DNA) may be included in a diagnostic PCR. This will allow comparison of numbers of target copies with those in a given standard. To determine whether the target copy number is too low would require an internal standard because the conditions of amplification are not predictable in patient or other analytical samples (see chapter 16 for quantitative assays).

Standard positive control samples (PC)

The analysis of human genomic sequences or retroviral integrated sequences requires the quantification of genomic DNA. This is achieved photometrically with a purified DNA extract (see chapter 7 for DNA preparation). An OD_{260nm} of 1 corresponds to 50µg/ml dsDNA. If the DNA is not badly degraded and does not have PCR-inhibitory properties, the most suitable amount of sample DNA for PCR may be determined with this method.

If no purified extracts are taken for analysis (see chapters 6 and 7), whole cells may be counted prior to lysis. Lysates from several cell numbers may be tested independently to find the optimum number of cells to use.

In many diagnostic assays for infectious agents, it is useful to quantify the copy number of the particular standard PC target sequence. This is achieved through semiquantitative fluorescence analysis of DNA fragments in a gel after gel electrophoresis (see chapter 10.1.4 for semiquantitative gel analysis). Suitable DNA fragments for gel analysis are linearized plasmids, plasmid inserts or PCR products themselves.

For PCR, dilutions of these PCs are mixed with an equal amount of genomic DNA (e.g., 50ng for 25µl reactions).

First experiment
(PC = positive control sample)

Choose the best conditions from 2.1.1 (e.g., 100µM dNTP, 0.5µM primers, 1U Taq; annealing 20sec 60°C).

Tube No.   PC copies, + 50ng genomic DNA each

1. 100,000
2. 10,000
3. 1,000
4. 100
5. 10
6. 1
7. 0.1
7. 0.01
8. 0 (!)
9. 0 (!) without genomic DNA

Sometimes it becomes obvious that specificity is not fully optimized (especially for very low copy numbers). If the detection of very low copy numbers is necessary, it may be possible to optimize for more dilute samples of PC. **This does not always lead to better results for samples with high target numbers.** In addition, it is useful to consider increasing the total cycle number for this particular purpose (as in paragraph 2.1.1.C). Again a southern blot analysis should be performed to prove the specificity of borderline signals and to check if a specifically amplified product is present but not detectable in the gel. In addition, the southern blot is an important contamination control. This is of extreme importance in diagnostics (see chapter 5).

The following optimization strategies should be tested:

- Increase in annealing temperature.
- Increase in annealing time in the first 5 cycles.
- Decrease in annealing temperature.
- Modify [primers].
- Modify [Taq].
- Modify [dNTP].
- Modify [$MgCl_2$].
- Check several co-solvents as additives (see chapter 4).
- Increase total cycle number.

2.2. Preparative PCR

In preparative PCRs, it is mainly the efficiency of DNA amplification which has to be optimized. Reamplification of PCR products with the same primers used in the intial PCR, or with nested primers, has to be optimized for high product yield and quality. Hybridization probes used to detect a PCR product should be amplified with nested primers internal to the product, in order to exclude the possibility that the probe may hybridize with the primers (and primer-containing unspecific artifacts).

2.2.1. Reamplification (see Method 1)

In principle, each specific amplification product may be used for probe synthesis. It is often useful to reamplify specific PCR products to yield sufficient template DNA for dsDNA and ssDNA probe synthesis from a single stock (Finckh 1991).
It is crucial that there is no excess of dNTPs (as discussed in chapter 1.1.4). With 20-40µM dNTPs, the maximum yield will probably not be achieved, but it is easier to exclusively synthesize the specific product. Smears should neither be used for further reamplification nor for probe synthesis.
Often, reamplification with nested primers seems to work better than reamplification with the same primers. However, the carryover of the external primers and external product may lead to significant synthesis of the longer sequence. In addition, for synthesis of single-stranded DNA, any carryover of primers should be avoided.
For many assays, it will be possible to reamplify directly from unpurified post-PCR samples. This often means a time-consuming optimization is needed in order to achieve the product quality required for

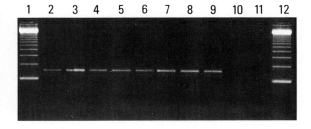

Figure 2.1: Amplification of a 185bp PDH DNA fragment from approx. 50ng genomic DNA in 0.4% final agarose. Gelled agarose stock solutions have been prepared with H_2O and added to the reaction mixtures after melting. 25µl total reaction volume, 10µl PCR product per lane. Lanes **1, 12:** 1µg 123bp ladder (Gibco BRL). The following agarose types are used (lanes **2 - 6**), **1:** Ultrapure™ agarose (Gibco BRL #5510); **2:** Agarose SERVA (Serva #11404); **3:** Agarose Low Melt (BioRad #9012-36-6); **4:** NuSieve™ GTG agarose (FMC BioProducts #50084); **5:** Agarose Standard Low - m (BioRad #162-0100); **6:** NuSieve™ 3:1 Agarose (FMC BioProducts #50092). Lanes **7, 8:** no agarose added; lanes **10, 11:** non-DNA contamination control samples. Note: **3 and 4** are low melting agaroses; **2, 5, 6** are normal agaroses for DNA electrophoresis. Buffer:: GeneAmp™ 10xPCR Buffer (Perkin-Elmer Cetus). Primers PDH-1 and PDH-2, 0.4µM. See chapter 1.5.2 for primer sequences. dNTPs 200µM, 1 U Taq polymerase. Machine: GeneAmp PCR System 9600 (Perkin-Elmer Instruments). Tubes: 500µl Eppendorf Safelock™. Thermoprofile: 3min 95°C initial denaturation; 35 cycles with 20sec 94°C, 20sec 62°C, 20sec 72°C; 10min 72°C final extension. 10µl PCR product per lane.

reamplification. Alternatively, it is possible to reamplify target sequences directly from agarose (Zintz and Beebe 1991; White and Blake 1991). We have observed good PCR amplifications with a 0.4% agarose concentration in the reaction tube (see fig. 2.1). Thus, even from a PCR in which more than a single fragment was produced, a particular fragment of interest may be reamplified directly after excising it from a suitable agarose gel (see methods 1 and 2). Primer carryover should not be a problem with such amplification.

Applications of agarose pieces in preparative PCR:

1. Quick ssDNA and dsDNA probe synthesis. A new assay may be checked immediately with hybridization techniques.
2. Reamplification of particular bands to increase template for sequencing reactions. If the band contains 20-100ng product, even ssDNA may be amplified efficiently.

2.2.2. Incorporation of label with Taq (see Method 2)

It makes no real difference if incorporation of labels in a PCR is done after the first amplification or after an additional reamplification. This will mainly depend on the available specific amplification product.

For synthesis of hybridization probes, it is possible to replace dNTPs completely or partially with the following labeled nucleotides:

labeled nucleotide	analog	Ref.:
Biotin-11-dUTP	dTTP	Lo 1988, Weier 1990
Biotin-16-dUTP	dTTP	
Biotin-21-dUTP	dTTP	see fig. 2.2 and 2.3
Digoxigenin-11-dUTP	dTTP	Lanzillo 1990; Lion and Haas 1990; Finckh 1991,1992
[α-^{32}P]dNTPs	dNTP	Bednarczuk 1991
[α-^{35}S]dATP	dATP	Stürzl and Roth 1990
[α-^{35}S]dCTP	dCTP	Stürzl and Roth 1990

Through the incorporation of [α-^{32}P]dNTPs during an analytical PCR, the amplification products may be analyzed directly with very high sensitivity. Usually, this is done with autoradiography of a polyacrylamide gel after electrophoresis (e.g., see 10.4). In addition, radioactive signals may be quantified more accurately with scintillation counting or scanning autoradiographs. In this section, we will focus on the PCR incorporation of nonradioactive labels for hybridization probe synthesis. Again, the labeling PCR is done with an unpurified template cut out from an agarose gel. We usually take agarose pieces containing 20-100ng template DNA fragments from a previous PCR. This is enough for labeling and amplification of dsDNA probes or ssDNA probes in a nonexponential PCR. In the presence of the biotin-dUTP (see figs. 2.2, 2.3) or

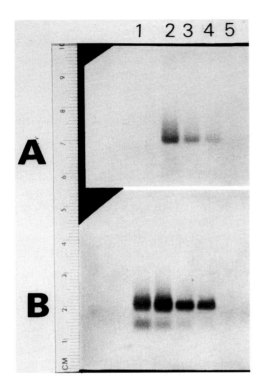

Figure 2.2: Reamplification of a 198bp CMV IE-DNA fragment in the presence of different biotin-21-dUTP/TTP ratios. The reamplification is much more efficient with high template amount (here, 50ng in **B**) than with low amount (0.5pg in **A**) in the presence of 100% biotin-21-dUTP (Bio-21). Possibly, Taq prefers unlabeled template, or the label interferes with primer annealing.
20μM dNTP concentration, where TTP is partially or completely replaced by Bio-21. Lane **1:** 100% Bio-21; **2:** 75% Bio-21, 25% TTP; **3:** 50% Bio-21, 50% TTP; **4:** 35% Bio-21, 65% TTP; **5:** TTP only. **A:** 0.5pg template DNA fragment, **B:** 50ng template DNA fragment. Direct blot of the samples from an 1.4% agarose gel on a nylon membrane (Hybond N+™, Amersham). Detection of the biotin label with a 1:1,000 dilution of a streptavidine alkaline-phoaphatase complex. The basic protocols and methods are described by Finckh et al (1992, p A37 this volume), in this chapter, and in chapter 10. 5μl from a 100μl PCR product are loaded on each lane.

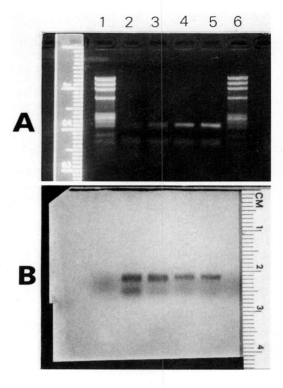

Figure 2.3: Reamplification of a 198bp CMV IE-DNA fragment in the presence of different biotin-21-dUTP/TTP ratios. In **A**, a 1.4% agarose gel and, in **B** the direct blot of the gel from A on a nylon membrane (Hybond N+™, Amersham) are shown. Molecular weight markers: Lane **1:** 1μg phiX174 Hae III digest (Clontech); lane **6:** 2μg phiX174 Hae III digest (see chapter 10.1.4). Lane **2:** 100% Bio-21; **3:** 75% Bio-21, 25% TTP; **4:** 50% Bio-21, 50% TTP; **5:** 35% Bio-21, 65% TTP. 5μl from a 100μl PCR product are loaded on lanes **2-5**. Template input: 50ng amplification product. Note: The label seems to reduce the overall amplification efficiency, as can be seen from the gel in **A**. On the other hand the signal from the label on the blot is the strongest in lane 2, suggesting a detectable significantly higher labeling rate with increasing Bio-21 concentrations. Interestingly, the same phenomenon can be observed with the primer-related artifacts (running faster). Detection of the biotin label with a 1:1,000 dilution of a streptavidine alkaline-phoaphatase complex. The basic protocols and methods are described by Finckh et al (p A37 this volume), in this chapter and in chapter 10.

digoxigenin-dUTP (see page A40, figure 1) organic labels, there must be enough unlabeled template for optimal efficiency of probe synthesis.

These nonradioactive probes have been shown to be suitable for DNA-DNA *in situ* hybridization (Weier 1990, see also Finckh et al. pp A37) and filter hybridization after southern blot (see fig. 1.13) or dot blot transfer of PCR products (Finckh *et al.*, unpubl.). See chapter 10 for agarose gel electrophoresis and hybridization protocols. We routinely use these probes directly, without further purification.

Procedure	Comments

Method 1: Reamplification of PCR products

1. Prepare 1.5% agarose gel: Buffer: 20ml 1xTris-acetate, add 1/10 vol H_2O if excessively boiled. Agarose: 1.4g When the gel is homogeneous after boiling, add 1µl ethidium bromide, mix well, cast at approx. 70°C (in cold lab if possible). 2. Mix 20-100ng (1-10µl) PCR product with 10 x gel loading buffer (GLB) and run electrophoresis until sufficient fragment separation is achieved. 2.a) Alternatively mix up to 3 µg PCR product (100-200µl) with GLB and run a preparative gel with a long slot (see figure 2.4). 3. Place the gel on a saran wrap on a 302nm UV-transilluminator; cut out band of interest. Store the gel piece in the reaction tube in which the reamplification will be carried out (at -20°C).	1. Stock: 50 x Tris-acetate (2M Tris-acetate; 242g/l Tris base, 57.1ml/l glacial acetic acid, pH 8.0). 20ml is appropriate e.g., for the BioRad Babygel electrophoresis system. Nusieve GTG™ (FMC), a low-melting agarose. Ethidium bromide stock: 10mg/ml; this compound is extremely mutagenic and should not be boiled. 2. See chapter 10.1.4 for semiquantitative product analysis. Note: None of the components of the gel neither loading buffer (GLB) nor ethidiumbromide, seems to affect the reamplification. See chapter 10.1.2 for composition of GLB. 3. Transilluminate as briefly as possible, to minimize UV-damage to DNA. Do not crosscontaminate fragments, use different disposable scalpels for different fragments. Freezing helps to elute the DNA from the agarose

Procedure (cont.)   **Comments (cont.)**

3.a) Cut out the long agarose slice completely and place it in a 1.5 ml Eppendorf tube. Melt gel slice in a heating block (70-95°C) and aliquot approx. 50ng into those reaction tubes in which the reamplification will be carried out.

3.a) This alternative method is very suitable for generation of identical template samples for probe labeling (Method 2).

4. Example:
Prepare a PCR master mix which contains all the reaction components but the template DNA in the gel piece:
      H_2O
      10 x reaction buffer
      100µM dNTP
      0.4µM primer 1
      0.4µM primer 2

      2 U Taq DNA polymerase.

4. For a PCR set-up, see chapter 1. volumes/tube(100µl reaction volume):

      70.6µl
      10µl
      1µl; stock 10mM
      4µl; stock 10µM
      4µl; stock 10µM
The nested primers that are exclusively designed for probe synthesis should be used.

      0.4µl; stock: 5U/µl

5. Pipet 90µl master mix onto the frozen gel piece in the reaction tube and immediately place the tube into the preheated thermal cycler.

6. Thermal cycling profile:
initial denaturation: 95°C, 5min
35 cycles
  denaturation step: 95°C, 20sec
  annealing step: 60°C, 20sec
  elongation step: 72°C, 20sec
final extension: 72°C, 5min

7. Store at -20°C.

Method 2 : PCR synthesis of double- and single-stranded probes

1. Prepare agarose gel as in Method 1.

2. Load product of a PCR with the nested primers that where designed for probe synthesis.

3. Cut out and store band as described in Method 1.

Procedure (cont.)

4. Example:
Prepare a PCR mastermix which contains labeled nucleotides and all the other reaction components but the template DNA in the gel piece

H_2O	
10 x reaction buffer	
40µM dATP	
40µM dCTP	
40µM dGTP	
27µM dTTP	
13µM Digoxigenin-11-dUTP	
or: 13µM Biotin-11-dUTP	
or: 13µM Biotin-16-dUTP	
or: 13µM Biotin-21-dUTP	
0.4µM primer 1	
0.4µM primer 2	

2 U Taq DNA polymerase.

5. Pipet 90 µl mastermix onto the frozen gel piece in the reaction tube and immediately place the tube into the preheated thermal cycler.

6. Thermal cycling profile:
initial denaturation: 95°C, 5min
45-70 cycles
 denaturation step: 95°C, 20sec
 annealing step: 60°C, 20sec
 elongation step: 72°C, 20sec
final extension: 72°C, 5min

7. Check probe purity in a 1-3% agarose gel (Agarose 3:1 NuSieve™, FMC).
Electrophoresis buffer: 1 x TBE
Prepare gel with ethidium-bromide as described in Method 1.
For details, see chapter 10.

8. Load 2µl probe/slot, load non-labeled amplification products in another slot.

Comments (cont.)

4. For a PCR set-up, see chapter 1, Method.

volumes/tube(100µl reaction volume):

55.6µl
10µl
4µl; stock 1mM
4µl; stock 1mM
4µl; stock 1mM
2.7µl; stock 1mM
1.3µl;stock 1mM (Boehringer)
1.3µl; stock 1mM (Enzo)
1,3µl; stock 1mM (Boehringer)
2.6µl (!); stock 0.5mM (Clontech)
4µl; stock 10µM
4µl; stock 10µM

The nested primers that are exclusively designed for probe synthesis should be used.
Note: If only one of the two primers is used in this step, a single stranded probe will be synthesized.

0.4µl; stock: 5U/µl

6. After PCR, the probe is ready for use without further purification.
Store at -20°C.

7. All labels mentioned in 4., except Biotin-21-dUTP, will retard the fragment in the gel compared with the same fragment without label.
10 x TBE: 0.9M Tris-borate, 0.01M EDTA; 108g Tris base, 55g boric acid, 20ml 0.5M EDTA, pH 8.0 (Sambrook 1989).

Procedure (cont.)	*Comments (cont.)*
9. Incubate the gel after electrophoresis and photodocumentation in 1,5M NaCl/0.5M Tris-HCl, pH 5.0 for 10min.	9. This corresponds to the neutralizing buffer for a southern blot transfer (see chapter 10.2.1). Denaturation is not recommended, because no hybridization is done.
10. Blot transfer of gel onto a nylon membrane (DuralonUV™, Stratagene; Nylon membrane positively charged, Boehringer) as described in chapter 10.	10. Blotting buffer: 1.5M NaCl/0.5M Tris-HCl, pH 5.0.
11. UV crosslinking: place the moist membrane in UV crosslinker, energy: 120mJ (Stratalinker™, Stratagene).	11. Alternatively: place the membrane with the DNA onto a 302nm UV transilluminator for 40sec.
12. Immunological detection immediately follows, or the membrane is air-dried and stored at RT for later detection.	12. Detection procedure is as described for filter hybridization; protocol see chapter 10.

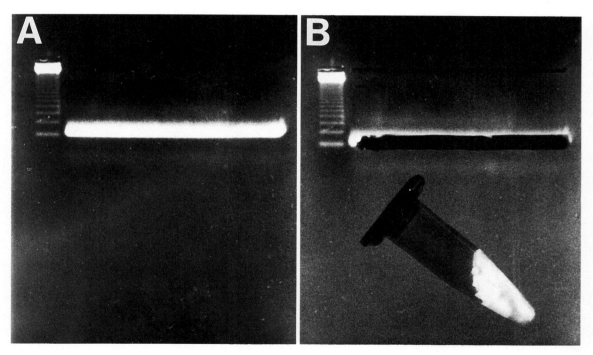

Figure 2.4: Preparative 1% NuSieve GTG™ agarose gel. Amplification of a nested 139bp CMV-LA fragment (for details see figure 1.7, legend) from a preamplified external 282bp CMV-LA fragment (for details see figure 1.13, legend). 160µl reaction product from 4 different tubes have been pooled (approx. 4µg DNA) and loaded into the preparative slot. Electrophoresis buffer: 1 x TA. Marker: 1µl 123bp ladder (Gibco BRL). For melting, the fragment completely cut out with a scalpel is stored in a 1.5ml Eppendorf tube. Melted aliquots have been used for probe synthesis as described in method 2.

References

1. Abramson RD, Stoffel S, Gelfand DH. 1992, J Biol Chem (in press)

2. Bednarczuk TA, Wiggins RC, Konat GW. Generation of high efficiency single-stranded DNA hybridisation probes by PCR. 1991, BioTechniques 10, 478.

3. Chou Q, Russel M, Birch DE, Raymond J, Bloch W. Prevention of pre-PCR mis-priming and primer dimerization improves low-copy-number amplifications. 1992, Nucl Acids Res 20, 1717-1723.

4. Finckh U, Lingenfelter PA, Myerson D. Producing single-stranded DNA probes with the *Taq* DNA polymerase: A high yield protocol. 1991, BioTechniques 10, 35-39.

5. Lanzillo J J. Preparation of digoxigenin-labeled probes by the polymerase chain reaction. 1990, BioTechniques 8:621-22.

6. Lion T, Haas OA. Nonradioactive labeling of probe with digoxigenin by polymerase chain reaction. 1990, Anal Biochem 188, 1-3.

7. Lo YD, Mehal WZ, Fleming KA. Rapid production of vector-free biotinylated probes using the polymersae chain reaction. 1988, Nucl Acids Res 16, 8719.

8. Stürzl M., Roth W.K.: "Run-off" synthesis and application of defined single-stranded DNA hybridisation probes. 1990, Anal Biochem 185, 164-69.

9. Weier HG, Segraves R, Pinkel D, Gray JW. Synthesis of Y chromosome-specific labeled DNA probes by *in vitro* DNA amplification. 1990, J Histochem Cytochem 33, 421-26.

10. White H, Blake N. DNA amplification in remelted agarose. 1991, Amplifications A forum for PCR users 6, 8-9.

11. Zintz CB, Beebe DC. Rapid re-amplification of PCR products purified in low melting point agarose gels. 1991, BioTechniques 11, 158-162.

3. General Applications of PCR

3.1. Asymmetric PCR

PCR-generated single-stranded DNA can be used as a strand-specific hybridization probe or as a template for sequencing reactions (Mazars 1991, Wilson 1990). The aim of asymmetric PCR is to amplify single-stranded DNA fragments of a specific length. This can be achieved by using two different primers, of which one is completely consumed during amplification. Only the extension product of the remaining primer will be amplified during subsequent cycles.

As soon as there is only one primer to be extended, the amplification process will no longer be exponential but linear. Asymmetric PCR can be performed by using (1) unequal primer ratios right from the beginning (Gyllensten and Erlich 1988) or (2) one primer only to reamplify one DNA strand of pre-existing double-stranded PCR fragments (two-step amplification procedure) (Finckh 1991).

A drawback of the first procedure is that it can only be performed with a limited primer concentration, which significantly reduces maximum yield. Furthermore, in the presence of free dNTPs and a lack of primers, specific fragments and nonspecific PCR by-products might start to prime each other, as described in chapter This method requires a large number of cycles, and is a potential source of incorporated errors (for details see chapter 21.6). Finally, it has often been the case that only one strand can be sequenced easily.

The second method makes it possible to start with a controllable and very high number of template DNA copies of the desired length. This is advantageous because maximum synthesis yield per cycle corresponds to the input amount of template DNA when the amplification kinetics are linear. Carry-over of undesired primers and by-products is prevented by directly cutting the template DNA from an agarose gel. This procedure will amplify several pmol of ssDNA. Such high yields of single-stranded (ss)DNA can be analyzed by means of ethidium bromide staining of agarose gels (see chapter 2.2, Method 2 and Finckh et al., p A37 this volume). However, the two physically separated steps required in this procedure might increase the problem of contamination.

There are some alternative protocols for producing single-stranded DNA, such as the use of biotin-tagged primers and streptavidin-coated paramagnetic particles (Dynabeads, Dynal Ltd. Oslo), which readily produce templates suitable for automated sequencing (for details see chapter 14).

3.2. Allele-specific amplification (ASA, PASA, ASP, ARMS)

Specific and efficient priming of DNA synthesis in PCR is mainly determined by the sequence of the last 1-2 nucleotides at the 3' end of the primers. While the desired allele is effectively amplified, the other alleles are less readily amplified as a result of the mismatch at or near the 3' end (Sarkar 1990). For allele-specific amplification - also called PCR amplification of specific alleles (PASA), allele-specific PCR (ASP) or amplification refractory mutation system (ARMS) - , where allele discrimination relies exclusively on the 3' end base of a primer (Wu 1989), short primers may be advantageous because of the high relative impact of a single base mismatch on T_m in short hybrids (in addition to the sometimes crucial role of 3' end complementarity) (see also chapter 1, 1.3. and 1.5 as well as chapter 16). It is important to make sure that the polymerase used for an allele-specific amplification lacks 3'-5' exonuclease/proofreading activity (see chapter 21). Each allele may be amplified in a separate reaction tube. Thus ASA should be performed with an internal standard DNA co-amplification to check the samples for "allele-specific inhibition". This is crucial to this method because the absence of a product has the same diagnostic meaning as its presence. The results of the studies by Kwok et al. (1990) are of importance for selecting primers with appropriate 3' ends. When using Taq polymerase, only A-G, G-A and C-C mismatches at the 3´terminus of a primer ensure to a high degree that there will be no effective elongation of the primer. Elongation in spite of a mismatch could give false-positive amplification results. Potential primer 3´ terminal G-T mismatches should be avoided because of their relative stability. For more details see chapter 13.

3.3. Nested PCR

Nested primers are primers annealed internally in a pre-existing amplification fragment. Chapter 2 (method 2) describes a procedure using a pair of product-internal nested primers for hybridization probe synthesis.

Extremely high sensitivy is to be expected when using a nested PCR. In addition, the nested primers serve as a specificity control for the external PCR fragment. For routine diagnostic procedures, however, the nested assays have the major drawback of introducing a high contamination risk (see chapter 5). Quantitative artifacts from the external PCR will be enhanced during the nested PCR, thus impeding quantitative assays. These drawbacks may be partially circumvented by designing a "one-tube nested PCR" using two primer pairs of different melting points (T_m) in one reaction mixture. Annealing of the nested primers during the first cycles is prevented by their low T_m.

Example of a one-tube nested PCR:

1. Long external fragment amplification

T_m of the external primers: 80°C. First 15-20 cycles. Two-temperature-step PCR: denaturation 95°C for 20sec; primer annealing/extension 72°C for 30sec. Concentration of external primers: 0.1µM.

2. Intermediate length, residual external and nested fragment length amplification

T_m of the nested primers: 45°C. Another 16 cycles. Three-temperature PCR: denaturation at 92°C for 20sec; 20sec annealing with reduction of the annealing temperature by 2°C after every second cycle starting at 66°C; nested primer annealing (+ external primer annealing); primer extension at 72°C for 20 sec. Concentration of nested primers: 0.4µM.

3. Short nested fragment amplification

37-45 cycles. Three-temperature PCR: 20 sec at 88°C for denaturation of only the nested PCR fragment; primer annealing: 20sec, 50°C; primer extension: 20sec, 72°C.

A difference in T_m of the external and nested fragment makes it possible to perform an exclusively internal PCR in the late cycles. The longer external fragment, which may have a higher G:C content than the nested fragment, will only be denatured at a slightly higher temperature than the nested fragment (according to formula [2] presented in chapter 1.5.2). This difference in denaturation temperature has to be determined accurately prior to performing analytical assays. In addition, the G:C content of the external fragment may be increased through the introduction of multiple G:C pairs ("GC-clamp") at the 5'-ends of the external primers. If a GC-clamp is used, the annealing temperature in the early cycles has to be low enough not to exceed the lower T_m of the external primers without the GC-clamp. After the initial cycles, GC-clamp sequences are introduced into the extension products, allowing for significantly higher annealing temperatures. In summary, "drop-in, drop-out nested priming" can be performed by limiting outer primer concentrations and using external fragments and primers with a higher T_m (Erlich 1991).

A similar procedure for producing single-stranded DNA for subsequent direct sequencing was reported by Mazars et al. (1991). The authors performed a pre-amplification step of 25 cycles with two primers (A, B) at an annealing temperature of 55°C. This was followed by the synthesis of the single-stranded DNA in the same tube by means of a third primer (C) (T_m +10°C). The latter step was performed at a higher annealing temperature (64°C), which led to the drop-out of the first two primers (A, B). According to the authors, the amount of specific DNA thus produced was similar to that obtained with the procedure published by Gyllensten (1988).

It is worthwile to note at this point that for synthesis of short PCR fragments (in one-tube nested PCR: the internal amplification product) lower denaturation temperatures give a higher yield of the intended product. Yap and McGee (1991) showed that short PCR fragments (110bp) can be amplified more effectively at denaturation temperatures between 87° and 90°C, while temperatures above 90°C reduce the yield. Larger fragments (500bp), on the other hand, require the usual denaturation temperatures (92°-95°C).

3.4. Multiplex PCR

With this method, several genomic regions from one infectious agent or from an eukaryotic gene of interest can be amplified simultaneously in one tube using a set of different primer pairs. In genetic analysis the absence of one or more of the fragments might indicate a sequence deletion (Chamberlain 1988). The procedure appears to be less suitable for diagnostic purposes (e.g. detection of coliform bacteria and *Escherichia coli* [Bej 1991]), especially when used for the detection and differentiation of infectious agents in patient samples. The different amplification products are not influenced in the same way by potential inhibiting factors of the patient sample. This may lead to false-negative results for some amplification products, depending on which unknown factor is present in the patient sample. The problem of false-negative PCR results is discussed in chapter 5. For more details about multiplex PCR see chapter 12.

3.5. Differential PCR

Differential PCR is based on the possibility of amplifying the target gene and a reference fragment in a single reaction vessel. The co-amplification of a quantified reference fragment and a fragment with an unknown copy number in one reaction tube might enhance quantitative differences to detectable levels. Frye et al. (1989), for instance, reported the suppression of single copy gene PCR amplification by an added standard DNA or a tumor tissue internal standard, when an amplified oncogene was present in the tumor tissue but not when the oncogene was absent. This suppression seems to result from competition for enzyme and substrates during PCR, since it occurred consistently only when the two different primer pairs were used in a single tube but not when the two amplifications were performed in separate tubes (Frye 1989). Neubauer et al. (1990) investigated whether the loss of chromosome 9p22 - the locus of the alpha- and beta- interferon genes - plays a role in the conversion of chronic phases of lymphocytic leukemia to blast crisis. The authors performed differential PCR with the alpha-interferon gene (84bp) on chromosome 12 as a reference fragment and an amplification target size for ß-interferon of 170pb. They showed that the sensitivity of the system and its ability to discriminate heterozygotic and homozygotic loss of the target gene is crucially dependent on the concentration of primers, while the number of PCR cycles and the fragmentation of DNA by sonication (average DNA size < 300bp) have no effect. The procedure seems to be sufficiently sensitive to detect gene copy ratios of 2:1 and 3:2 (reference:target gene). For details see also Neubauer et al., p A11 this volume. Nevertheless, this method might be susceptible to false-negative and false-positive results due to sample-inherent differences in the inhibition of amplification ("differential inhibition").

3.6. Competitive PCR

Competitive PCR is the basic principle of quantitative assays (Perrin 1990, Gilliland 1990). Different competition situations may be designed:
1. Identical primers with addition of a different (mutated) "competing" standard DNA template of the same length (restriction site differences, more complex sequence differences for the simultaneous hybridization with differently labeled probes, or different capture probes in different micro-titer plate wells).
2. Different primer sequences and labels (Gibbs 1989) and competing standard template DNA with a identical or different internal sequence and identical length, so that there will only be substrate and enzyme competition but no primer competition. Simultaneous hybridization with an identical (or different) capture probe in a single micro-titer plate well. Amplification of an internal standard to check the amplifiability of a sample and comparison of the signal intensity of amplified target with a standard intensity (see chapter 16).

When competitive PCR is used for detecting allelic differences in heterozygous carriers by means of restriction enzymes or allele-specific hybridization and the alleles of interest are located in a relatively "central" position of the amplification product, the following phenomenon may occur: Incomplete elongation of a primer on one allele and switch to the other template in a subsequent cycle may produce hybrid sequences, which contribute to the false interpretation of results (see also chapter 3.2).

When using competing oligonucleotides, attention must be paid to the fact that the efficiency of discriminating point mutations increases with decreasing primer size. Ideally, short oligonucleotides with 12 - 16 bp are used. It is obvious that DNA polymerases with proofreading activity cannot be used in such assays. Under these conditions, Gibbs et al. (1989) found that competitive primers can correctly detect a point mutation even if the concentration of the mismatched primer is 100 times higher than that of the primer showing correct binding.

Note that it is probably impossible to imitate the crucial situation during the first couple of cycles, the so-called "genomic screening" (see chapter 1, 1.2.2.) with a competing standard DNA (for details see also chapter 16). Thus the final aim of quantitative PCR must be the direct quantification of a PCR fragment using added standard DNA with as few cycles as possible.

3.7. Amplification of unknown sequences

Regarding the amplification of "unknown sequences", a distinction is to be made between genes of which parts have been identified completely, while others (e.g., the 5'- or 3'-end) are unknown, and gene sequences that are entirely unknown and must therefore be identified on the basis of membership in multigene families or known corresponding sequences of other species. Major aspects of the first constellation (RACE, "panhandle PCR", targeted gene walking) are discussed in chapter 15. This section will focus on the amplification of corresponding regions of one gene in different species by means of multiple sequence alignments to generate highly degenerate oligonucleotide primers ("universal primers").

Another strategy is to design primers from peptide sequences. The back-translation from a peptide sequence to the corresponding DNA coding sequence is complicated by the fact that few peptides (C, D, E, F, H, K, M, N, Q, Y) are encoded by only one or two possible codons, while most amino acids are defined by more than one codon. Thus, primers derived from a given peptide sequence generally have to reflect the full redundancy.

1. Peptide sequence	L	A	T	N	N
2. Corresponding codons	CTG	GCA	ACT	AAT	AAT
	CTA	GCT	ACA	AAC	AAC
	CTT	GCC	ACC		
	CTC	GCG	ACG		
	TTA				
	TTG				

3. Resulting primer sequence: [C,T]T[A,C,T,G]-GC[A,C,T,G]-AC[A,C,T,G]-AA[T,C]-AA[T,C]

As a result of the necessity to incorporate all possible codon permutations into a primer, relatively short primer sequences of 15bp already have 512 different permutations. Thus, only 1/512 of total primers would be expected to show specific annealing in a subsequent PCR assay. He et al. (1989) have recently cloned new POU-domain cDNA families using oligonucleotides of 196,608- and 32,768-fold complexity. A procedure to reduce the number of required sequence combinations has recently been published by Hooft van Huijsduijnen et al. (1992). Another solution is to use the universal base inosine in those sequence positions which would have to be occupied by three or four different bases (here: [A,C,T,G]). Inosine is a purine base which naturally occurs as a rare nucleotide in cellular tRNA and has the remarkable ability to match with all four bases (A, C, G, T). According to Sommer and Tautz (1989), inosine should not be used at the 3'-end of the primer. This recommendation is in contrast to our own observations, which suggest that primers with inosine at the 3'-end can successfully be utilized to prevent false-negative results by 3'-mismatching (see also Batzer 1991). The high variability of individual base positions is of particular importance at the critical 3'-end of the PCR primer, since a mismatch in this position might prevent primer elongation, even if all other bases show ideal annealing. It is therefore recommended to always select primer sequences with the 3' base in a maximally preserved segment of the gene. No specific reaction conditions are required when using highly degenerate primers (Coloma 1991), though a reduction of the annealing temperature may be necessary in some cases.

3.8. Application of PCR for genetic examinations, DNA amplification fingerprinting (DAF)

Every individual is characterized by a unique hereditary composition. The only exception are identical twins, who possess the same genotype, but, due to consequences of complex developmental events, differ slightly in their phenotype. Moreover, the DNA of a specific individual is the same everywhere, regardless of whether it is obtained from his blood cells, hair, or organ cells. Numerous genetic diseases arise from a limited number of mutated alleles or gene variations. These divergent sequences can be used to screen for carrier status and in fetal diagnosis, e.g., phenylketonuria or sickle-cell disease. Mostly, these diseases are caused by very few single nucleotide differences. Others are characterized by large deletions, e.g., Duchenne muscular dystrophy. For the identification of such changes in gene sequence, various methods are available. Large deletions can be detected by pulsed-field gel electrophoresis (den Dunnen 1987). Today point mutations or smaller deletions can be easily and reliably detected by PCR. For example, the hypoxanthine-guanine phosphoribosyltransferase gene (defective in Lesch-Nyhan syndrome) can be amplified from genomic DNA by PCR, and the point mutation can then be identified through sequencing (Gibbs 1989).

The analysis of genetic linkage is based on the exchange of genetic information (recombination) between the pairs of maternally and paternally derived chromosome homologs during the meiotic cell divisions. Sequence polymorphisms appear in the genome every few hundred nucleotides, mostly as a consequence of single-nucleotide substitutions, which sometimes alter the site of cleavage by restriction enzymes. Alterations in the positions of cleavage sites result in DNA fragments that occur in different sizes in different individuals. These different forms are called "restriction fragment length polymorphisms" (RFLPs) and may constitute a valuable genetic linkage marker. One type of RFLP is caused by the presence of variable numbers of tandem repeat DNA sequences (VNTRs).

Eukaryotic cells contain about 100 times more non-protein-coding DNA than coding DNA. This noncoding DNA consits largely of repeating sequences. The human genome is composed of repetitive sequences, the Alu family alone representing 5% of total DNA (see also chapter 15.2). Alu sequences are mostly localized in regions between single genes and only rarely in the intron region. Thus, the mammalian genome is characterized on the one hand by single-copy DNA for most of the enzyme- and structural protein-coding genes and on the other hand by non-coding sequences interspersed with repetitive segments of varying length. A concentration of satellite repetitive DNA occurs in the heterochromatic region near the chromosome centromeres and near the telomeres.

Hypervariable regions of the genome (HVR), to which no function can so far be attributed, are arrays of short, usually GC-rich units, which are repeated in tandem. In these tandem repeats, a molecular basis of genetic variability can be found. Cloned HVR loci can be used for the production of probes. The complex patterns of hypervariable bands resulting from these probes in the course of hybridization yield an individual-specific DNA fingerprint. It is important to note that these fingerprint bands are inherited in a Mendelian fashion. The evolutionary instability causing the hypervariability in these gene regions is not great enough to interfere with segregation analysis. Therefore, DNA fingerprinting is to be recommended in linkage studies. The disadvantage of classical fingerprinting are the relatively large DNA amounts required, up to 5µg per lane in the gel. In contrast, the PCR is capable of analyzing minute amounts of DNA, even it is degraded (e.g. 1ng). The fingerprint analysis with the PCR is based on the analysis of either a length polymorphism (VNTR region) or a sequence polymorphism. The amplification of VNTR regions is carried out with the help of two primers that are complementary to a unique sequence flanking the tandem repeat region (Tautz 1989). The allelic variations can then be distinguished by the differences in size of the PCR products. Jeffreys et al. (1988) describe the amplification of hypervariable minisatellites, which sometimes have lengths of up to 5-10kb. The authors demonstrate the ability to perform a DNA fingerprint analysis from single cells with the use of the PCR. Horn et al. (1989) have published the same procedure for the VNTR segment, which is detected by the pYNZ22 probe (HGm locus D17S30) and identifies one of the most highly polymorphic regions. More than 10 alleles have so far been demonstrated using the southern blot hybridization. The PCR amplification products described by the authors, with a length of 170bp to 870bp (1 to 11 repeat units between the primers), follow the Mendelian pattern of inheritance. The amplified DNA fragments are separated by high-resolution polyacrylamide-gel electrophoresis (PAGE). After electrophoresis, the DNA fragments are made visible by silver staining. This technique allows the detection and distinguishability of DNA fragments differing in length by 10bp or less (Allen 1989).

In 1990, Jeffreys et al. demonstrated that, with the help of the PCR, allelic variations within a minisatellite locus can be analyzed. This approach, called "minisatellite variant repeat" (MVR), dramatically increased the number of different alleles of each minisatellite locus detectable in the population. Jeffreys et al. demonstrated this procedure by the example of the hypervariable locus D1S8 (probe MS32) at region 42-43 on the long arm of chromosome 1. About half of the repeats showed an A to G transition, which created a HaeIII restriction site. Using allele-specific primers that differ at their 3' ends (Jeffreys 1991), these HaeIII+ and HaeIII- repeat units can be detected and distinguished in a PCR (so-called MVR-PCR). The MVR-PCR also shows that a very high level of allelic variability exists within the human minisatellite sequence. This provides evidence that recombination is involved in the generation of ultravariability.

The disadvantage of all hitherto mentioned methods that use the PCR for fingerprinting is that the sequence of the gene region flanking the minisatellite or VNTR must be known, since the primers for the PCR must be synthesized complementary to it. In contrast, DNA amplification fingerprinting (DAF) offers a possibility of demonstrating DNA polymorphisms with the use of a single arbitrary primer without knowledge of flanking DNA sequences (Caetano-Anolles 1991). The primers used by Williams et al. (1991) and by Welsh (1991) have a length of at least 8 base pairs and a GC content of over 40%. The exchange of a single base in the sequence of the primer (e.g., 5'TGG TCA CTG A 3' vs. 5'TGG ACA CTG A 3') yields a completely different band pattern in agarose gel or silver stain. The amplification conditions differ from the usual PCR assays in that the annealing temperature is considerably lower (usually between 34°C and 40°C). The RAPD (random amplified polymorphic DNA) markers produced using this method are well suited for genetic mapping and DNA fingerprinting, particularly for studies in population genetics. As with other molecular markers, the information content of a single RAPD marker is low. Only in comparison with many other DNA samples investigated are they useful. Their essential advantage in the use for linkage studies is the fact that they require no preparation, like the isolation of cloned probes, DNA sequencing or filter hybridization, and while they admit a high degree of automation, making possible the simple identification of many bacterial strains. Nevertheless, the hot-start PCR will be essential - especially for this procedure - to minimize nonspecific results (see also chapter 1 and 2).

3.9. Amplification with consensus primers

A promising method is the application of "consensus" primers that prime the amplification of sequences from different types of organisms or different alleles from one genomic locus. After amplification with a single primer pair, the product(s) can be differentiated by several methods (e.g. differences in length, restriction sites).

Examples	Differentiation	Reference
Enteroviruses	hybridization	Chapman 1990
Mycobacteria	hybridization	Brisson 1989
VNTR	polyacrylamide gel	Richards 1991
T-cell receptor	sequencing	Yokota 1991
RAS	dot blot hybridization	Enomoto 1991
Human papillomavirus	endonucleases	Rodu 1991

The use of fluorescence-labeled primers and hybridization of the amplified products to solid phase-bound capture probes might allow automation, differentiation and quantification of the specifically bound products (Sninsky, personal communication). This would be of great importance for the detection and differentiation of infectious agents. Such a procedure may eventually lead to the development of diagnostic tests which simultaneously "screen" patient samples for different infectious agents or alleles.

3.10. Expression PCR

Using a universal promoter sequence expression PCR allows synthesis of functional proteins by direct in-vitro translation of PCR-generated fragments without cloning (Kain 1991). A suitable template for in-vitro translation can be generated by splicing a universal promoter sequence (T7 bacteriophage promoter: 5' TAA TAC GAC TCA CTA TA 3') with the target DNA to be expressed. Kain et al. initially amplified the target DNA by means of a 5'primer with an homology to the 3'-end of the universal promoter (5' CCA AGT TTC TAA TAC GAC TCA CTA TAG GGT TTT TAT TTT TAA TTT TCT TTC AAA TAC TTC CAC C [ATG] 3´ : bases 10 - 26 universal T7 promoter sequence, bases 27 - 64 untranslated leader sequence, ATG start site). The amplified product and the universal promoter sequence are then mixed and re-amplified. Overlapping of the 5'-end of the target DNA and the 3'-end of the promoter sequence results in the formation of an overlapping hybrid following denaturation of the mixture. In a subsequent PCR assay, this hybrid is first completed in both directions and then amplified by addition of primers. It can thus be transcribed and translated in vitro without further processing. Expression PCR has the advantage of not requiring special transcription vectors, cloning procedures, plasmid isolation or creation of special restriction sites. This procedure also provides a simple means for the synthesis of mutant proteins by alteration of the DNA template.

3.11. Detection of infectious agents or rare sequences

For the detection of an unknown number of target sequences in a DNA or cDNA sample, for example infectious agents, long primers (20-30 bases) may provide better conditions than short ones because of the higher annealing temperature and the lower relative impact of point mutations within the annealing site sequence (see also chapter 13.2). In samples with very low target concentrations, a marked improvement of the amplification result can also be achieved by increasing the annealing time of the first 3 - 5 cycles to 2 - 4 min (see also figure 1.6). Prolonged annealing probably enhances DNA template screening by the primers present in the assay (Ruano 1991). Other study groups have reported that a considerably prolonged single initial denaturation step of 30 min at 95°C also increases amplification efficiency in samples with low target concentrations. But on the other hand, especially when rare sequences are to be amplified or cloning of the PCR fragments is planned, thermally induced mutations of the target DNA might be a drawback (see also chapter 21). Ruano et al. (1989) described a booster PCR assay including the following steps: In the first 20 cycles, the primers are diluted to an initial 10^7-fold molar excess relative to the template. The first step is followed by a second phase (30 - 50 cycles) with oligonucleotide concentrations of 0.1 µM (about 4×10^{10} molecules). This procedure can be used to amplify low target amounts, since it reduces the formation of primer dimers, which may result from very low target concentrations. The system can be further improved by utilizing nested primers and increasing the Taq concentration during the second phase.

D'Aquila et al. (1991) report that the addition of the denatured target DNA into an aliquoted mastermix reaction assay preheated to temperatures above the annealing temperature increases the product yield as well as the specificity of the PCR. This preamplification heating - a variant of the hot-start PCR (see chapters 1 and 2) - may provide for a more stringent annealing of the primers and possibly prevent the formation of "primer-dimer complexes" (see chapter 20.1) and "primer self-annealing".

If highly polymorphic target sequences are to be amplified, a set of primers slightly shifted on the target DNA, e.g. sequences with different 3'termini (Weber-Rolfs unpublished observation), or the use of 3'-inosine (Linz 1990) might be helpful. Alternatively, a DNA polymerase with proofreading activity might be suitable in such cases (see chapter 21).

Table 3.1.: List of pathogens for which PCR detection assays have been established (the abbreviation "p" stands for the probe)

Pathogen	Primer sequence (5'- 3')	PCR product	Reference
Hepatitis A virus	gtt ttg ctc ctc ttt atc atg cta tg gga aat gtc tca ggt act ttc ttt g p: tca aca aca gtt tct aca ga	229bp	Margolis 1990
Hepatitis B virus	ctg gga gga gtt ggg gga gga gat t ggc gag gga gtt ctc ctt cta ggg g p: gga aag aag tca gaa ggc aa	632bp	Carman 1989
	gct ttg ggg cat gga cat tga ccc gta taa ctg act act aat tcc ctg gat gct ggg tct	270bp	Kaneko 1989
	aga cca cca aat gcc cct atc cgt ctg cga ggc gag gga	101bp	Lo 1989
Hepatitis C virus	gca tgt cat gat gta t aca ata cgt gtg tca p: cct tca cca ttg aga caa tca cgc tcc- ccc agg atg ctg t		Weiner 1990
Hepatitis D virus	tat tct tct ttc cct tct aga agt tag agg aac tgc p: ttg tcg gtg aat cct ccc ctg aga ggc- ctc ttc cta ggt c	359bp	Zignego 1990
Cytomegalovirus	cca agc ggc ctc tga taa cca agc c cag cac cat cct cct ctt cct ctg g p: gag gct att gta gcc tac act ttg g	435bp	Demmler 1988
	ccc gac ttt acc atc cag ta aag acg aag agg aac tat ct p: ggg tga agg agt cga aa		Stanier 1989
	gct atg ttt cag atg tcg ccg cc ccc acc tcg ggc tca aac ac	215bp	Kouzarides 1987
Epstein-Barr virus	cag gct tcc ctg caa ttt tac aag cgg ccc aga agt ata cgt ggt gac gta ga p: gat gat aag gtg tcc aa	288bp	Saito 1989

Pathogen	Primer sequence (5'- 3')									PCR product	Reference
Epstein-Barr virus	cca	cca	gca	gca	cca	gca	ca			89bp	Sixbey 1989
	ggt	ggc	cac	cat	ggt	ggc	cc				
	p: tta	cat	cat	cta	ccc	tcg					
	cct	gta	ggg	gaa	gcc	gat				387bp	Ambinder 1990
	caa	tgg	tgt	aag	acg	aca	tt				
	p: gga	gaa	ggc	cca	agc	act	gg				
Human Herpes Virus 6	ccc	att	tac	gat	ttc	ctg	cac	cac ctc		245bp	Buchbinder 1988
	cga	cat	gct	caa	tga	cat	aac	ggt ccc	tga a		
	p: ccg	taa	aaa	att	tac	acc	tcc	att	tca tct t		
Herpes simplex virus 1+2	gcg	aga	tat	cgg	ccg	ggg	ag			124bp	Boerman 1989
	tgc	ggg	ccc	aca	gcc	tcc	c				
	cag	tac	ggc	ccc	gag	ttc	gtg	acc ggg		330bp	Kimura 1991
	ggc	gta	gta	ggc	ggg	gat	gtc	gcg			
	p: atg	gtg	aac	atc	gac	atg	tac	gg			
Varizella zoster	cgt	cac	ata	tta	tgc	aaa	cat	g		224bp	Davison 1983
	cgt	ttt	taa	tat	tac	aaa	tcc	cgc			
Human papillomavirus 6	tag	tgg	gcc	tat	ggc	tcg	tc			280bp	Melchers 1989
	tcc	att	agc	ctc	cac	ggg	tg				
	p: cat	taa	cgc	agg	ggc	gcc	tga	aat tgt	gcc		
Human papillomavirus 6-11	gac	cag	ttg	tgc	aag	acg	ttt	aat c		398bp	Ferre 1989
	ctt	cca	tgc	atg	ttg	tcc	agc	ag			
	p HPV6: ctg	ttt	cga	ggc	ggc	tat	cca	ta			
	p HPV11: gca	cac	tct	gca	aat	tca	gtg	cg			
Human papillomavirus 16	aat	gct	agt	gct	tat	gca	gc			153bp	Cornelissen 1989
	att	tac	tgc	aac	att	ggg	tac				
	p: gca	aac	cac	cta	tag	ggg	aac	act ggg	gca		
Human papillomavirus 18	tgg	tgt	ata	gag	aca	gta	tac	ccc a		248bp	Ferre 1989
	gcc	tct	ata	gtg	ccc	agc	tat	gt			
	p: att	caa	cgg	ttt	ctg	gca	ccg	ca			

Pathogen	Primer sequence (5'- 3')	PCR product	Reference
Picornaviruses	aag cac ttc tgt ttc c cat tca ggg gcc gga gga p 1: ggc cgc caa cgc agc c p 2: ggc agc cac gca ggc t	298bp	Hyypia 1989
HIV-1 (env)	gta gta ttg gta aat gtg a ctt aat ttg cta tct p: cta tat cag ttt ata aag	815bp	McKeating 1990
	agc agc agg aag cac tat gg cca gac tgt gag ttg caa cag p: acg gta cag gcc aga caa tta ttg tct ggt ata gt	122bp	Ou 1988
HIV-1 (gag)	cag gga gct aga acg at ctt ctg atc ctg tct ga p: aat cct ggc ctg tta gaa aca tca gaa g	107bp	Carman 1989
HIV-1 (LTR)	act agg gaa ccc act gct ggt ctg agg gat ctc ta p: acc aga gtc aca caa cag acg ggc aca cac tac t	105bp	Ou 1988
HIV-1 (nef)	atg ctg att gtg cct ggc ta tga att agc cct tcc agt cc p: aag tgg cta aga tct aca gct gaa t	151bp	Murakawa 1988
HIV-1 (tat)	ctt agg cat ctc cta tgg ca cgg gcc tgt cgg gtt ccc tc	2472bp	Hart 1988
HIV-2 (LTR)	agg agc tgg tgg gga acg gtg ctg gtg aga gtc tag ca p: ttg agc cct ggg agg ttc tct cca gca- gta gca ggt ag	165bp	Rayfield 1988
HTLV-1 (gag)	cga ccg ccc cgg ggg ctg gcc gct ggt act gca gga ggt ctt gga gg p: gat ccc gtc ccg tcc cgc gcc a	535bp	Reddy 1989

General Applications of PCR

Pathogen	Primer sequence (5'- 3')	PCR product	Reference
HTLV-1 (LTR)	ccc ggg ggc tta gag cct ccc agt gaa ttc tct cct gag agt gct ata p: tca ggt agg gcg gcg ggc gcg tga agg-aga gat gcg agc c	718bp	Greenberg 1989
HTLV-2 (tax)	tgg ata ccc cgt cta cgt gt gag ctg aca acg cgt cca tcg p: agg tga gtt ggt gct ctg gac agg tgg-cca gga ggg cat	159bp	Kwok 1988
Rotavirus	ggc ttt aaa aga gag aat ttc cgt ctg g ggt cac atc ata caa ttc taa tct aag	1062bp	Gouvea 1990
Borrelia burgdorferi	cga aga tac taa atc tgt gat caa ata ttt cag ctt p: aat cag ttc cca ttt gca	371bp	Rosa 1989
Legionella pneumophila	gtc atg agg aat ctc gct g ctg gct tct tcc agc ttc a p: gtc cgt tat ggg gta ttg atc acc a	700bp	Starnbach 1989
Mycoplasma pneumoniae	gaa gct tat ggt aca ggt tgg att acc atc ctt gtt gta agg p: cgt aag cta tca gct aca tgg agg	468bp	Bernet 1989
Plasmodium falciparum	ggc tta gtt acg att aat ag aca ctt tca tcc aac acc ta p: acg aaa gtt aag gga gtg aag acg a	212bp	Jaureguiberry 1990
Toxoplasma gondii	gga act gca tcc gtt cat gag tct tta aag cgt tcg tgg tc p: ggc gac caa tct gcg aat aca cc	194bp	Burg 1989
Candida albicans	cat aac tca ata tgg cta tt ctt ttg acg aca tgc ttc ga	245bp	Buchman 1990
Pneumocystis carinii	gat ggc tgt ttc caa gcc ca gtg tac gtt gca aag tac tc p: ata agg tag ata gtc gaa ag	346bp	Wakefield 1990

References

1. Allen RC, Graves G, Budowle B. Polymerase chain reaction amplification products separated on rehydratable polyacrylamide gels and stained with silver. 1989, BioTechniques 7, 736-744

2. Ambinder RF, Lambe BC, Mann RB, Hayward SD, Zehnbauer B, Burns WS, Charache P. Oligonucleotides for polymerase chain reaction amplifiction and hybridization detection of Epstein-Barr virus DNA in clinical specimens. 1990, Mol Cell Probes 4, 397-407

3. Batzer MA, Carlton JE, Deininger PL. Enhanced evolutionary PCR using oligonucleotides with inosine at the 3'terminus. 1991, Nucl Acids Res 19, 5081

4. Bernet C, Garret M, de Barbeyrac B, Bebear C, Bonnet J. Detection of Mycoplasma pneumoniae by using the polymerase chain reaction. 1989, J Clin Microbiol 27, 2492-2496

5. Boerman RH, Arnoldus EP, Raap AK, Bloem BR, Verhey M, van Gemert G, Peters AC, van der Ploeg M. Polymerase chain reaction and viral culture techniques to detect HSV in small volumes of cerebrospinal fluid: an experimental mouse encephalitis study. 1989, J Virol Methods 25, 189-197

6. Brisson-Noel A, Gicquel B, Lecossier D, Levy-Febrault V, Nassif X, Hance AJ. Rapid diagnosis of mycobacterial DNA in clinical samples. 1989, Lancet II, 1069-1071

7. Buchbinder A, Jospehs SF, Ablashi D, Salahuddin SZ, Klotman ME, Manak M, Krueger GR, Wong-Staal F, Gallo RC. Polymerase chain reaction amplification and in situ hybridization for the detection of human B-lymphotropic virus. 1988, J Virol Methods 21, 191-197

8. Buchman TG, Rossier M, Merz WG, Charache P. Detection of surgical pathogens by in vitro DNA amplification. Part I: Rapid identification of Candida albicans by in vitro amplification of a fungus-specific gene. 1990, Surgery 108, 338-346

9. Burg JL, Grover CM, Pouletty P, Boothroyd JC. Direct and sensitive detection of a pathogenic protozoan, Toxoplasma gondii by polymerase chain reaction. 1989, J Clin Microbiol 27, 1787-1792

10. Caetano-Anolles G, Bassam BJ, Gresshoff PM. DNA amplification fingerprinting using very short arbitrary oligonucleotide primers. 1991, BioTechnology 9, 553-557

11. Carman WF, Jacyna MR, Hadzizyannis S, Karayinnis P, McGravey MJ, Makris A, Thomas HC. Mutation preventing formation of hepatitis B e antigen in patients with chronic hepatitis B infection. 1989, Lancet II, 588-591

12. Carman WF, Kidd AH. An assessment of optimal conditions for amplification of HIV cDNA using Thermus aquaticus polymerase. 1989, J Virol Methods 23, 277-289

13. Chamberlain JS, Gibbs RA, Ranier JE, Ngyen PN, Caskey C Th. Deletion screening of the Duchenne muscular dystrophy locus via multiplex DNA amplification. 1988, Nucl Acids Res 16, 11141-11156

14. Chapman NM, Tracy S, Gauntt CJ, Fortmueller U. Molecular detection and identification of enteroviruses using enzymatic amplification and nucleic acid hybridization. 1990, J Clin Microbiol 28, 843-850

15. Coloma MJ, Larrick JW, Ayala M, Gavilondo-Cowley JV. Primer design for the cloning of immunoglobulin heavy-chain leader-variable regions from mouse hybridoma cells using the PCR. 1991, BioTechniques 11, 152-156

16. Cornelissen MT, van den Tweel JG, Struyk AP, Jebbink MF, Briet M, van der Noordaa J, ter Schegget JT. Localization of human papillomavirus type 16 DNA using the polymerase chain reaction in the cervix uteri of women with cervical intraepithelial neoplasia. 1989, J Gen Virol 70, 2555-2562

17. D'Aquila RT, Bechtel LJ, Videler JA, Eron JJ, Gorczyca P, Kaplan JC. Maximizing sensitivity and specificity

of PCR by preamplification heating. 1991, Nucl Acids Res 19, 3749

18. Davison AJ. DNA sequence of the US component of the Varicella zoster virus genome. 1983, EMBO J 2, 2203-2209

19. Demmler GJ, Buffone GJ, Schimbor CM, May RA. Detection of cytomegalovirus in urine from newborns by using polymerase chain reaction DNA amplification. 1988, J Infect Dis 158, 1177-1184

20. den Dunnen JT, Bakker E, Breteler EG, Pearson PL, van-Ommen GJ. Direct detection of more than 50% of the Duchenne muscular dystrophy mutations by field inversion gels. 1987, Nature 329, 640-642

21. Enomoto T, Inoue M, Peratoni AO, Buzard GS, Miki H, Tanizawa O, Rice JM. K-ras activation in premalignant and malignant epithelial lesions of the human uterus. 1991, Cancer Res 51, 5308-5314

22. Erlich HA, Gelfand D, Sninsky JJ. Recent advances in the polymerase chain reaction. 1991, Science 252, 1643-1651.

23. Finckh U, Lingenfelter PA, Myerson D. Producing single-stranded DNA probes with the *Taq* DNA polymerase: A high yield protocol. 1991, Biotechniques 10, 35-39.

24. Frye RA, Benz CC, Liu E. Detection of amplified oncogenes by differential polymerase chain reaction. 1989, Oncogene 4, 101-105.

25. Gelfand DH, White TH J. Thermostable DNA polymerases. In: PCR protocols. A guide to methods and applications. Eds.: MA Innis, DH Gelfand, JJ Sninsky, Th J White. 1990, Academic Press, San Diego, pp129-141

26. Gibbs RA, Nguyen PN, McBride LJ, Koepf SM, Caskey CT. Identification of mutations leading to the Lesch-Nyhan syndrome by automated direct DNA sequencing of in vitro amplified cDNA. 1989, Proc Natl Acad Sci USA 86, 1919-1923

27. Gibbs RA, Ngyen PN, Caskey C Th. Detection of single DNA base differences by competitive oligonucleotide priming. 1989, Nucl Acids Res 17, 2437-2448

28. Gilliland G, Perrin S, Blanchard K, Bunn HF. Analysis of cytokine mRNA and DNA: detction and quantitation by competitive polymerase chain reaction. 1990, Proc Natl Acad Sci USA 87, 2725-2729

29. Gouvea V, Glass RI, Woods P, Taniguchi K, Clark HF, Forrester B, Fang ZY. Polymerase chain reaction amplification and typing of rotavirus nucleic acid from stool specimens. 1990, J Clin Microbiol 28, 276-282

30. Greenberg SJ, Ehrlich GD, Abbott MA, Hurwitz BJ, Waldman TA, Poiesz BJ. Detection of sequences homologous to human retroviral DNA in multiple sclerosis by gene amplification. 1989, Proc Natl Acad Sci USA 86, 2878-2882

31. Gyllensten UB, Erlich HA. Generation of single-stranded DNA by the polymerase chain reaction and its application to direct sequencing of the HLA-DQA locus. 1988, Proc Natl Acad Sci USA 85, 7652-7657.

32. Hart C, Schochetman G, Spira T, Lifson A, Moore J, Galphin J, Sninsky J, Ou CY. Direct detection of HIV RNA expression in seropositive subjects. 1988, Lancet II, 596-599

33. He X, Treacy MN, Simmons DM, Ingraham HA, Swanson LW, Rosenfeld MG. Expression of a large family of POU-domain regulatory genes in mammalian brain development. 1989, Nature 340, 35-41

34. Hoof van Huijsduijnen RAM, Ayala G, DeLamarter F. A means to reduce the complexity of oligonucleotides encoding degenerate peptides. 1992, Nucl Acids Res 20, 919

35. Horn GT, Richards B, Klinger KW. Amplification of highly polymorphic VNTR segment by the polymerase chain reaction. 1989, Nucl Acids Res 17, 2140

36. Hyypia T, Auvinen P, Maaronen M. Polymerase chain reaction for human picornaviruses. 1989, J Gen Virol 70, 3261-3268

37. Jaurequiberry G, Hatin I, d'Auriol L, Galibert G. PCR detection of Plasmodium falciparum by oligonucleotide probes. 1990, Mol Cell Probes 4, 409-414

38. Jeffreys AJ, MacLeod A, Tamaki K, Neil D, Monckton DG. Minisatellite repeat coding as a digital approach to DNA typing. 1991, Nature 354, 204-209

39. Jeffreys AJ, Neumann R, Wilson V. Repeat unit sequence variation in minisatellites: a novel source of DNA polymorphism for studying variation and mutation by single molecule analysis. 1990, Cell 60, 473-485

40. Jeffreys AJ, Wilson V, Neumann R, Keyte J. Amplification of human minisatellites by the polymerase chain reaction: towards DNA fingerprinting of single cells. 1988, Nucl Acids Res 16, 10953-10971

41. Kain KC, Orlandi PA, Lanar DE. Universal promoter for gene expression without cloning: expression-PCR. 1991, BioTechniques 10, 366-373

42. Kaneko S, Feinstone SM, Miller RH. Rapid and sensitive method for the detection of serum hepatitis B virus DNA using the polymerase chain reaction technique. 1989, J Clin Microbiol 27, 1930-1933

43. Kimura H, Futamura M, Kito H, Ando T, Goto M, Kuzushima K, Shibata M, Morishima T. Detection of viral DNA in neonatal herpes simplex virus infections: frequent and prolonged presence in serum and cerebrospinal fluid. 1991, J Infect Dis 164, 289-293

44. Kouzarides T. Sequence and transcription analysis of the human cytomegalovirus NA polymerase gene. 1987, J Virol 61, 125-133

45. Kwok S, Kellogg D, Ehrlich G, Poiesz B, Bhagavati S, Sninsky JJ. Characterization of a sequence of human T cell leukemia virus type 1 from a patient with chronic progressive myelopathy. 1988, J Infect Dis 158, 1193-1197

46. Kwok S, Kellogg DE, McKinney N, Spasic D, Goda L, Levenson C, Sninsky JJ. Effects of primer-template mismatches on the polymerase chain reactioion: human immundefciency virus type 1 model studies. 1990, Nucl Acids Res 18, 999-1005

47. Linz U, Delling U, Rübsamen-Waigmann H. Systematic studies on parameters influencing the performance of the PCR. 1990, J Clin Chem Clin Biochem 28, 5-13

48. Lo YM, Mehal WZ, Fleming KA. In vitro amplification of hepatitis B virus sequences from liver tumour DNA and from paraffin wax embedded tissues using the polymerase chain reaction. 1989, J Clin Pathol 42, 840-846

49. Margolis HS, Nainan OV. Identification of virus components in circulating immune complexes isolated during hepatitis A virus infection. 1990, Hepatology 11, 31-37

50. Mazars GR, Moyret C, Jeanteur P, Theillet CG. Direct sequencing by thermal asymmetric PCR. 1991, Nucl Acids Res 19, 4783

51. McKeating JA, Griffiths PD, Weiss RA. HIV susceptibility conferred to human fibroblasts by cytomegalovirus-induced Fc receptor. 1990, Nature 343, 659-661

52. Melchers W, van den Brule A, Walboomers J, de Bruin M, Burger M, Herbrink P, Meijer C, Lindeman J, Quint W. Increased detection rate of human papillomavirus in cervical scrapes by the polymerase chain reaction as compard to modified FISH and southern blot analysis. 1989, J Med Virol 27, 329-335

53. Murakawa GJ, Zaia JA, Spallone PA, Stephens DA, Kaplan BE, Wallace RB, Rossi JJ. Direct detection of HIV-1 RNA from AIDS and ARC patient samples. 1988, DNA 7, 287-295

54. Neubauer A, Neubauer B, Liu E. Polymerase chain reaction based assay to detect allelic loss in human DNA: loss of ß-interferon gene in chronic myelogenous leukemia. 1990, Nucl Acids Res 18, 993-998

55. Ou CY, Kwok S, Mitchell SW, Mack DH, Sninsky JJ, Krebs JW, Feorino P, Warfield D, Schochetman G. DNA amplification for direct detection of HIV-1 in DNA of peripheral blood mononuclear cells. 1988, Science 239, 295-297

56. Perrin S, Gilliland G. Site-specific mutagenesis using asymmetric polymerase chain reaction and a single mutant primer. 1990, Nucl Acids Res 18, 7433-7438

57. Rayfield M, de Cock K, Heyward W, Goldstein L, Krebs J, Kwok S, Lee S, McCormick J, Moreau JM, Odehouri K et al. Mixed human immunodeficiency virus (HIV) infection in an individual: demonstration

of both HIV type 1 and type 2 proviral sequences by using polymerase chain reaction. 1988, J Infect Dis 158, 1170-1176

58. Reddy EP, Sandberg-Wollheim M, Mettus RV, Ray PE, DeFreitas E, Koprowski H. Amplification and molecular cloning of HTLV-1 sequences from DNA of multiple sclerosis patients. 1989, Science 243, 529-533

59. Richards B, Horn GT, Merrill JJ, Klinger KW. Characterization and rapid analysis of the highly polymorphic VNTR locus D4S125 (YNZ32), closely linked to the Huntington disease gene. 1991, Genomics 9, 235-240

60. Rodu B, Christian C, Synder RC, Ray R, Miller DM. Simplified PCR-based detection and typing strategy for human papillomaviruses utilizing a single oligonucleotide primer set. 1991, BioTechniques 10, 632-637

61. Rosa PA, Schwan TG. A specific and sensitive assay for the Lyme disease spirochete Borrelia burgdorferi using the polymerase chain reaction. 1989, J Infect Dis 160, 1018-1029

62. Ruano G, Fenton W, Kidd KK. Biphasic amplification of very dilute DNA samples via "booster" PCR. 1989, Nucl Acids Res 17, 5407

63. Ruano G, Brash DE, Kidd KK. PCR: The first few cycles. 1991, Amplifications A Forum for PCR users 7, 1-4

64. Saito I, Servenius B, Compton T, Fox RI. Detection of Epstein Barr virus DNA by polymerase chain reaction in blood and tissue biopsies from patients with Sjogren's syndrome. 1989, J Exp Med 169, 2191-2198

65. Sarkar G, Cassady J, Bottema CDK, Sommer SS. Characterization of polymerase chain reaction amplification of specific alleles. 1990, Anal Biochem 186, 64-68

66. Sixbey JW, Shirley P, Chesney PJ, Buntin DM, Resnick L. Detection of a second widespread strain of Epstein-Barr virus. 1989, Lancet II, 761-765

67. Sommer R, Tautz D. Minimal homology requirements for PCR primers. 1989, Nucl Acids Res 16, 6749

68. Stanier P, Taylor DL, Kitchen AD, Wales N, Tryhorn Y, Tyms AS. Persistence of cytomegalovirus in mononuclear cells in peripheral blood from blood donors. 1989, BMJ 299, 897-898

69. Starnbach MN, Falkow S, Tompkins LS. Species-specific detection of Legionella pneumophila in water by DNA amplification and hybridization. 1989, J Clin Micorbiol 27, 1257-1261

70. Tautz D. Hypervariability of simple sequences as a general source for polymorphic DNA markers. 1989, Nucl Acids Res 17, 6463-6471

71. Wakefield AE, Pixley FJ, Banerji S, Sinclair K, Miller RF, Moxon ER, Hopkin JM. Detection of Pneumocystis carinii with DNA amplification. 1990, Lancet II, 451-453

72. Weiner AJ, Kuo G, Bradley DW, Bonino F, Saracco G, Lee C, Rosenblatt J, Choo QL, Houghton M. Detection of hepatitis C viral sequences in non-A, non-B hepatitis. 1990, Lancet I, 1-3

73. Welsh J, Petersen Ch, McClelland M. Polymorphisms generated by arbitrarily primes PCR in the mouse: application to strain identification and genetic mapping. 1991, Nucl Acids Res 19, 303-306

74. Williams JGK, Kubelik AR, Livak KJ, Rafalski JA, Tingey SV. DNA polymorphisms amplified by arbitrary primers are useful as genetic markers. 1990, Nucl Acids Res 18, 6531-6535

75. Wilson RK, Chen C, Hood L. Optimization of asymmetric polymerase chain reaction for rapid fluorescent DNA sequencing. 1990, BioTechniques 8, 184-189

76. Wu DY, Ugozzoli L, Pal BK, Wallace RB. Allele-specific enzymatic amplification of ß-globin genomic DNA for diagnosis of sickle cell anemia. 1989, Proc Natl Acad Sci USA 86, 2757-2760.

77. Yap EPH, McGee O'D. Short PCR product yields improved by lower denaturation temperatures. 1991, Ncul Acids Res 19, 1713

78. Yokota S, Hansen-Hagge TE, Bartram CR. T-cell receptor delta gene recombination in common acute lymphoblstic leukemia: preferential usage of V delta 2 and frequent involvement of the J alpha cluster. 1991, Blood 77, 141-148

79. Zignego AL, Deny P, Feray C, Ponzetto A, Gentilini P, Tiollais P, Brechot C. Amplification of hepatitis delta virus RNA sequences by polymerase chain reaction: a tool for viral detection and cloning. 1990, Mol Cell Probes 4, 43-51

4. Substances Affecting PCR: Inhibition or Enhancement

PCR amplification can be adversely or advantageously affected by a large number of factors. In the chapter dealing with optimization of PCR it has already been pointed out that altering any one of the basic parameters of the polymerase chain reaction - be it physical or chemical - will influence the reaction. Among the most influential changes introduced into a certain PCR assay are those brought about by altering Mg^{2+}-ion and/or dNTP concentration, Taq concentration or the cycle temperature profile, especially the annealing temperature. In brief, 10mM $MgCl_2$ inhibits Taq polymerase activity 40-50% and concentrations of monovalent ions exceeding 75mM KCl inhibit activity (Gelfand 1990). Due to their interaction with magnesium ions, elevated concentrations of dNTPs in PCR also influence Taq polymerase activity. Even oil overlay can affect the efficiency of PCR (Mezei 1990). A good optimization strategy of these parameters will in most cases increase specificity and thus sensitivity of the PCR assay being established. However, if the PCR assay being established still yields unsatisfactory results despite optimization, further components of the assay must be considered. These include the nature of the native material, the method employed to isolate template DNA, reagents used to isolate DNA and inadvertantly introduced into the PCR as well as sequence features of the target DNA. These, as well as a handful of further interesting observations regarding the use of additives in PCR are summarized in this chapter.

4.1. Inhibition introduced by native material

The pivotal starting point is to reassure oneself that inhibitory substances in the native material are not being introduced into the PCR in effective concentrations. Typical sources of DNA templates for diagnostic PCR are urine, peripheral blood cells, cell smears, sputum, cells of the cerebrospinal fluid and biopsy material. Although the precise inhibitory substances have not been discerned, urine seems to contain several. Protocols using urine which has simply been boiled for 10 minutes in order to liberate DNA from cellular material and/or from infectious particles (e.g. viral particles) by hydrolysing structural proteins have shown that it is often necessary to dilute the urine sample to obviate inhibition in PCR (Demmler 1988). However, diluting the sample can artificially lower the number of infectious agents to such an extent that detection of the target DNA by PCR is jeopardized. The interpretation of negative PCR results is then rather difficult. Performing PCR in reaction mixtures with unknown inhibitory substances always requires good controls which will allow the examiner to estimate the actual sensitivity of the assay. This is best realized by setting up serial dilution assays of both the native material itself as the background of the PCR and of exogenously added target DNA sequence which can be readily obtained, if an infectious agent is of interest. The PCR results from the experimental serial dilutions together with those obtained using sample material directly at a given dilution can yield helpful information regarding the interpretation of negative and positive results. If there is evidence that there are inhibitory substances in the native material, then negative results must be judged critically because they could reflect false negatives. Positive results in native material which has been substantially diluted must also be viewed critically, since a higher risk may ensue that a contamination has led to the positive result. In this case it is absolutely mandatory to run a number of stringent controls which allow judging of extraneous contamination.

4.1.1. Blood

Using whole blood as a source for template DNA sometimes poses problems. Fortunately, they can easily be circumvented. First, blood samples should be collected in tubes containing EDTA (1mg/ml) as an anticoagulant but not heparin (standard conditions, 14.3 U/ml of blood). Both Beutler et al. (1990) and Holodniy et al. (1991) conclude that heparin can cause attenuation or complete inhibition of target DNA amplification during PCR. As little as 0.05 U of heparin per reaction tube suppresses PCR (Holodniy 1991). It is interesting to note that the effect of heparin in the isolated DNA fraction could not be reversed by a large number of treatments. Neither boiling the DNA, filtering on Sephadex G-75, nor acidification or alkalinization followed by gel filtration, had an effect. Repeated ethanol precipitations or titration with protamine sulfate were also insufficient (Beutler 1990). Only incubation of the DNA with either heparinase I or II according to standard protocols abolished the negative effect. Heparinase treatment of a whole blood preparation can initially be circumvented by separating the leucocytes from the heparinized blood by centrifugation followed by at least two washings in a saline buffer.

Furthermore, all DNA extractions from whole blood must eliminate contaminations with porphyrin compounds derived from heme, since these are regarded as the most inhibitory substances in blood preparations for PCR (Higuchi 1989). This is best achieved by subjecting the red blood cells to lysis and then selectively pelleting the leucocytes (see chapter 6). Often two incubations in a red cell lysis buffer are necessary followed by 1-2 washing steps in a saline buffer. Alternatively, a buffer lysing all cells may also be employed, and the nuclei pelleted, if no RNA preparation is intended (Buffone 1985).

4.1.2. Fixed Paraffin-Embedded Tissue

While DNA preparations of fresh tissue are readily amenable to PCR, DNA preparations from fixed tissues exhibit limitations. Thus, not all PCR assays using DNA extracted from paraffin-embedded tissue can be amplified. First, the extent of DNA modification or cross-linking induced by the fixative used or the fixation time (Dubeau 1986, Greer 1990 and Greer 1991) can invariably reduce amplification efficiency. The most comprehensive analysis of the effect of various fixatives as well as fixation times on DNA which was to serve as a template for amplification products ranging from 110 to 1327 bp was reported by Greer et al. (1990 and 1991). Eleven different fixatives were examined at three different fixation times (1, 4 and 24hrs) and 4 fixatives were examined after long-term fixation (2hrs, 24hrs, 8 days and 30 days). In all assays, standard fixation protocols were carried out prior to embedding in paraffin. In the first investigation addressing short-term fixation up to 24 hrs, acetone and 10% (v/v) buffered neutral formalin (BNF) yielded good results for all amplification products up to 1327 bp. Amplification products up to 989 bp were obtained after fixation for 24 hrs either in Zamboni's, Clarke's, paraformaldehyde, formalin-alcohol-acetic acid, alcoholic formalin or methacarn. Amplification was increasingly compromised in Carnoy's, Zenker's and Bouin's fixative after 24 hrs. Here, the largest amplifiable DNA fragment was 268bp, 110bp and no amplicon, respectively. In the second investigation addressing long-term fixation up to 30 days, tissue fixed in 95% ethanol and acetone were amenable to PCR yielding 1327 and 989 bp amplicons, respectively, after 30 days. Results obtained after fixation in

OmniFix (American Histology Reagent Co., Stockton, CA) were comparable to those obtained in acetone, however, slightly compromised. Amplification efficiency of DNA fixed in 10% BNF was reduced in a time-dependent fashion successively yielding shorter PCR products. Thus, after 30 days, only the 268 bp fragment could be amplified. Second, aside from a number of fixatives which are also currently being investigated with regard to Taq polymerase inhibition (Wright 1990), time-dependent physical degradation of DNA in paraffin-embedded tissue considerably limits the length of a fragment which can successfully be amplified using PCR to between 100 and 200 bp. Goelz et al. (1985) reported that the size of a DNA fragment prepared from samples 4 to 6 years old was often smaller than the size of DNA from samples less than two years old. There is also evidence that DNA from tissue fixed in 10% BNF and 5 years or older is less readily amplifiable. However, occasional amplification of ancient DNA up to 600 bp has been described (Pääbo 1989). These observations must be kept in mind when working with fixed paraffin-embedded tissue, especially if a retrospective study of material collected over a longer period of time should yield trustworthy results.

4.2 Inhibition introduced by reagents during DNA isolation: Detergents, Proteinase K and Phenol

4.2.1. Detergents

The isolation or liberation of DNA for PCR often makes use of detergents for cell lysis and denaturation of proteins enveloping nucleic acids. Detergents can very generally be categorized as non-ionic or ionic detergents. Nonidet P-40, Tween 20, Triton-X-100 and N-octylglucoside belong to the former and sodium desoxycholate, sarkosyl and sodium dodecyl sulfate belong to the latter group. The use of a non-ionic detergent as opposed to that of an ionic detergent in isolating DNA for PCR has several advantages: It has been demonstrated that non-ionic detergents generally do not inhibit Taq polymerase in end concentrations <5% (v/v) accept for N-octylglucoside which inhibits PCR at concentrations exceeding 0.4% (w/v) (Weyant 1990). Thus, it is not necessary to phenolize a cell lysate which was subjected to proteinase K digestion following lysis with a non-ionic detergent before introducing the sample to PCR - this saves time. Moreover, the probability of cross-contaminations due to excessive sample handling is also significantly reduced. In acccordance with the results reported by Weyant et al. (1990), Kawasaki (1990) found that Laureth 12 and Tween 20 at 0.5% (v/v) do not inhibit Taq polymerase activity. Further, although the presence of up to 1% nonidet P40 (NP40) works well with reverse transcriptase, it has been observed that NP40 may inhibit Taq polymerase activity even at such low levels as 0.1% (v/v). This suggests that effective inhibitory concentrations may vary from one PCR assay to another rendering it necessary to run pilot experiments when establishing a new PCR assay.

In contrast, ionic detergents used for cell lysis and protein denaturation must be removed by phenolization and ethanol precipitation of the DNA prior to PCR. This is in part due to the fact that most detergents are employed in concentrations higher than those which could be compatible with PCR. A very effective ionic detergent, sodium dodecyl sulfate (SDS) e.g., is often used in end concentrations up to 2.0% (w/v). Table 1 summarizes effective PCR inhibitory concentrations of well known ionic detergents reported by Weyant et al. (1990).

Table 4.1.: Taq polymerase inhibition by ionic detergents

Ionic detergent	Inhibitory Concentration	
Sodium desoxycholate	>0.06%	(w/v)
Sarkosyl	>0.02%	(w/v)
Sodium dodecyl sulfate	>0.01%	(w/v)

The effect of different concentrations of SDS on PCR was more closely looked at by Gelfand (1989). While 0.001% SDS can have a marginal stimulatory effect on PCR, 10- and 100-fold concentrations distinctly depress Taq activity to 10% and <0.1%, respectively. The inhibitory effects of low SDS concentrations can, however, be reversed by certain non-ionic detergents: 0.5% each Tween 20/NP40 will counteract the inhibitory effect of 0.1% SDS, and 0.1% each is sufficient to counteract the inhibitory effect of 0.01% SDS. As mentioned above, an alternative to reversing the inhibitory effect of SDS is to remove SDS from the DNA sample prior to performing PCR by phenolization and ethanol precipitation. In a very simple assay, we demonstrated that SDS is sufficiently removed by phenol/chloroform extraction. SDS contamination of an aqueous solution was judged by precipitation of SDS at 4°C. A serial dilution of SDS down to 0.005% precipitated at 4°C. The same serial dilutions in a panel of DNA extraction samples were than phenol/chloroform extracted and the aqueous phase kept at 4°C for several hours. No precipitate was seen in an aqueous phase which had initially contained 5% (w/v) or less SDS. Interestingly, an initial concentration of 10% SDS (w/v) made phase separation impossible. Nevertheless, standard working concentrations of SDS seem to be removed sufficiently by phenolization. In addition, ethanol precipitation using 0.2M sodium chloride instead of ammonium acetate before adding ethanol will allow SDS to remain soluble and not to coprecipitate with the nucleic acids (Wallace 1987).

4.2.2. Proteinase K

Many detergents are used in combination with proteinase K to denature and subsequently digest proteins. Because the Taq polymerase is very susceptible to proteolytic degradation, care must be taken to inactivate proteases. Proteinase K is sufficiently inactivated by heat-treatment of the cell lysate or of the purified DNA sample at 95°C for 10 min.

4.2.3. Phenol

Residual phenol can inhibit the DNA polymerase. A final extraction with chloroform-isoamylalcohol (49:1) after phenolization steps have been performed removes trace amounts of phenol contaminating the aqueous phase (see Proteinase K digest). Subsequent DNA precipitation is carried out using salts which should be removed by washing the DNA pellet with 80% ethanol.

4.2.4. Salts and buffer systems

The effects of salt concentrations on Taq polymerase activity were reported by Gelfand (1989): 50mM ammonium chloride or ammonium acetate or sodium chloride lead to mild inhibition, no effect or slight stimulation (25-30%), respectively. Thus, it is important to keep in mind that salts coprecipitated with the target template DNA can affect Taq polymerase activity. Other ions introduced into the PCR, e.g. potassium, can have an effect on the Tm of the primer. This is expressed in the following equation already mentioned in the introductory chapter (1.5.2):

$$T_m = 81.5 + 16.6(\log_{10}[J^+]) + 0.41(\%G+C) - (600/l) - 0.63(\%FA)$$

A very recent investigation with regard to the effect of different buffer compositions on successful amplification of long DNA fragments demonstrated that the complete omission of KCl and the substitution of 100mM Tris-HCl by 300mM Tricine in the reaction buffer yielded the best results (Ponce 1992). Only 10 cycles were needed to visualize an array of PCR products ranging from 2 - 6kb on an ethidium bromide stained agarose gel, when the initial template amount ranged from 100ng to 1µg. Two variations of the standard 10 x buffer supplied by Perkin Elmer Cetus (100mM Tris-HCl pH, 8.3, 500mM KCl, 15mM $MgCl_2$, 50mM ß-mercaptoethanol, 0.01% gelatin and 1% Thesit) designated II and III worked best:

	II	III
Tris-HCl pH 8.5	300mM	
Tricine pH 8.4		300mM
MgCl$_2$	20mM	20mM
ß-Mercaptoethanol	50mM	50mM
Gelatin	0.1%	0.1%
Thesit	1%	1%

In vitro amplification of long DNA fragments was carried out using the following temperature profile after initial denaturation at 94°C for 5min: 1min at 94°C, 35sec of transition to 55°C, 1min at 55°C, 1min of transition to 72°C and 5min at 72°C. After 10 cycles, final extension was at 72°C for 10min.

4.3. Additives influencing the efficiency of PCR

The mechanisms underlying the effect of additives or cosolvents on PCR are largely unknown. It has been proposed that they may affect the melting temperature of primers, the thermal activity profile of the Taq DNA polymerase, the degree of product strand separation (Gelfand 1989) or facilitate primer annealing by altering primer secondary structure (Pomp 1991). Recently, the effect of certain cosolvents on the half-life of Taq polymerase at different temperatures has been demonstrated (Sninsky 1992). It must be emphasized, however, that no single cosolvent reported to enhance PCR at a given concentration in a certain assay can unequivocally be employed in a second PCR set up to achieve the same effect. Each PCR set up remains a unique reaction. In the following section, a summary is made of a number of cosolvents successfully employed to promote PCR.

4.3.1. Dimethyl sulfoxide (DMSO)

DMSO is a strong denaturant. Both Smith et al. (1990) and Pomp et al. (1990) describe PCR assays which only worked in the presence of this cosolvent probably due to more complete denaturation of the target DNA template. One assay describes the successful amplification of G/C-rich viral genomes of herpes simplex virus 1 and 2 by the addition of DMSO to yield a final concentration of 3% (Smith 1991). The second example demonstrated that while no amplification of a sheep metallothionein transgene by PCR was observed in the absence of DMSO, an end concentration of 5% DMSO clearly allowed detection (Pomp 1991). In this case, the authors suggest that the addition of DMSO possibly assisted in eliminating primer secondary structure. In addition, DMSO lowers Tm by 5-6°C. In both cases, the final concentration of DMSO did not exceed 10%. Empirically, concentrations exceeding 10% are known to inhibit Taq DNA polymerase activity by 50% (Gelfand 1990).

4.3.2. Glycerol

The same PCR assays as described above could also be promoted by the addition of glycerol to give an end concentraion of 10-15%. The mode of function may also be the same as suggested above: 1) more complete denaturation of the target DNA template and 2) elimination of primer and/or template secondary structure. Moreover, there seems to be some evidence that glycerol stabilizes protein structure, thus, having an influence on the Taq polymerase (personal communication Sninsky). In both assays a similar concentration was empirically determined to be most effective. While concentrations between 10-15% can enhance PCR, end concentrations exceeding 20% tended to inhibit PCR.

4.3.3. Formamide

There are several reports describing the advantageous effect of formamide on PCR. Formamide has been used to improve the correctness, fidelity and reproducibility of DQ alpha typing results. In this case, the addition of formamide (final concentration 5%) to the PCR reliably reversed previous false negative results (Comey 1991). In a second case, the addition of formamide in end concentrations between 1.25 and 10% clearly increased the specificity of the amplification of a GC-rich target DNA sequence of the human dopamine D2 receptor gene (Sarkar 1990). It is interesting to note that in this experiment, whilst 2.5-10% DMSO increased the sensitivity of the PCR assay and only an end concentration of 15% had a marked effect on specificity, even low concentrations of formamide already increased both sensitivity and specificity. Empirically, end concentrations of formamide below 10% are not known to inhibit Taq DNA polymerase activity (Gelfand 1989). Examination of the half-life of Taq polymerase in different end concentrations of glycerol and/or formamide and at different temperatures (Sninsky 1992) showed that the half-life of recombinant Taq polymerase (rTaq) in 10% glycerol at 95°C was increased by one half. The half-life ($T_{1/2}$) of rTaq at 95°C is approximately 40 min. In the presence of 5% and 10% formamide $T_{1/2}$ of rTaq was reduced to approximately 35% and 5%, respectively. The combination of 10% glycerol with 5% and 10% formamide reduced $T_{1/2}$ to 60% and 10%, respectively. Again, these results suggest that glycerol may have a stabilizing effect, since the $T_{1/2}$ of rTaq in the presence of both glycerol and formamide is clearly elevated as opposed to $T_{1/2}$ of rTaq in the presence of formamide alone. At 97.5°C, $T_{1/2}$ of rTaq under all conditions stated above was distinctly decreased. (Data presented by Sninsky at the Perkin Elmer Symposium in Berlin, March 1992).

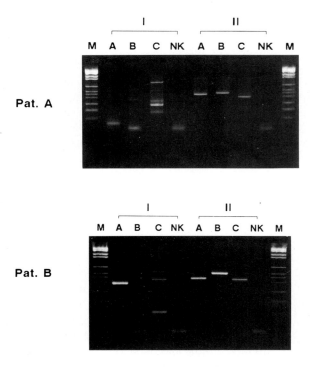

Figure 4.1.: Effect of Tween 20 on the efficacy of the amplification of three overlapping DNA regions within the env-region of the HIV genome using nested PCR in two HIV - positive patients. The outer PCR was designed to amplify a 1067 bp fragment from position 5470 to 6537 (BH10 nomenclature) and carried out without (I) or with Tween 20 (II) at a final concentration of 1% (w/w). The nested PCR was carried out using 1µl from the outer PCR "I" or "II" in 100µl reaction volume and standard conditions. The following DNA regions were amplified: A position 5545 - 5947, B 5764 - 6187 and C 6074 - 6429. Due to 5' tagging, the resulting amplicons were 440, 461 and 393 bp long, respectively. The results show that while an array of non-specific products were obtained in all three nested PCRs using 1µl from the outer PCR without Tween 20 (I), nearly only specific product was obtained in each nested PCR performed using 1µl from the outer PCR supplemented with Tween 20 (II).

4.3.4. Polyethylene glycol (PEG)

Not very many trials have been reported using PEG as a cosolvent. Pomp et al. (1991) were, however, able to demonstrate that detection of the metallthionine transgene by PCR was also promoted in the presence of PEG. They assert that PEG enhances and maintains amplification at concentrations between 5 and 15%. Efficiency decreases at higher concentrations, and is inhibited at concentrations exceeding 20%.

4.3.5. Tween 20

As mentioned above, Tween 20 is a non-ionic detergent capable of reversing the inhibitory effects of certain ionic detergents such as SDS. An incubation of the DNA sample at 37°C for 40 min in the presence of Mg^{2+} is sufficient (Gelfand, 1989) prior to performing PCR. We have used Tween 20 to greatly improve the efficiency of nested PCR amplification of HIV-1 provirus DNA in patient samples by directly supple-menting the reaction with 1% Tween 20. Tween 20 was used only in the first PCR reaction. A second PCR was performed using nested primers (see figure 4.1). The advantageous effects of cosolvents in establishing assays which are then characterized by good reproducibility justify their use. The selection of cosolvents described above with regard to inhibition or enhancement independent of whether Taq polymerase activity, annealing or denaturation is being affected are compiled in the table below:

Table 4.2. Concentrations of cosolvents affecting PCR

Cosolvent	Inhibition	Enhancement
DMSO	>10%	5%
PEG	>20%	5-15%
Formamide	>10%	5%
Glycerol	>20%	10-15%
Tween 20	n.d.	0.1-2.5%

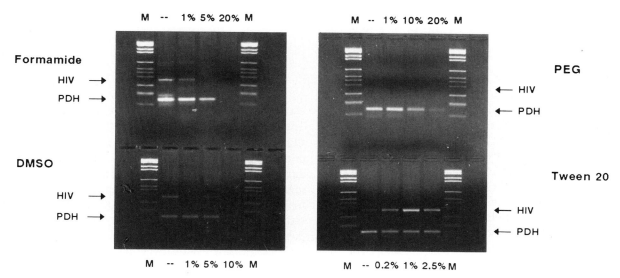

Figure 4.2.: The effect of a variety of additives in increasing concentrations on amplification efficacy are shown. Two different genomic DNA regions were amplified from one sample in separate reaction tubes: 1) ß-subunit of the pyruvate dehydrogenase gene (PDH) from position 4297 to 4481 (185 bp) and 2) a region of HIV proviral DNA from position 7698 to 8025 in correspondence to the BH10 nomenclature). While amplification of the 185 bp PDH fragment reflects a highly optimized faithful PCR assay, amplification of proviral DNA is often cumbersome and often without any result at all. The reaction buffer was either used directly or supplemented with an additive at the final concentration denoted. First, the results demonstrate that the amplification of the proviral HIV fragment is not always reproducible. Second, while formamide, DMSO and PEG (6000) had no enhancing or stabilizing effect on amplification, Tween 20 at a final concentration of 1% (w/w) showed enhancement. Third, the effect of the denoted additives on a stable PCR assay showed that the highest concentrations of formamide DMSO and PEG adversely affected amplification, while Tween 20 in all concentrations tested had virtually no negative effect - on the contrary, PCR efficiency was promoted.

Procedure	Comments
4.4. Evaluation of the effect of individual additives Additives can affect a large number of parameters in the PCR reaction. If an additive is used in a certain assay, it is often fairly difficult to pin-point the exact mechanism of action, e.g. whether denaturation of template DNA is more efficient, whether secondary structure of the primers or the template DNA has been eliminated or whether the Tm of the primers has been	affected, just to state a few of the important issues. In contrast, probably only Taq polymerase activity can more readily be judged by measuring the incorporation of labeled dNTPs. Thus, if a PCR reaction has been positively influenced by an additive, in many cases the reasoning remains hypothetical. Altogether though, the overall effect of additives on a PCR reaction remains the sum of adverse and advantageous influences on each cycle step: the influence on denaturation, primer/template annealing and/or Taq polymerase activity.

Procedure	Comment

Method: Improving the efficiency of PCR amplification of HIV-1-provirus DNA from patient samples using a panel of additives

Procedure	Comment
Possibly due to low copy number or to features of the template DNA, certain regions of the HIV-1-provirus DNA are not readily amplified in vitro, even after optimization strategies have been followed. In order to assess the effect of different additives on PCR efficiency, we chose the following approach. Using one HIV- positive human genomic DNA, two different PCR assays were performed parallel in separate tubes without and with increasing concentrations of a given additive: amplification of 1) the ß-subunit of the pyruvate dehydrogenase gene (PDH) from position 4297 to 4481 (185 bp) and 2) a region of HIV proviral DNA corresponding to position 7698 to 8025 of the BH10 sequence. Amplification of the PDH fragment reflects the amplification of a single copy gene using highly optimized primer pair. Amplification of the specified HIV fragment from the env region only	occurred sporadically, making optimization difficult. The advantage of chosing a comparative approach - like using a highly optimized and a non-optimized primer pair - when testing different additives is that this approach may provide additional information with regard to the general effect of the additives, e.g. inhibition or enhancement. If the additive inhibits the stable PCR in the assay, then it is not very likely that a positive effect can be expected on the PCR assay yielding sporadic results. Even though different gene regions are being amplified with different primer pairs, the effect of the additive on the basic PCR set up with regard to the temperature profile can be judged, if the T_m values of the primers and the expected PCR fragment length are similar, and all other reaction components identical. Therefore,

Procedure(cont.)

1. Make a mastermix containing all PCR components except for the primer pairs and the additive, and be sure to always keep the mix on ice.

2. Divide the master mix into two equal volumes and add the appropriate amount of each primer pair.

3. Supplement equal volumes of the additive or dilutions of the additive to yield the intended final concentration and volume.

4. Overlay with mineral oil and place in a preheated thermal cycler (95°C) for initial denaturation. Then run the temperature profile commonly used for the stable PCR assay.
The results and the conclusions we drew are shown and described in figure 4.2.

Comments(cont.)

1. In our hands, the risk of obtaining non-specific products when all components are mixed together is clearly reduced, if the reagents and the individual reaction tubes are stringently kept on ice

4. As stated above, the characteristics of the two independent primer pairs should be similar, so that the likelihood of the temperature profile being suitable for both reactions is very high.

References

1. Beutler E, Gelbart T, Kuhl W. Interference of heparin with the polymerase chain reaction. 1990, BioTechniques, 9, 166.

2. Buffone GJ, Darlington, GJ. Isolation of DNA from biological specimens without extraction with phenol. 1985, Clin Chem, 30, 164-165.

3. Comey Theisen C, Jung JM, Budowle B. Use of formamide to improve amplification of HLA DQ alpha sequences. 1991, BioTechniques, 10, 60-61.

4. Demmler GJ, Buffone GJ, Schimbor CM, May RA. Detection of cytomegalovirus in urine from newborns by using polymerase chain reaction DNA amplification. 1988, J Infect Dis, 158, 1177-1184.

5. Dubeau L, Chandler LA, Gralow JR, Nichols PW, Jones PA. Southern blot analysis of DNA extracted from formalin-fixed pathology specimens. 1986, Cancer Res, 46, 2964-2969.

6. Gelfand DH. Taq DNA Polymerase. In: PCR Technology: Principles and applications for DNA amplification. Erlich HA (Ed.), (Stockton Press, New York, NY) 1989, 17-22.

7. Gelfand DH, White TJ. Thermostable DNA Polymerases. In: PCR Protocols: A guide to methods and applications. Innis MA, Gelfand DH, Sninsky JJ, White TJ (Eds.) (Academic Press, Inc., San Diego) 1990, 129-141.

8. Goelz SE, Hamilton SR, Vogelstein B. Purification of DNA from formaldehyde-fixed and paraffin-

embedded human tissue. 1985, Biochem Biophys Res Commun 130, 118-126.

9. Greer CE, Peterson SL, Kiviat, NB, Manos MM. PCR amplification from paraffin-embedded tissues: Effects of fixative and fixation time. 1990, Am J Clin Path 95, 117-124.

10. Greer CE, Lund JK, Manos MM. PCR amplification from paraffin-embedded tissues: Recommendations on fixatives for long-term storage and prospective studies. 1991, PCR Methods and Applications 1, 46-50.

11. Higuchi R. Rapid, efficient extraction for PCR from cells or blood, 1989, Amplifications A Forum for PCR Users 2, 1-3.

12. Holodniy M, Kim S, Katzenstein D, Konrad M, Groves E, Merigan TC. Inhibition of human immunodeficiency virus gene amplification by heparin. 1991, J Clin Microbiol 29, 676-679.

13. Kawasaki ES. Sample preparation from blood, cells, and other fluids. in PCR protocols: A guide to methods and applications, eds. Innis MA, Gelfand DH, Sninsky JJ, White TJ (Eds.), (Academic Press, Inc., San Diego) 1990, 146-152.

14. Mezei, L.M. Effect of oil overlay on PCR amplification. 1990, Amplifications A Forum for PCR Users 4, 11-13.

15. Pääbo S, Higuchi RG, Wilson AC. Ancient DNA and the polymerase chain reaction. The emerging field of molecular archeology. 1989 J Biol Chem 264, 9709-9712.

16. Pomp D, Medrano JF. Organic solvents as facilitators of polymerase chain reaction. 1991, BioTechniques 10, 58-59.

17. Ponce MR, Micol JL. PCR amplification of long DNA fragments. 1992, Nucl Acids Res 20, 623.

18. Sarkar G, Kapelener S, Sommer SS. Formamide can dramatically improve the specificity of PCR. 1990, Nucl Acids Res 18, 7465.

19. Smith KT, Long CM, Bowman B Manos MM. Using Cosolvents to enhance PCR amplification. 1990, Amplifications A Forum for PCR Users 5, 16-17.

20. Sninsky JJ. Perkin Elmer Symposium, Klinikum Steglitz, Free University Berlin, March 1992.

21. Weyant RS, Edmonds P, Swaminathan B. Effect of ionic and non-ionicdetergents on the Taq polymerase. 1990, BioTechniques 9, 308-309.

22. Wright DK, Manos MM. Sample preparation from paraffin-embedded tissues. In PCR Protocols: A guide to methods and applications. Innis MA, Gelfand DH, Sninsky JJ, White TJ (Eds.), (Academic Press, Inc., San Diego) 1990, 153-158.

5. PCR Contamination and Falsely Interpreted Results

Due to the fact that PCR is an enzymatic process with extreme sensitivity, the quality of diagnostic assays has to be monitored continuously. Polymerase inhibition or omission of reaction components are just as deleterious as contamination with any DNA.

The following example was published by Hughes (1990): Ten centers in North America and Europe received ten different samples prepared from leukemia cell lines. The presented results were "heterogeneous":

Phase I study to detect the presence or absence of BCR/ABL transcripts in CML and Non-CML cell lines

Sample material	total samples	correct result	* false-positive	* false-negative
positive undiluted	20	12	6	4
positive diluted	40	13	19	17
negative	38		15	23

* In some cases an incorrect result was classified as false-positive and false-negative because the correct transcript was not detected while another transcript was falsely identified.

Figure 5.1. The results from this table were reported by Hughes (1990). They reflect a particular PCR problem with which many laboratories using this method may be familiar.

Non-specific amplification by-products, whether identical in length to the specific product or not, should not be denoted as "contamination" or "false-positive results". Whether a "background amplification" results from lack of reaction specificity, specific or non-specific DNA contamination has to be checked through hybridization.

We sometimes observed serious problems with nested PCRs when performed sequentially in two reactions. Sometimes, it seemed that single samples can be contaminated sporadically with external or nested amplification product. Sporadic contaminations cannot be controlled systematically and therefore present a most deleterious event that must be prevented. Sporadic contamination events might be detected through repeated testing, because it is unlikely that such events occur the same way again (Kwok and Higuchi 1989). Generally, any reagent or lab material purchased might be contaminated with DNA if not certified "PCR-grade".

5.1. Control Experiments

No PCR without controls

Control experiments should be designed to detect contamination with extraneous DNA or PCR products, to check overall reaction quality, and to check single samples for inhibiting activity. Table 1 lists a number of controls. These are described below and denoted by a control number referred to after each explanation. In diagnostic assays, negative control samples should be subjected to the same extraction and purification procedures as the patient samples. For every sample preparation and extraction series, at least as many negative control samples have to be included as primer pairs used. Negative controls should be designed to check PCR reagents for contamination by (1) human DNA and/or (2) nonhuman target DNA, if infectious agents are to be detected for diagnostic purposes [Ctrl. No 1) and 2)].

For the detection of infectious agents, it is always necessary to check the patient sample for the presence of amplifiable DNA. This is done with primers that amplify a human target sequence [Ctrl. No3)]. If the PCR is contaminated with such a target sequence, it may wrongly be assumed that amplifiable patient DNA is present and then lead to a false negative result with regard to the present of an infectious agent. If cell-free samples are to be analyzed, such as serum, the potential inhibitory characteristics of the sample can only be observed through amplification of a previously added internal DNA standard (see chapter 4).

With specific positive controls (PC) for infectious agents (high and low copy numbers), mixed with human DNA, the overall quality of an assay must be checked for specificity and sensitivity [Ctrl. No 4) and 5)]. Ctrl. No 6) checks whether essential reaction components are missing or degraded. This is crucial in cases where unspecific signals are found or where many faint positive or negative samples are analyzed.

For amplification and diagnostics of DNA from infectious agents, it is advisable to amplify two different gene sequences from the infectious agent independently and to compare the results. This is a suitable control for the plausibility of positive and negative results, especially when considering the problems with post-PCR cross-contamination [Ctrl. No 7)]. A similar purpose is served by performing each amplification twice. This is simultaneously a control for reproducibility [Ctrl. No 8)]. Positive control DNA may be genomic DNA, a cloned sequence or even a PCR amplification product of the target region. If cloned-target sequences are used in the lab and serve as positive controls, then vector-specific primers can be used to identify this potential source of contamination (Nerenberg and Minor 1991).

The content and copy number of any positive control amplification products or plasmids can be estimated in an agarose gel (see chapter 10.1.4) and diluted to reflect the sensitivity of the PCR assay (see chapter 2.1.3)

In a "routine" PCR, the following controls must be included:

Ctrl No.	Control for	sample*	primers**
1)	- contamination with specific PCR product	non-DNA	specific
	- contamination with positive patient DNA	non-DNA	specific
	- contamination with PC-DNA	non-DNA	specific, possibly vector specific
2)	contamination with negative patient DNA	non-DNA	human
3)	presence of amplifiable DNA in sample	patient	human
4)	reaction specificity	NC-DNA	specific
5)	set-up, thermoprofile, reaction sensitivity	NC + specific PC-DNA	
6)	completeness of reaction mixture	PC-DNA or NC-DNA	specific or human

7) and 8), not necessarily in the same setting:

7)	plausibility of results	patient	different specific
8)	- reproducibility of results	patient	specific twice
	- occurrence of sporadic contaminations	patient	specific twice

Table 5.1: * PC-DNA = target specific positive control DNA, NC-DNA = target negative control DNA; ** specific human primers for the amplification of sequences being assessed in the particular assay, primers for the amplification of human sequences that are different from the specific amplification products. For further explanation, see text.

5.2. Sources of contamination

5.2.1. Pre-PCR contamination

A sample might be contaminated with DNA prior to reaching the diagnostic laboratory. Often routine sample collection methods have not yet been established for PCR-diagnostics. For example, clinical equipment may be sterile, but not necessarily free of DNA.

Further, the more people in the lab the more incalculable contamination risks become. Contaminating DNA may originate from any person's skin or hair, especially from the operator himself (Kitchin 1990). Door handles and any surface in the laboratory are potential sources of contamination (Cone 1990). Bad ventilation or shedded or dusty material carried by air might be the cause of sporadic contaminations of single samples. If the presence of an eventually minute human DNA amount from a patient has to be checked in a sample for assessment of the sample quality (e.g., CSF samples), these air-carried materials might be a serious problem, eventually leading to misinterpretation of PCR results (see previous paragraph).

It has already been mentioned that any reagent that is not certified as "PCR-grade" might be a source of unspecific or specific DNA contamination. Especially enzyme and recombinant or biological products are potential sources of extraneous DNA contamination. DNA contamination of procaryotic and eucaryotic origin in Taq polymerase lots from several manufactures has been reported (Schmidt 1991). A high risk of DNA contamination may be encountered in reagents such as gelatine, BSA (being often PCR components), antibodies, reverse transcriptase, DNA ligase, restriction enzymes, deoxynucleotide transferase.

The most potent source of contamination are PCR products from previous PCRs, especially when a diagnostic PCR is repeatedly performed for one particular genomic sequence. Procedures to minimize carryover are outlined in chapter 5.3.5. and 5.3.6..

5.2.2. Post-PCR contamination

As described in chapter 10, post-PCR cross-contamination might lead to false positives in hybridization assays. For example, through the pipetting of post-PCR samples into a flat HLA-typing plate, onto parafilm or similar devices, microdroplets can contaminate neighboring samples. If a positive sample contains only 1ng/10µl specific product (which is not detectable in agarose gel electrophoresis), and if only 0.01 µl (= 1pg) of this sample spits into another, possibly negative sample, this might have two deleterious effects (1 pg is detectable with non-radioactive detection systems):

1. Creation of false positives.
2. Contamination of negative control samples that would prohibit further diagnostic conclusions from the whole PCR.

Note: This cannot be overcome through positive displacement pipets. Such droplets cannot be controlled through pipetting alone; therefore, we prefer deep 96-well titer plates or reaction tubes for post-PCR sample handling.

Similar problems have to be expected during gel loading or dot blot procedures.

These problems gain rising importance, because the post-PCR product handling and analysis becomes more and more a bottleneck for PCR diagnostics and is subject of intense research and industrial activity. Electronic fluorescence and luminescence detection and quantification systems are highly sensitive (approx. 1-100fg product detection), thus making post-PCR contamination even more hazardous. Robotic workstations will be necessary to cope with the huge numbers of minute samples. Eventually, a new principle of handling small volumes by transferring droplets through capillary forces and surface charges or adhesion forces instead of pipetting them might overcome these problems. This will be crucial for robotic workstations.

Table 5.2: Potential sources of contamination

- patient body surface
- sample collector or collection equipment
- laboratory environment
- air-conditioning system or filters
- operators' body suface
- autoclave
- tissue homogenizer and other DNA extraction equipment
- liquid nitrogen
- ice
- pipets (aerosol from inside; outer pipet surface)
- pipet tips
- tubes
- reagents (especially: ethanol, phenol, chloroform)
- enzymes and other recombinant or biological products (e.g., BSA, gelatin)
- hood filters
- vacuum centrifuges
- microtome blades
- glassware
- pH-meter
- tap water (especially legionellae)
- water-bath water
- heating blocks
- thermocycler
- anything that has come into contact with amplification products (e.g., freezer shelves and door handles, room door handles)
- post-PCR cross-contamination (handling of the amplicon, pipetting, gel loading, dot blot procedure, etc.)

5.3. Prevention and elimination of contamination

5.3.1. Laboratory architecture

Separate rooms on different floors and different operators for pre- and post-amplification procedures will probably prevent most contamination problems. However, never store or handle any positive control (PC) DNA in the pre-PCR lab rooms. PC DNA must be added to the reaction mixture in a separated environment (with otherwise identical conditions). When many patient samples are to be prepared and handled, a third lab room exclusively for sample preparation should be available.

5.3.2. Autoclave

Contamination during autoclaving may be possible through fragmented specific DNA (Porter-Jordan 1990), especially, if the autoclave is used for decontamination of cell culture material. Such fragmented molecules might create overlapping structures with specific sequences and protruding 5´ends which can be elongated by Taq. Via a "jumping PCR" (Pääbo 1989), Taq might extend the rising mosaic structures during the next cycles, which could lead to longer, again overlapping molecules with specific primer annealing sites. These could be amplified exponentially. Therefore, a separate (e.g., tabletop) autoclave exclusively for pre-PCR equipment and reagents should be used.

5.3.3. Working place and equipment

A laminar air flow work bench class II (DIN 12950; DIN 58956; NSF/No.49; references 6, 7, 15) with built in UV lamps provides a suitable dust-free environment for setting up the reaction. Approx. 10% of the air circulating in the bench is continuously exchanged. The newly incomimg air passes the built in filter system prior to circulation. However, it seems to be unknown to what extent and how safely DNA is retained by the filters. So, it is not clear at the moment whether it is better or not to pipet a PCR with running air circulation.

Whenever possible, reagents should be weighed out on a balance by pouring directly from the original container into a PCR-grade reaction vessel. Metal and glass devices, such as spoons, spatulas, Pasteur pipets, etc., are usually not part of the PCR equipment, but if used, they should be flamed, e.g., with a Bunsen burner with a foot switch.

Personal pipet and reagent sets for each operator should be the rule. Positive displacement pipets are advantageous for the handling of patient and control samples. Usually, the patient samples are initially

delivered in 10- to 15-ml tubes or even larger vessels (urine, sputum ...) or syringes. For transfer of parts of the samples, reagents or pellets (see chapter 6) from these deep vessels into smaller tubes, long disposable plastic pipets (available as single- unit 1-, 2-, 5-, 10- and 25-ml pipets, e.g., Falcon; Greiner) must be used. Always wear gloves and change them often. Gloves without powder are preferable. The use of disposable mob caps, masks and safety goggles might be necessary, depending on individual circumstances (Kitchin 1990, Chou 1992).

All PCR reagents except the DNA polymerase stock should be aliquoted to volumes that are suitable for single experiments and stored at < -20°C.

Commercially available distilled *aqua ad injectabilia* (purified water) has proven to be "PCR-grade".

5.3.4. Influence of contamination risks on experimental design and handling

Due to the frequent change of vessels and the use of DNA-preserving reagents in high volumes (chloroform, phenol, ethanol), alternative methods to DNA extraction or purification should be used whenever possible (see chapter 7).

Master-mix or hot-start setup techniques (see chapter 1.9) should be applied. Tubes with the complete ,mreaction mixture should not be reopened prior to thermal cycling. Vapor barriers, such as light mineral oil or paraffin (AmpliWax™), used as reaction overlays might help to prevent cross-contamination.

The reaction tubes have to be kept closed as much as possible. Reagents in pre-PCR and post-PCR tubes must be spun down before opening tube. Especially during opening of the sometimes tightly closed tubes, splashes might contaminate the gloves or anything in the surroundings.

Instead of two-tube nested PCR protocols, one-tube nested protocols as described in chapter 3.3 should be tried. This seems to be crucial for diagnostic situations as described in the initial paragraph of this chapter.

5.3.5. Decontamination procedures

5.3.5.1. UV irradiation

Due to the fact that DNA is susceptible to damage by UV-light irradiation, it is possible to convert contaminating DNA in reaction tubes or in the surroundings to an unamplifiable structure. The UV sensitivity of particular DNA sequences is not fully predictable and depends on various factors, some of which are listed in table 5.3. UV irradiation leads to pyrimidine dimer formation, DNA strand breakage and certain other damage. See Cimino et al. (1990) for further discussion and references. Generally, dry and undissolved DNA necessitates much longer UV irradiation times for PCR-inactivation than DNA in solution (Fairfax 1991). Compared to inhibition of the amplification of a 750bp fragment through 5-20min UV irradiation of a liquid sample in a 500µl polypropylene tube on a 254nm transilluminator (Sarkar and Sommer 1990), 8-10hrs of direct UV irradiation for dry DNA is recommended for PCR inactivation (Fairfax 1991). Generally, the susceptibility of PCR to UV inactivation increases with target sequence length. For unknown reasons, short sequences are sometimes more suceptible to UV damage than expected (Sarkar and Sommer 1991). Taq polymerase and oligonucleotides with neighboring thymidine bases are susceptible to UV damage, but not dNTPs (Ou 1991).

For PCR decontamination, the following is reported:
- incubation for >10min with 100µJ/min UV energy (254nm) in a UV box (Stratalinker 1800™, Stratagene) for decontamination of reaction tubes and all parts of the reaction mix except Taq polymerase, primers and sample DNA (Ou 1991).
- incubation for >8hrs with 400µW/cm^2 UV energy in a work bench (distance <1m) for decontamination of the bench (Fairfax 1991).

Table 5.3.: Parameters influencing UV-dependent DNA damage and PCR inactivation

- DNA pyrimidine content and content of consecutive pyrimidines
- Nucleotide sequence next to potential pyrimidine dimer site
- Target sequence length
- Irradiation distance
- Irradiation time
- Wavelength
- Energy

5.3.5.2. Chemical and enzymatic DNA degradation

Inactivation of PCR amplification of fragments as small as 76bp has been reported by treatment of test samples with 10% v/v sodium hypochlorite for 5min. This compound was much more effective in DNA decontamination than 2N HCl (Prince and Andrus 1992). After decontamination of working areas with 10% sodium hypochlorite, metal surfaces should be rinsed with water due to the corrosive properties.

When there are restriction sites in the target DNA, reagents can be decontaminated through restriction enzyme pretreatment. However, this method is not universal and sometimes has the drawback of introducing salts required for the restriction enzyme, but negatively influencing the PCR (DeFilippes 1991). Generally, enzyme incubation procedures are time- and work-intensive and harbor contamination risks.

5.3.6. Chemical modification of PCR products to prevent carryover of amplifiable fragments

dUTP may substitute dTTP during PCR, thus leading to a modified DNA that does not occur naturally. This modified DNA can be digested with the enzyme uracil N-glycosylase (UNG). If UNG (e.g., Uracil DNA Glycosylase, Gibco BRL #510-8054SA) is added to a PCR mixture (without Taq), carried-over fragments are digested, but not the sample DNA. After placing on ice and addition of Taq, the PCR can be started as usual (Longo 1990). This is the principle of a commercially available carryover prevention kit (Perkin-Elmer #808-0068).

Recently, a promising "post-PCR sterilization" procedure was reported that relies on the photochemical adduction to DNA of isopsoralen compounds after PCR (Cimino 1991, Isaacs 1991). These angular compounds (4'-AMDMIP, 6-AMDMIP) form monoadducts to DNA through a photoreaction primarily with pyrimidines under long-wave UV irradiation (300-400nm). They do not form interstrand crosslinks, as do some other psoralens, and thus do not interfere with post-PCR hybridization assays for PCR product analysis. They are added to the reaction mixture with the master mix, and the reaction tube is UV-irradiated after PCR for 15min before it is opened. The created monoadducts cannot serve as a template for DNA polymerases anymore, thus, eliminating product carryover as a contamination source. One drawback of this method seems to be the negative influence on the PCR amplification efficiency by the chemical additives, requiring a modification of the PCR protocol (addition of glycerol or DMSO) (Isaacs 1991).

References

1. Chou Q, Russell M, Birch DE, Raymond J, Bloch W. Prevention of pre-PCR mis-priming and primer dimerization improves low-copy-number amplifications. 1992, Nucl Acids Res 20, 1717-1723.

2. Cimino GD, Metchette KC, Tessman JW, Hearst JE, Isaacs ST. Post-PCR sterilization: a method to control carryover contamination for the polymerase chain reaction. 1991, Nucl Acids Res 19, 99-107.

3. Cimino GD, Metchette KC, Isaacs ST, Zhu YS. More false-positive problems. 1990, Nature 345, 773-774.

4. Cone RW, Hobson AC, Huang M-LW, Fairfax MR. Polymerase chain reaction decontamination: the wipe test. 1990, Lancet II 686-687.

5. DeFillippes FM. Decontaminating the polymerase chain reaction. 1991, BioTechniques 10, 26-30.

6. DIN 12950. Sicherheitswerkbänke für mikrobiologische und biotechnologische Arbeiten. 1984, Beuth-Verlag, Berlin.

7. DIN 58956. Medizinisch-Mikrobiologische Laboratorien -Klassifizierung, Abgrenzung der Arbeitsstätten, Räumlichkeiten - Sicherheitstechnische Anforderungen und Prüfung. 1990, Beuth-Verlag, Berlin.

8. Fairfax MR, Metcalf MA, Cone RW. Slow inactivation of dry PCR templates by UV light. 1991, PCR Methods and Applications 1, 142-143.

9. Hughes T. False positive results with PCR to detect leukaemia-specific transcript. 1990, Lancet II, 1037-1038.

10. Isaacs ST, Tessman JW, Metchette KC, Hearst JE, Cimino GD. Post-PCR sterilization: development and application to an HIV-1 diagnostic assay. 1991, Nucl Acids Res 19, 109-116.

11. Kitchin PA, Szotyori Z, Fromholc C, Almond N. Avoidance of false positives. 1990, Nature 344, 201.

12. Kwok S, Higuchi R. Avoiding false positives with PCR. 1989, Nature 339, 237-238.

13. Longo MC, Berninger MS, Hartley JL. Use of uracil DNA glycosylase to control carry-over contamination in polymerase chain reactions. 1990, Gene 93, 125-128.

14. Nerenberg MI, Minor T. Detection of plasmid contamination in PCR samples. 1991, BioTechniques 11, 332-333.

15. NSF/No.49. Standard No.49 for class II (laminar flow) biohazard cabinetry. 1976, The National Sanitation Foundation, Ann Arbor, Michigan.

16. Ou C-Y, Moore JL, Schochetman G. Use of UV irradiation to reduce false positivity in polymerase chain reaction. 1991, BioTechniques 10, 442-446.

17. Pääbo S, Higuch RG, Wilson AC. Ancient DNA and the polymerase chain reaction. 1989, J Biol Chem 264, 9709-9712.

18. Porter-Jordan K, Rosenberg EI, Keiser JF, Gross JD, Ross AM, Nasim S, Garrett CT. Nested polymerase chain reaction assay for the detection of cytomegalovirus overcomes false positives caused by contamination with fragmented DNA. 1990, J Med Virol 30, 85-91.

20. Prince AM, Andrus L. PCR: How to kill unwanted DNA. 1992, BioTechniques 12, 358-360.

21. Sarkar G, Sommer SS. Parameters affecting susceptibility of PCR contamination to UV inactivation. 1990, BioTechniques 9, 590-594.

22. Schmidt TM, Pace B, Pace NR. Detection of DNA contamination in Taq polymerase. 1991, BioTechniques 11, 176-177.

6. Biological Material Amenable to PCR

6.1. Sample preparation and storage

Clinical samples for PCR are not usually fixed or dried and are transported native or in isotonic saline solutions. This makes them sensitive to degradation and/or bacterial overgrowth. Especially, RNA will degrade, depending on tissue type and time delay. If there is any time delay, the material should be stored at 4°C. Generally, the sample material should be as fresh as possible, considering PCR "conditions" from the first step on, to avoid contamination. Precautions must be taken to reduce material degradation to a minimum. Cellular material should be stored at -70°C or in liquid nitrogen until nucleic acid isolation is performed.

For enrichment and isolation of tissue or blood DNA, the cells are usually purified and concentrated prior to lysis.

PCR detection of infectious agents, which are not always obligatory intracellular pathogens, is possible from "cell-free" samples (e.g. serum, urine, supernatant).

The DNA content of several tissues and samples varies considerably (see table 1). Nevertheless, even the smallest amounts of biological material have yielded more than sufficient amounts of DNA for PCR. 1µl of human blood (5,000 leucocytes) contains approx. 35ng DNA. Whether sufficient copies of target DNA sequences are amplifiable or not, will depend on the state of the sample, the sample preparation, and DNA isolation procedure.

Source	DNA content	genome size (bp)	Copies/µg
human diploid cell	~7pg	6.6×10^9	1.4×10^5
human plucked hair	0.3µg		
Yeast	22fg	2×10^7	0.5×10^8
E.coli	4.6fg	4.2×10^6	2.2×10^8
MTB	2.75pg	2.5×10^9	3.6×10^8
HBV	3.52ag	3.2×10^3	2.8×10^{11}
CMV	0.25fg	2.3×10^5	4.0×10^9
HSV	0.17fg	1.5×10^5	5.9×10^9
1 kb ~ 1.1 ag			

Table 6.1

6.1.1. Peripheral blood leucocytes

The following procedures are suitable for unclotted blood (EDTA, heparin, Na-citrate). Note: For some hematologic questions it is necessary, to obtain blood from an intravenous catheter and not a syringe that might contain some skin and tissue cells.

If it is planned to isolate RNA it will be essential to separate the leucocytes as quick as possible and to immediately continue with the RNA extraction (see chapter 8). For preferential separation of either lymphozytes, polymorphnuclear leucocytes or all leucocytes, Methods 1, 2, or 3 is recommended, respectively.

The selective elimination of red blood cells when preparing leucocytes for the isolation of template DNA for PCR helps avoid possible PCR inhibition. Since porphyrin compounds derived from heme are known to inhibit Taq polymerase activity (Higuchi 1989), selective and complete elimination of red blood cells as well as supernatants containing liberated porphyrin compounds is essential. It must be kept in mind that any DNA template isolated from blood cells which cannot be amplified in vitro by PCR may potentially be contaminated with porphyrin compounds. This may lead to false negative results.

Selective lysis of red blood cells and preparation of intact leucocytes can be achieved by certain buffer systems. This is necessary if the aim of the experiment is to isolate DNA as well as RNA from white blood cells. The buffer routinely used in our laboratory contains NH_4Cl to achieve selective red blood cell lysis. Alternatively, Buffone et al. (1985) described a buffer using Triton X-100 which dissolves the cytoplasmic membrane of all cells. This eliminates inhibitory porphyrin compounds derived from heme. A disadvantage of this method is that cytoplasmic RNA and DNA are removed with the supernatant leaving exclusively white blood cell nuclei for DNA isolation.

Procedure	Comments

Method 1: Selective lysis of red blood cells

Procedure	Comments
1. Collect EDTA-blood and mix well.	

2. Mix 1 volume of blood with a double volume of red blood cell lysis buffer in a 50ml Falcon tube.	2. Lysis Buffer 10mM $KHCO_3$
	                        155mM NH_4Cl
	                        0.1mM EDTA
	Adjust pH to 7.4.
	Dissolve in appropriate amount of double distilled autoclaved water. Pass through a sterile 0.22µm filter unit. Avoid autoclaving the buffer since the development of gases can cause the bottle to explode. Store buffer at 4°C.

Procedure(cont.)

3. Place on ice for 15-30 min.

4. Pellet white blood cells at 300-400g in a Beckman CPKR centrifuge for 10 min at 10°C.

5. Remove and discard supernatant.

6. Wash cells by gently resuspending in 10ml 1 x PBS, and subsequently pellet cells at 300-400g in the same centrifuge as before.

7. Repeat previous step.

8. Resuspend cells in 1 x PBS and count cells in a Fuchs-Rosenthal chamber or hemacytometer.

9. Subject the appropriate amount of cells to lysis by proceeding to the lysis protocol of choice. This may require to repellet the cells in order to remove excess volume (e.g., for alkaline lysis) or to keep the cells resuspended as is the case for automated DNA extraction system.

Comments(cont.)

5. If the white blood cell pellet is highly contaminated with red blood cells, repeat steps 2.-4.

6. 10 x PBS is commercially supplied by Gibco BRL.

Method 2: Buffy coat

1. Mix the blood sample (3-10ml) gently and place the tube vertically. After 20-30min a leucocyte and plasma containing upper phase and an erythrocyte containing lower phase will be formed.

2. Gently take off the upper phase gently with a pasteur pipette, without touching the erythrocyte phase. Collect in centrifugation tube.

3. Repeat step 1. and 2. once or twice. Mix gently and take 10µl for cell counting.

4. Centrifuge at 350g for 10min.

1. In most cases this may be done with the original sample tube. Depending on leucocyte count, a faint greyish layer of leucocytes will be visible on top of the erythrocyte phase.

4. If the pellet contains no visible erythrocytes, it can be transferred into an Eppendorf reaction tube with 1ml 0.83% NH_4Cl.

Procedure(cont.)	*Comments(cont.)*
5. Decant supernatant (plasma), resuspend cell pellet with 5-10ml 0.83% NH_4Cl and place on ice for 20-30min.	5. Plasma may be collected for other purposes. NH_4Cl will selectively lead to lysis of erythrocytes. 0.83% NH_4Cl (final concentration 157mM)
6. Centrifuge at 350g for 10min.	6. Step 5.and 6. may be repeated if pellet contains erythrozytes.
7. Resuspend cell pellet in 1 ml 0.83% NH_4Cl and spin down in a 1,5ml Eppendorf tube 5min at 350g.	7. Aliquots of $1-2 \times 10^7$ cells are recommended for final storage. This allows the use of small portions at a time without exposing the rest of the preparation.
8. Remove supernatant completely including the red edge on top of the pellet with an Eppendorf pipet.	
9. Resuspend the cells with 50μl PCR-grade H_2O	9. Cells are ready for DNA or RNA extraction (see chapters 7 and 8).
10. Store at -70°C.	

Method 3: Isolation of mononuclear cells using FICOLL-PAQUE

This method exploits an erythrocyte aggregating agent of low viscosity (Ficoll) to separate lymphocytes from other blood cells (Boyum 1964). Granulocytes and aggregated red blood cells pass through Ficoll combined with sodium diatriazole of the proper density and osmotic strength, while lymphocytes collect at the boundary between Ficoll and plasma upon centrifugation. Recovery of lymphocytes is approximately 50±15%. This method can be used for varying amounts of blood. Very small amounts can be subjected to a microprocedure (Fotino 1971), and up to 15ml blood can be processed in a 50ml Falcon tube.

Procedure	Comments
(FICOLL-PAQUE Protocol, Pharmacia)	
1. Collect blood using heparin, EDTA, citrate or acid citrate dextrose as anticoagulant. Mix well.	

2. Dilute blood 1:1 in 0.14M NaCl (0.9%). Mix gently by drawing blood and buffer in and out of a Pasteur pipette. Place on ice.

2. Dilution and low temperature will both improve the yield and purity of the lymphocyte fraction. Both lower the degree of red cell aggregation causing less trapping and sedimentation of lymphocytes to the Ficoll phase upon centrifugation.

3. Invert Ficoll-Paque bottle several times to ensure thorough mixing.

4. Layer one half volume into a 50ml Falcon tube.

4. If the volume of the diluted blood is 20ml, then 10ml Ficoll.

5. Layer the blood sample on the Ficoll-Paque taking care not to mix the sample with the Ficoll-Paque.

5. Choice of tube: Since the height of the blood sample determines the amount of red cell contamination and influences the time of separation, it is advisable to maintain a ratio of 2.4cm Ficoll-Paque to 3cm sample. The diameter of the tube does not affect separation.

6. Centrifuge at 400g for 30-40min at 18-20°C.

6. This narrow temperature range has proven to be the optimum and reflects a compromise. High temperatures (37°C) accelerate the aggregation of red blood cells and thus reduce the time needed for separation at the expense of a lowering yield of lymphocytes. Low temperatures would achieve the opposite.

7. After centrifugation carefully remove plasma with a clean Pasteur pipet leaving the lymphocyte layer undisturbed.

8. Transfer lymphocyte layer to a clean centrifuge tube. Careful aspiration will help avoid contamination with the Ficoll-Paque phase.

9. Wash lymphocytes in at least 3 volumes of 1 x PBS or in the recommended balanced salt solution. Suspend cells and centrifuge at 100-300g for 10 min at 18-20°C.

9. Balanced salt solution:
    0.1% anhydrous D-glucose
    0.05mM $CaCl_2\ 2H_2O$
    0.98mM $MgCl_2\ 6H_2O$
    5.4mM KCl
    145mM Tris-HCl
Adjust pH to 7.6 using a 10N HCl stock solution.

10. Remove supernatant and resuspend cells in 6-8ml balanced salt solution and proceed as in step 9.

Procedure(cont.)   *Comments(cont.)*

11. Resuspend the recovered cell pellet in a balanced salt solution and count cells to estimate the fraction needed for subsequent procedures.

6.1.2. Pharyngeal and mouthwashes

Several µg DNA may be isolated from oropharyngeal mucus (Tobal 1989) by two vigorous mouthwashes.
Whenever possible, the washes should be done with 0.9% NaCl (10ml), to prevent hypotonic cell disruption. If this is not tolerated, the wash may be done with dH_2O immediately spit into a container with 0.9% NaCl.
For many diagnostic questions it is essential not to clean the oropharynx prior to the wash.
Depending on volume, 1-50ml of sample are centrifuged at 350g for 10-30min. Sometimes no pellet forms and higher centrifugation may be necessary. Decant supernatant. Pellet may be washed with 1-3ml 0.9% NaCl or PBS and spun down in a smaller centrifugation tube (350g, 5min) if desired. Resuspend pellet in 50-200µl double distilled water and store suspended pellet and an aliquot of the supernatant at -70°C.

6.1.3. Sputum, bronchoalveolar fluids

When preparing these materials it is necessary first to establish the optimal conditions for the following centrifugation step to be effective. To achieve this goal, the N-Acetyl-L-Cystein/sodium-hydroxid preparation (NALC/NaOH) is the recommended method (Salfinger 1991, Anonymous) for the liquefaction of the mucus and subsequent detection of mycobacterial DNA. Other methods for the disruption of intracellular bacteria have been published using mutanolysin (Fliss 1991) or other media, e.g., diatomer for separation of the liberated DNA to avoid contaminations with PCR-inhibiting phenol (Boom 1990).
1. Add the same volume of 20 mM NaOH, 0,5% w/v

Method 4: Preparation of mycobacterial DNA from sputum

Generally, preparation of mycobacterial DNA is performed following the same basic methods as described in chapter 7. The constitution of the sample on the one hand and difficulties due to the special structure of rigid mycobacterial cell walls on the other hand demand some modifications of the standard protocols.

Like in convential microbiological methods, it is necessary to first concentrate mycobacterial particles by centrifugation. However, different procedures are necessary for different materials.

Because mycobacteria are facultative intracellular pathogens they may be concentrated with peripheral blood leucocytes according to the methods in paragraph 6.1.1.

Procedure	Comments
1. Add the same volume of 20mM NaOH, 0.5% w/v NALC solution to the sample.	1. If the mucus-lysis seems to be incomplete add more NaOH/NALC. If bacterial decontamination of the samples seems to be unnecessary, a reagent containing only NALC can also be used. It is possible to perform DNA extraction followed by PCR from the same material prepared for mycobacterial culture with both the NALC method and an anti-bacterial drug mixture which inhibits growth of other microbiological agents (Beige unpublished). Solid tissues, biopsies: To extract DNA from tissue repeated freeze-and-thaw procedures are very useful. The number of the repetitions depends on the constitution of the sample, 5-10 fold repetition is minimum. The volume of the tissue should not exceed 1-2 mm^3 Use liquid nitrogen and a boiling water bath or a micro-wave oven and proceed with a screw-cap (Falcon™) microfuge tube. Although cell disruption is incomplete, the resulting crude suspension is effectively lysed with proteinase K in the following step.
2. Vortex vigorously, at least 5 min, to complete lysis of any mucus.	

Procedure(cont.)

3. If the volume of the material after homogenisation and decontamination is smaller than 5ml, double distilled water should be added to a final volume of 10ml to reach optimal conditions for the following centrifugation, 20min at 3,000g. In materials with only few cells or with possible mycobacterial cell fragments it is very useful to save the supernatant of the first centrifugation and centrifugate this in a second step at high speed and for a long time (10,000g, 45min) to sedimentate cell fragments, as well. Both pellets from these two steps are now resuspended in 100µl water, unified and then undergo further preparation.

4. Next step is the extraction of DNA from the pretreated samples with or without precipitation using the methods previously described. Modifications for mycobacteria see below.

a) Proteinase K lysis, followed by phenol extraction: Useful modification for preparation of mycobacteria. After the regular incubation at 37°C with Proteinase K (24 hours) increase the temperature to 60°C to denaturate remaining proteins and lysate mycobacteria completly.

b) Alternatively, alkaline lysis (see chapter 7.1) can be used. Modification for mycobacteria: Operate in general with 100 mM NaOH instead of 50 mM NaOH. Neutralization with 1 M Tris -HCL after lysis will be done with 16/50 of the NaOH-volume (instead of 8/50). Use higher concentrations of NaOH if the sample is cell-rich in order not to exceed a final volume of 300µl. Highly diluted target DNA might cause difficulties in the PCR reaction.

Generally, prepared samples should be stored at -20°C and for any longer period at -70°C. If samples are to be used right after preparation they may be stored at 4°C to avoid DNA degradation. Bear in mind, that any residual proteinases in the samples might degrade the Taq polymerase in the PCR assay. Therefore it is necessary to avoid contact of the sample with the PCR assay at room temperature.

Comments(cont.)

3. Centrifugation of the sample produces a concentration of mycobacterial particles in the sediment.

4. Proteinase K lysis with subsequent phenol extraction is a very effective method with a good yield of highly purified DNA. Repeated changing of reaction tubes (see protocol in chapter 5) frequently causes contamination problems.

Ultrasonication methods are alternative and effective procedures for disruption of mycobacteria (Sabbor 1992, Ralphs 1991, Parra 1991). Nevertheless, they are time-consuming, and systems which are in direct contact with the sample bear contamination risks. This problem has not yet been clarified. Buck et al. (1992) studied different methods for treating mycobacteria to release DNA for PCR amplification. The presented results were not satisfactory and many questions remained unanswered.

6.1.4. Cerebrospinal fluid

Cerebrospinal fluid usually contains less than 5 cells/µl, and for PCR diagnostics often only a small fraction is available.

If only approximately 1ml is available, this should be centrifuged as fresh as possible in a 1.5ml Eppendorf tube at 350g for 10min.

If no pellet is visible, the supernatant should be removed carefully and stored seperately, leaving about 20µl on the bottom. Only visible pellets should be washed with PBS once. Supernatant and pellet are stored at -70°C.

6.1.5. Urine

Sometimes, urine contains PCR inhibiting substances. This has to be controlled as described in chapter 8 1. 1-50ml urine are centrifuged directly at 350g for 10-30min, depending on volume. Wash pellet once with 1ml 0.9% NaCl and spin down in 1.5ml Eppendorf reaction tube (350g, 5min). Resuspend the pellet, depending on pellet volume in 10-100µl aqua bidest. Store suspended pellet and an aliquot of the supernatant at -70°C.

6.1.6. Plasma, serum and other samples without cellular DNA from host

For detection of infectious agents that may be distributed extracellularly, a direct treatment of the sample with proteinase K (as described in chapter 5.3) is recommended.

6.1.7. Biopsies and solid tissue samples

Tissue samples should be placed in a cold isotonic saline solution and brought to the laboratory as quickly as possible. The sample should be separated from the isotonic solution immediately, transferred into a clean tube and submerged in liquid nitrogen.

6.1.8. Formalin-fixed and paraffin-embedded tissue (see also chapters 4.1, 7.3 Method 3)

Tissue sections may be amenable to PCR after extraction of the paraffin with an organic solvent (e.g. xylene). Depending on sample age and on quality of fixatives, the length of the amplifiable DNA fragment will usually be limited to < 650 bp (Wright and Manos 1990).

For more details see chapters 4.1 and 7.3.

The protocol described by Wright and Manos (1990) continues with a proteinase K digest (after organic treatment), and the sample is to be used for PCR without further DNA extraction procedures.

Heller et al. (1991) describe a method using sonication after paraffin extraction. The sample incubation buffer contains 2-5mg of cleaned glass beads and proteinase K and the sample is placed in a sonicating water bath. Note: Usually the embedded tissue is not collected for PCR diagnostics. Therefore it is likely that no contamination precautions are being taken.

References

1. Anonymous: Tuberkulosediagnostik.1988,Medizinische Mikrobiologie, Normen und weitere Unterlagen, 119-168.

2. Boom R, Sol CJ, Salimans MM, Jansen CL, Wertheim van Dillen PM, van der Noordaa J. Rapid and simple method for purification of nucleic acids. 1990, J Clin Microbiol 28, 495-503.

3. Boyum A. Isolation of mononuclear cells and granulocytes from human blood. 1968, Scand J Clin Lab Invest 21, 77-89.

4. Boyum A. Separation of white blood cells. 1964, Nature 204, 793-794.

5. Brisson-Noel A, Lecossier D, Nassif X, Gicquel B, Levy-Frebault V, Hance AJ. Rapid diagnosis of tuberculosis by amplification of mycobacterial DNA in clinical samples. 1989, Lancet II, 1069-1971.

6. Buck GE, O'Hara LC, Summersgill T. Rapid, simple method for treating clinical specimens containing Mycobacterium tuberculosis to remove DNA for polymerase chain reaction. 1992, J Clin Microbiol 30, 1331-1334.

7. Buffone GJ, Darlington, GJ. 1985, Isolation of DNA from biological specimens without extraction with phenol. Clin Chem 30, 164-165.

8. Eisenach KD, Cave MD, Bates JH, Crawford JT: Polymerase chain reaction amplification of a repetitive DNA sequence specific for Mycobacterium tuberculosis. 1990, J Infect Dis 161, 977-981.

9. Fliss I, Emond E, Simard RE, Pandian S. A rapid and efficient method of lysis of listeria and other gram-positive bacteria using mutanolysin. 1991, Biotechniques 11, 453-456.

10. Fotino M, Merson EJ, Allen FH. Micromethod for rapid separation of lymphocytes from peripheral blood. 1971, Ann Clin Lab sci 1, 131-133.

11. Heller MJ, Burgart LJ, TenEyck CJ, Anderson ME, Greiner TC, Robinson RA. An efficient Method for the extraction of DNA from formalin-fixed, paraffin-embedded tissue by sonication. 1991, Biotechniques 11, 372-377.

12. Hermans PWM, Schuitema ARJ, van Soolingen D, Verstynen CP, Bik EM, Thole JE, Kolk AH, van Embden JD. Specific detection of Mycobacterium tuberculosis complex strains by polymerase chain reaction. 1990, J Clin Microbiol 28, 1204-1213.

13. Jiwa NM, Van Gemert GW, Raap AK, Van de Rijke FM, Mulder A, Lens PF, Salimans MMM, Zwaan FE, Van Dorp W, Van der Ploeg M. Rapid detection of human cytomegalovirus DNA in peripheral blood

leukocytes of viremic transplant recipients by the polymerase chain reaction. 1989, Transplantation 48, 72-76.

14. Parra CA, Londono LP, del Portillo P, Pattaroyo ME: Isolation, characterization, and molecular cloning of a specific Mycobacterium tuberculosis antigen gene; identification of a species specific sequence. 1991, Infect Immunity 59, 3411-3417.

15. Ralphs NT, Garett S, Morse R, Cookson JB, Andrew PW, Boulnois GJ: A DNA primer/probe system for the rapid and sensitive detection of Mycobacterium tuberculosis-complex pathogens. 1991, J Appl Bacteriology 70, 221-226.

16. Saboor SA, Johnson N McI, Mc Fadden J. Detection of mycobacterial DNA in sarcoidosis and tuberculosis with polymerase chain reaction. 1992, Lancet I, 1012-1015.

17. Salfinger S. Microbiological diagnosis of mycobacteria. "Charite Microbiological Symposium", 18.10.1991.

18. Sjöbring U, Mecklenburg M, Andersen AB, Miörner H. Polymerase chain reaction for detection of Mycobacterium tuberculosis. 1990, J Clin Microbiol 28, 2200-2204.

19. Tobal K, Layton DM, Mufti GJ. Non-invasive isolation of constitutional DNA for genetic analysis. 1989, Lancet II, 1281-1282.

20. Wright DK, Manos MM. Sample preparation from paraffin-embedded tissues. In: PCR Protocols: A Guide to Methods and Applications, Eds. Innis MA, Gelfand DH, Sninsky JJ, White TJ. 1990, Academic Press, San Diego, pp153-158.

7. Isolation of DNA from Cells and Tissue for PCR

Purity, homogeneity and DNA content of samples may vary considerably (see also chapter 1.7) - largely depending on the native material itself and the method chosen to isolate or purify DNA. Many protocols have been described that yield DNA suitable for PCR. Criteria strongly influencing which protocol will ultimately be chosen are:
- Expenditure of time and manpower
- Diagnostic reliabilit
- Contamination risks
- Yield of amplifiable sample DNA

For samples containing less than approximately 70ng DNA, the DNA purification through Phenol/Chloroform and the final ethanol precipitation step bear the risk of significant loss. For isolation of viral DNA from patient samples it is crucial that there is sufficient "carrier" DNA from the patient to coprecipitate with the viral DNA. Otherwise no DNA extraction procedure should be performed.

On the other side, purified DNA will be the best storage form for further analyses. Nonpurified samples after crude cell lysis cannot be quantified photometrically, but are useful to prevent loss of DNA. If DNA breakdown is a critical factor, as e.g. in forensic or environmental samples with minimal DNA content, the chelating resin Chelex^R 100 might provide better amplifiable DNA yield (Singer-Sam 1989). For detailed Chelex^R protocols see Walsh *et al.* (1991). In this chapter we describe several protocols in detail. All of them have proved to be suitable for amplification of human DNA or DNA from infectious agents.

7.1. Alkaline lysis

In our hands, the alkaline lysis technique has proved to be a very suitable rapid method for isolating DNA amenable to PCR from a wide variety of DNA sources. Even solid tissue and, in particular, needle biopsies can be treated according to this method. With regard to needle biopsies, one advantage becomes distinctly clear, namely, that minute samples may be prepared without loss of the small amount of DNA - this would very likely be the case if lengthy extraction procedures were followed.

We routinely use this method to isolate DNA from nearly all body fluids and tissue for diagnostic purposes, e.g., the detection of cytomegalovirus DNA. Recently, in our laboratory this method provided succesful preparation of patient samples for PCR detection of mycobacterial DNA (Beige unpublished). A further advantage of using the alkaline lysis technique is definitely the lower risk of cross-contamination. First, the sample remains in one single tube throughout the procedure and second, the sample is covered with mineral oil providing a physical barrier. The following procedure was similarly reported by Jiwa *et al.* (1989) for amplification of CMV DNA and contains essential suggestions from P. Lingenfelter and D. Myerson, Seattle.

Procedure	Comments

Method 1: Isolation of DNA using alkaline lysis

1. Add approx. identical volume dH_2O from material. Freeze-thaw solid tissue, nondissolved cell pellets and biopsies twice. This is done quickly with the sample in a Eppendorf tube, liquid N_2 and hot water. If the tissue is very solide, disrupt its structure mechanically with disposable pipets, scalpels ore else.

2. Overlay tissue homogenate or sample cell preparation (as described in 1.) with 10 - 500 µl 50 mM NaOH in a 1.5ml eppendorf reaction tube.

2. 10µl for up to 10^5 cells, 100µl for up to 5×10^6 cells, but at least the volume of the cell suspension or tissue.

3. Vortex vigorously. Cell pellets have to be suspended completely.

4. Spin down briefly

5. Overlay with 150 ml light mineral oil.

5. E.g., Sigma #M-5904

6. Place on 95°C heating block for 10 min

7. Neutralize with 1 M Tris-HCl, pH 7.0. Pipet the correct amount underneath the oil. Note: The hot sample may contaminate your pipet.

7. Take 8µl 1 M Tris-HCl, pH 7.0 for 50 µl NaOH.

8. Store at -70°C

8. Sample ready for PCR.

7.2. Guanidinium rhodanid method (GuSCN)

DNA suitable for PCR can also be recovered from the organic and interphase after RNA extraction (chapter 8, Method 1).
Procedure: Do not discard the organic phase and the interphase after preparation of RNA (ca.600µl). Add 300µl 3M Tris-base (pH ca. 10.0) and mix vigorously. Spin with 2000rpm in an Eppendorf centrifuge for 10min to separate the phases. Pipet the upper phase (ca. 300µl) into a new 1.5ml Eppendorf tube. If there was a visible opaque interphase, an additional phenol/chloroform extraction using phenol (pH >7.8) should be performed. This is described in 7.3. Method 1, step 9 - 12. After this additional extraction, or if there was no visible interphase, the procedure is continued with step 13.

7.3. Proteinase K digestion for the isolation of DNA

Traditional protocols using proteinase K digestion and a number of often lengthy subsequent steps after cell lysis were designed to isolate high quality, high molecular weight DNA for cloning procedures and for establishing DNA libraries. The demands that PCR places on the DNA template are different. As long as the DNA isolated is not extensively fragmented or nicked, so that the two primers employed in the PCR are not physically separated, the designed PCR should succeed. Proteinase K is still widely used in protocols describing the isolation of DNA for PCR. However, the time needed to obtain the desired template for PCR has been reduced considerably. The procedures which take a day for DNA isolation contain phenol extraction steps. The quick procedures omit these steps and also yield a DNA accessible to PCR. Whichever procedure is employed, care must be taken to eliminate substances known to inhibit PCR or at least to keep them at ineffective concentrations. Further, all measurements required to avoid extraneous contamination or cross-contamination must be realized. The procedures outlined below can be used for cells isolated acccording to one of the methods described in chapter 6 or for small amounts of tissue (biopsy material). One procedure for the isolation of DNA from infectious viral agents in serum is also presented.

Procedure	Comments

Method 2: Proteinase K/phenol-chloroform extraction

Procedure	Comments
1. Resuspend cell pellet in 1 x PBS, a balanced salt solution, or 0.9% NaCl adjusted to approximately 10,000 cells/µl.	
2. Add 1 volume of 2 x lysis buffer. Tissue material: Cover fresh tissue material with a slight excess of buffer and mechanically shred by	2. Because of the high risk of contamination, the use of tissumizers can not be recommended, especially in PCR for diagnostic purposes.

Procedure(cont.)

drawing in and out through a disposable positive displacement pipet to avoid contamination. Frozen tissue can be initially pulverized using a clean glass rod and adding 1ml 1 x lysis buffer/100mg tissue (wet weight).

3. Vortex until a viscous homogenous lysate is obtained.

4. Spin down briefly to remove liquid in or around the cap.

5. Add proteinase K to yield an end concentration of 100µg/ml for cells and up to 500µg/ml for tissue depending on the solubility of the tissue.

6. Mix well by vortexing, and incubate at 37°C overnight or at 56°C for at least 1 hour.

7. If microfuge tubes have been used, inactivate the protease by incubating at 95°C for 10 min on a thermal block.

Comments(cont.)

- 2 x Lysis Buffer
- 20mM EDTA
- 20mM Tris-HCl
- 300mM NaCl
- 0.4% sodium dodecyl sulfate (SDS) (w/v)

The first three components make up the stock buffer which is either autoclaved or passed through a sterile filter before use. The stock lysis buffer containing salts is stored at 4°C. Since SDS precipitates at temperatures < 10°C, it is advisable to prepare a 10% SDS stock solution (PCR-grade) and to supplement the appropriate amount to the salt buffer needed. Do not inhale or allow SDS powder to come in contact with skin.

5. Proteinase K: Always use fresh proteinase K. Prepare a stock solution at a concentration of 10-20mg/ml in water. Aliquot in suitable portions and store at -20°C. The optimal reaction buffer for catalytic activity contains 10mM Tris (ph 7.8), 5mM EDTA and 0.5% SDS. Although higher EDTA concentrations remove Ca^{2+} from the enzyme and thus reduce catalytic activity, residual activity is sufficient to degrade proteins contaminating nucleic acid preparations. The advantage of higher EDTA concentrations resides in the more complete inhibition of Mg^{2+}-dependent nucleases (Sambrook 1989).

6. Progression of proteinase K digestion of tissue samples should be controlled at intervals. Vortex occasionally. This will sometimes finally homogenize remaining tissue particles. If digestion is slow, consider the addition of some more proteinase K and continue digestion.

Procedure(cont.)

8. Spin down condensed water collected in the caps.

9. Add an equal amount of Tris-saturated phenol (pH > 7.8)/chloroform/isoamyl alcohol mixed in the following ratio according to volume (25:24:1). Gently vortex the mixture for 1 min until a fine emulsion is created.

10. Separate the organic phase from the aqueous phase by centrifuging at full speed in a Beckman CPKR centrifuge or a microfuge for 5-10 min at room temperature.

11. Transfer upper aqueous phase to a new clean tube without disturbing the interphase.

12. Extract once with an equal volume of chloroform, mix and centrifuge as described above.

13. Add 1/10 volume of 3M sodium acetate or of 2M sodium chloride and 2 volumes of cold pure ethanol. Mix well and allow the DNA to precipitate at -20°C for at least 1 hour.

14. Sediment precipitated DNA by centrifuging at

Comments(cont.)

9. Phenol must be equilibrated to a pH > 7.8 prior to use because DNA partitions to the organic phase at acid pH. Phenol is best prepared according to the guidelines given in Sambrook et al. (1989) by saturating phenol with a 0.5M and subsequently with a 0.1M Tris-HCl (pH 8.0) solution (PCR-grade). The addition of 0.1% hydroxyquinoline gives a yellow color to the organic phase and thus assists in detection. It is also an antioxidant and can be used to judge phenol oxidation (yellow to pink). Phenol oxidation products can breakdown phosphodiester bonds or cross-link RNA and DNA! Liquid phenol should be stored at -20°C. Equilibrated phenol can be stored in an opaque bottle for up to 1 month at 4°C.

11. If the interphase is very thick, phenolize the aqueous and interphase a second time to avoid DNA loss to the interphase. Repeat steps 9. to 12.

12. Residual phenol must be removed in order to avoid denaturation of enzymes in subsequent steps.

13. Using 2M sodium chloride instead of 3M sodium acetate will allow residual SDS to remain soluble in order to avoid coprecipitation (Wallace 1987).

Guidelines for precipitating DNA (Wallace 1987):
a) Small volumes less than 1ml containing >10µg/ml DNA in the original sample can be precipitated at -70°C for 15 min - recovery figuring 80%.
b) If large volumes are to be precipitated at -70°C, then more time is needed to allow temperature equilibration of the sample: 30 min for a 30ml sample.
c) DNA concentrations <10ng/ml in the original sample can be effectively recovered by precipitating overnight at -20°C and best if a carrier is added.

14. This holds true for precipitates of at least 1 µg/ml.

Procedure(cont.)   *Comments(cont.)*

12,000 rpm for 20-30 min at 4°C in a Sorvall centrifuge, or if precipitation has been carrried out in an Eppendorf tube, then centrifuge at full speed in a bench top centrifuge for 20-30 min at 4°C.

                                      Smaller amounts in the nanogram range can also be efficiently recovered using a microcentrifuge as long as a carrier (tRNA or ultra pure glycogen) is added.

15. Suspend DNA pellet in autoclaved double distilled water or in 1 x TE buffer by vortexing gently and incubating at 37°C until the pellet is completely dissolved.

                                      15. For quantifying assays complete dissociation is absolutely mandatory. The content of the DNA sample can be determined spectrophotometrically at 260nm. An optical density (OD) reading of 1 is equivalent to 50ug/ml. This value can be used to adjust the concentration of DNA per microliter.

10 x TE Buffer   100mM Tris-HCl
                      10mM EDTA
                      adjusted to pH 8.0

EDTA is a chelator and helps inhibit nuclease activity.

16. Store DNA samples at 4°C or at -70°C for long term storage.

Method 3: PCR-adapted proteinase K method for leucocytes or whole blood (Kawasaki 1990)

1. Thoroughly mix 100µl of whole blood with 0.5ml 1 x TE buffer in a microfuge tube. Spin for 10 sec at 13,000g. Resuspend the pellet in 0.5ml 1 x TE buffer by vortexing and pellet again. This is repeated twice until a clean nuclei pellet is obtained.

                    or

Isolate cells from 1-2ml blood by Ficoll-Paque density gradient centrifugation or by selective lysis of red blood cells. Count cells in a hemacytometer and pellet an aliquot of the cell suspension to yield 5×10^5 cells by centrifugation.

2. Resuspend cell nuclei or 5×10^5 in 100µl lysis buffer K by vortexing.

                                      2. Lysis buffer K (Kawasaki 1990):
                                                1 x PCR buffer
                                                1% Laureth 12 or 0.5% Tween 20
                                                100µg/ml fresh proteinase K.

Procedure(cont.)   *Comments(cont.)*

Preparation of a proteinase K stock solution is described under step 5. in Method 1.

3. Spin down briefly and incubate at 56°C for 45 min.

4. Inactivate protease at 95°C for 10 min.

5. Spin down briefly and use 10µl of the cell/nuclei lysate in a 100µl reaction volume for PCR. This amount of DNA is equivalent to sampling 25-50,000 cells.

Method 4: DNA isolation from paraffin-embedded tissue (Modification of the method described by CC Impraim)

Successful isolation of DNA from formalin-fixed, paraffin-embedded tissue allows retrospective analysis of patient material collected over a longer period of time by PCR. Direct analysis of preserved material without high grade DNA extraction has been described (Shibata 1988). However, high-grade DNA extractions from preserved tissue can be stored for several weeks without substantial degradation, so that purified DNA can be repeatedly subjected to analysis. An approach using proteinase K followed by phenol/chloroform extraction has proven to be a good method for isolating DNA from preserved tissue. The following procedure is a personal communication from Frank Tiecke.

Procedure   Comments

1. Place one 5-10µm section in a 1.5ml Eppendorf tube.

2. Remove paraffin by treating with 400µl xylene. Vortex vigorously.

3. Centrifuge at full speed in a bench top centrifuge for 5 min at room temperature.

4. Remove xylene carefully with a pipette.

                     4. Make sure not to disturb the loose tissue pellet at the bottom of the tube.

5. Repeat steps 2.-4.

Procedure(cont.) *Comments(cont.)*

6. Remove residual xylene by gently mixing the tissue pellet with 400µl of absolute ethanol.

7. Centrifuge at full speed in a bench top centrifuge for 5 min at room temperature.

8. Carefully remove ethanol with a pipette.

8. Pay attention not to disturb the loose tissue pellet at the bottom of the tube.

9. Repeat steps 6.- 8. once.

10. Allow ethanol to evaporate by incubating in an oven at 37°C for 10-15 min.

10. Tissue pellet should remain slightly moist in order to facilitate resuspension.

11. Resuspend tissue pellet in 50µl proteinase K buffer.

11. Proteinase K buffer: 50mM Tris-HCl, pH 8.7
10mM NaCl, 0.1% Triton-X 100
Add the appropriate amount of a fresh solution of proteinase K so that the end concentration is 500µg/ml.

12. Incubate lysis mixture at 50°C over night.

12. An additional aliquot of proteinase K may be added to the lysis mixture after several hours to reassure more complete protein digestion.

13. Spin down briefly to remove any condensated water in the lid.

14. Add one volume phenol/chloroform/isoamyl alcohol (25:24:1). Vortex vigorously and separate the organic phase from the aqueous phase by centrifuging at full speed as described above.

15. Transfer upper aqeous phase to a clean 1.5 Eppendorf tube.

16. Reextract the organic phase by adding 100µl TE-buffer. Vortex vigorously and separate the organic phase from the aqueous phase by centrifuging at full speed as described above.

17. Transfer this aqeous phase to the aqueous phase collected previously .

18. Precipitate the DNA from the aqueous phase by adding 1/10 volume of 3M Na-acetate pH 5.2 and 2.5

Procedure(cont.)   *Comments(cont.)*

volumes of pure ethanol. Mix well.

19. Incubate overnight at -20°C.

20. Centrifuge at full speed for at least 30min at 4°C in a bench top centrifuge.

21. Carefully remove supernatant and allow any residual ethanol to drain away by inverting the tube.

22. Wash DNA pellet with 200µl of 70% ethanol and centrifuge at full speed for 10 min at 4°C.

23 Remove supernatant and dry DNA pellet in an oven at 37°C.

24. Resuspend in 20µl TE-buffer and store at -20°C.

24. Approximately 400ng of DNA can be recovered from one 10µm section (3mm x 4mm x 10µm.)

Method 5: Detection of viral DNA from serum (Ishigaki 1991)

1. Free serum samples of cells by passing through a sterile 0.45um filter.

2. Mix 100µl cell-free serum with 100µl lysis buffer B.

2. Lysis buffer B: 100mM KCl
　　　　　　　　　20mM Tris-HCl (pH 8.3)
　　　　　　　　　5mM $MgCl_2$
　　　　　　　　　0.2mg/ml gelatin
　　　　　　　　　0.9% Tween 20

3. Add fresh proteinase K to a final concentration of 60µg/ml.

3. Preparation of a proteinase K stock solution is described under step 5. in Method 1.

4. Incubate for 1 hour at 55°C.

5. Inactivate the protease by heating at 95°C for 10 min.

6. Centrifuge at 12,000g for 10 min and add 10µl to a 100µl PCR.

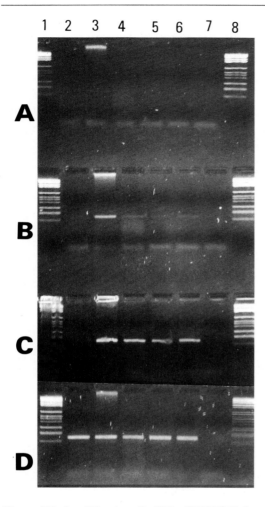

Figure 7.1: Amplification of a 185bp PDH DNA fragment from genomic DNA. To a solid tissue sample (prostate tumor), four different DNA extraction methods were applied. Lane **2**: Guanidium rhodanid method (see 7.2), sample: approx. 250ng DNA extract. Lane **3**: Proteinase K digestion and phenol/chloroform extraction (see 7.3), sample: approx. 250ng DNA extract. Lane **4**: Direct treatment of the tissue sample with guanidium rhodanid for 20min instead of Proteinase K and extraction with phenol/chloroform (see 7.3), sample: approx. 250ng DNA extract. Lane **5**: Alkaline lysis (see 7.1), sample: 1µl from a 250-300µl total volume. Lane **6**: As lane 5, but 2.5µl sample. Premixed reaction mixtures, including the DNA samples, were aliquoted, and the PCR was performed with the respective aliquots for 20 (**A**), 25 (**B**), 30 (**C**) and 35 (**D**) cycles. Primers and procedure: see legend to fig. 2.1.

7.4. Automated DNA extraction

The development of the Applied Biosystems GENEPURE™ 341 Nucleic Acid Purification System introduced the automization of the isolation of nucleic acids. The method of isolation adapted for automization is based on the proteinase K/phenol-chloroform extraction method. Properly prepared samples are added to a preheated lysis buffer. Lysed material is digested with proteinase K at 60°C, extracted twice with 70% phenol/water/chloroform and once with chloroform. This is followed by conventional isopropanol precipitation. The precipitated nucleic acid is finally rescued on a filter mounted on one end of the vessel. Nucleic acid isolation takes place in glass vessels pretreated with silane. Up to 8 samples can be processed simultaneously. Valves at both ends of the vessel regulate the flow of reagents to and wastes away from the vessel in a time dependent modus according to a method devised either by the manufacturer or the operator. Depending on the amount of DNA expected to be isolated, the operator can chose between a 14ml or 30ml vessel. Up to 800µg total nucleic acid can be rescued in the former and up to 1.5mg in the latter vessel.

The success of automated DNA extraction largely depends on the proper preparation of the sample. As stated in the manual, the sample must be homogeneous, free of particulate matter and readily dispersed when added into the reaction vessels. Second, it is necessary to load the proper volume of a sample defined by the number of cells or by tissue weight so that complete digestion of the sample can take place. Overloading the system can have consequences which are very cumbersome to deal with, especially if a line is obstructed. On the contrary, the purification of small amounts of genomic DNA (from $< 10^6$ cells) will yield varying results with regard to DNA recovery, if any at all using the standard protocol. The introduction of a new silica resin, BaseBinder™, and slight alteration of the precipitation step greatly improve the recovery of DNA. Using this altered method, it is possible to isolate DNA from as little as 50µl blood (ABI communication).

Advantages:
1. The automated DNA extraction system is fairly versatile. There are possibilities for additional reagents to be mounted so that individual protocols can be adapted to the system. Such protocols usually require additional enzymes for lysing bacteria, e.g. lysozym, lysostaphin or mutanplysin (Fliss 1991).
2. Previously time consuming procedures such as phenolization and ethanol precipitation of large numbers of samples can be carried out within 4-5 hours, while at the same time other routine laboratory assignments can be performed.
3. Minimal sample handling also significantly reduces risks of cross contaminating samples during manual manipulation. However, we highly recommend running controls to reassure oneself that no extraneous DNA is being carried over from successive preparations in the same vessel. In order to avoid DNA carry-over, it is absolutely necessary that the vessels are treated with silane. This must be done regularly. In addition, the manufacturers have designed an extensive purge program which must be performed after every extraction. In order to assess whether nucleic acids have been retained in the vessel system, it is advisable to run an extraction program and to simply substitute water for the sample volume. We have unfortunately noticed that an array of DNA products were amplified during PCR which could be faintly visualized on an ethidium bromide stained agarose gel. This is most likely due to binding of DNA fragments to one another which have not been completely rinsed out of the vessel and then are able to prime extension.
4. Compared to manual DNA preparation performed by different technicians, automated DNA extraction more readily realizes the standardization of a procedure, since it is less susceptible to the inaccuracy of the investigator.

REFERENCES

1. Fliss I, Emond E, Simard RE, Pandian S. A rapid and efficient method of lysis of Listeria and other Gram-positive bacteria using mutanolysin. 1991, BioTechniques 11, 453-457.

2. Impraim CC, Saiki RK, Erlich HA, Teplitz RL. Analysis of DNA extracted from formalin-fixed, paraffin-embedded tissues by enzymatic amplification and hybridization with sequence -specific oligonucleotides. 1987, Biochem Biophys Res Commun 142, 710-716.

3. Ishigaki S, Takeda M, Kura T, Ban N, et al. Cytomegalovirus DNA in the sera of patients with cytomegalovirus pneumonia. 1991, Brit J Haematol 79, 198-204.

4. Jiwa NM, van Gemert GW, Raap Ak, van de Rijke FM, Mulder A, Lens PF, Salimans MMM, Zwaan FE, van Dorp W, van der Ploeg M. Rapid detection of human cytomegalowirud DNA in peripheral blood leukocytes of viremic transplant recipients by the polymerase chain reaction. 1989, Transplantation 48, 72-76

5. Kawasaki ES. Sample preparation from blood, cells, and other fluids. In: PCR protocols: A guide to methods and applications. Eds. Innis MA, Gelfand DH, Sninsky JJ, White TJ. (Academic Press, Inc., San Diego) 1990, 146-152.

6. Sambrook J, Fritsch EF, Maniatis T. Molecular cloning: A laboratory manual (Cold Spring Harbor Lab, Cold Spring Harbor, NY) 1989.

7. Shibata DK, Arnheim N, Martin WJ. Detection of human papilloma virus in paraffin-embedded tissue using the polymerase chain reaction. 1988, J Exp Med 167, 225-230.

8. Singer-Sam J, Tanguay RL, Riggs AD. Use of Chelex to improve the PCR signal from a small number of cells. 1989, Amplifications A Forum for PCR Users 3, 11.

9. Wallace DM. Precipitation of nucleic acids. 1987, Methods Enzymol 152, 41-48.

10. Walsh PS, Metzger DA, Higuchi R. Chelex* 100 as a medium for simple extraction of DNA for PCR-based typing from forensic material. 1991, Biotechniques 10, 506-513.

8. Isolation of RNA from Cells and Tissue for PCR

8.1. General Preparations

Elimination of ribonuclease contamination is an essential prelude to any attempt to isolate undegraded RNA. Ribonucleases (RNases) are present in virtually all cells and released from cellular compartments upon disruption of the cell. They are resistant to heat and maintain activity even after being boiled, function over a wide pH range and hardly require any cofactors. Because of their stability, RNases are found in most solutions and on glassware. A major source of RNases which should not be underestimated are the fingers of the investigator. Thus, anything one touches can potentially be contaminated with ribonucleases.

A number of precautions help eliminate RNase contamination of utensils and solutions used in working with RNA: 1. New glassware should be set aside and exclusively used for RNA procedures. Prior to usage, glassware should be treated with a 0.1% solution of diethyl pyrocarbonate (DEPC) which is a non-specific inhibitor of ribonucleases. After adding the appropriate amount of DEPC to double distilled water, DEPC must be dispersed by either vigorous shaking or stirring for at least 10 min. Complete dispersion can be judged visually. Soak glassware in DEPC solution for at least 30 min, rinse in DEPC-treated, autoclaved water, and autoclave to break down residual DEPC into CO_2 and H_2O, and bake in an oven at 250°C for at least 4 hours. It is important to remove residual DEPC, since it inhibits in vitro translation reactions (Ehrenberg 1974). 2. Sterile disposable plasticware has proved to be free of contaminating RNases and should be used whenever possible. 3. Eppendorf tubes and pipet tips should be autoclaved twice before usage. 4. Solutions are prepared as usual and finally adjusted to 0.1% DEPC. DEPC must again be dispersed thoroughly and completely removed by autoclaving. The only exceptions are Tris buffers. These are prepared by directly using DEPC-treated, autoclaved water and then reautoclaved (Sambrook 1989). 5. Reagents for RNA preparations should be set aside and used solely for this purpose. 6. Last but not least, be sure to wear gloves and change them often in order to eliminate exogenous ribonuclease contamination.

8.2. Inhibition of endogenous RNases

As stated above, RNases are released during cell disruption when the natural compartmentalization of RNases and RNA is destroyed. Nucleolytic degradation of RNA can be avoided if cellular proteins including RNases are denatured or RNase activity inhibited. The former demands that the rate of denaturation must exceed the rate of RNA hydrolysis by the liberated RNases (Chirgwin 1979). The amount of RNases found in different tissues varies considerably, and accordingly, many procedures have been developed in order to isolate intact RNA. They make use of either powerful

RNase inhibitors or of chaotropic agents which denature proteins. Potent specific inhibitors of RNases are vanadyl-ribonucleoside complexes (VCR) and RNasin. Detailed protocols are described by Berger (1987), de Martynoff (1980), and Wallace (1987). These can be used in combination with a phenol extraction. Phenol extraction leads to the deproteinization of the aqueous phase containing nucleic acids. The choice of pH of the extraction system determines whether DNA or RNA or both will be extracted. At pH 5-6 DNA is retained in the organic phase and interphase, while RNA remains in the aqueous phase. However, if phenol is used alone at pH values below 7.6, then a large amount of poly(A)-mRNA is also lost to the organic phase (Palmiter 1974). In combination with chloroform or sodium dodecyl sulfate (SDS), poly(A)-mRNA will efficiently partition to the aqueous phase (Perry 1974). The use of guanidinium chloride as a deproteinization agent for isolating RNA was first described by Cox (1968). The inefficiency of this approach to isolate good yields of undegraded RNA from ribonuclease enriched tissue was followed by further improvement. The combined application of a stronger denaturant, guanidinium thiocyanate, and of a reductant, 2-mercaptoethanol, to break protein disulfide bonds introduced by Chirgwin (1979) has become one of the most common methods for the isolation of intact RNA. Briefly, the guanidinium thiocyanate cell lysate is ultracentrifuged through a CsCl cushion and the RNA pellet washed to remove salts and other degradation products.

8.3 Methods for the isolation of RNA suitable for RT-PCR

PCR is unequivocally a method distinguished by its speed and efficiency in amplifying target DNA and cDNA fragments. In contrast, many standard methods for isolating nucleic acids are fairly time consuming. In line with saving time, a large number of "quick and easy" methods have been devised which yield DNA or RNA accessible to PCR. Since RNA cannot directly serve as a template for the Taq polymerase, RNA must be reverse transcribed to a cDNA prior to amplification. Thus, quick methods for isolating RNA must fulfill at least two requirements: 1. degradation of RNA must be obviated and 2. the preparation must be suitable for reverse transcriptase.

In one of the quickest methods 2×10^6 cells are resuspended in 100 µl freshly made 0.1% DEPC in double distilled water, boiled for 5 min, cell debris sedimented at 12,000g for 30 sec and an aliquot of the supernatant used for reverse transcription (Ferre 1989). Another method described for blood cells uses a detergent, nonidet P-40 (NP40), in an isotonic high pH buffer to lyse cells and freshly made DEPC to inhibit RNAses. Cell nuclei are selectively separated by centrifugation which definitely helps avoid DNA contamination of the RNA preparation, and the supernatant is heated for a short period to remove DEPC. The supernatant is then suitable for reverse transcription (Kawasaki 1990). These crude cell preparations, however, have some drawbacks. First, it is difficult to judge whether components in the lysate will inhibit reverse transcription or even subsequent PCR. The first very likely candidate is residual DEPC. Thus, if the first attempt was unsuccessful, then reheating the sample lysate might spell success. Second, the number of components which could possibly inhibit the Taq polymerase is large and largely unknown. In this case overcoming inhibition is fairly difficult and PCR optimization strategies might never work. A third difficulty which might be encountered when working with crude cell lysates is the fact that if the RNA transcript is only of low abundance, then background DNA could very likely render "successful RT-PCR" impossible. Fourth, since little is known about RNA degradation in a crude lysate after DEPC has been removed, such preparations will not be amenable to procedures requiring quantification. These aspects as well as the unknown extent of RNA degradation in initial and subsequent analyses make it hard to interpret "false negative" results. A positive result will undoubtly be valid as long as essential controls allow for such interpretation (see chapter 5).

Two methods have been devised which, according to our opinion, are amenable to most RT-PCR applications. The method reported by Chomczynski

(1987) provides a high purity preparation of intact RNA with a substantial yield and can be carried out within 4 hours. It combines the use of a powerful denaturant - guanidinium thiocyanate - with a phenol extraction in an acidic environment in a single step.

A large number of samples can be processed using this procedure and isolation of total RNA even from small quantities of cells or tissue is possible. The method described by Rappolee (1990) is a modification of the technique introduced by Chirgwin (1979). Both methods are outlined below. In addition, one quick method is also described

Procedure

Comments

Method 1: Acid guanidinium thiocyanate-phenol-chloroform extraction (Chomczynski and Sacchi 1987)

1. Pellet 5×10^6 to 1×10^7 cells in Eppendorf tubes at 300-400g for 12 min at 4°C.

1. Handling is easier if all steps can be performed using Eppendorf tubes. For this purpose the stated number of cells works well. If more material should be investigated, use 4 ml polypropylene tubes initially and finally precipitate RNA in Eppendorf tubes.

2. Place tubes on ice, remove and discard supernatants.

2. Keeping samples on ice will reduce nuclease activity if present.

3. Add 500µl of a 4M guanidinium thiocyanate stock solution (solution D) to each tube.

3. Solution D

    4M guanidinium thiocyanate
    25mM sodium citrate, pH 7.0
    0.5% sarcosyl
    0.1M 2-mercaptoethanol

Guanidinium is a hazard to health. Therefore, it is advisable to mix the guanidinium stock solution as described by Chomczynski. Prepare stock solutions of the individual components: 0.75 M sodium citrate (Merck), pH 7.0, and 10% sarcosyl. Add 293ml dd H_2O to 250g guanidinium thiocyanate (Fluka) in the original bottle, supplement with 17.6ml 0.75M sodium

Procedure(cont.) | *Comments(cont.)*

citrate and 26.4ml 10% sarcosyl and dissolve at 65°C. Storage is possible for at least 3 months at room temperature. Prior to usage, 50ml stock solution are supplemented with 0.36ml 2-mercaptoethanol (assists denaturation by breaking down disulfide bonds). This can be stored 1 month at room temperature.
Guideline: for 100mg tissue use 1 ml stock solution and 100µl for 10^6 cells.

4. Vortex vigorously in order to completely homogenize the cell pellet in the shortest time possible.

4. The rate of protein denaturation must exceed the rate of RNA hydrolysis. The homogenate should be clear and viscous.

5. Briefly spin tubes in order to remove fluid from lids.

5. This is absolutely important in order to avoid cross contamination during handling. PCR is a very sensitive method and theoretically, one molecule will suffice to yield a positive result.

6. Add 50µl of 2M sodium acetate, pH 4.0. Vortex and spin down briefly.

6. At pH 5.0-6.0, DNA is selectively retained in the organic phase and interphase, while RNA remains in the aqueous phase (Wallace 1987). The addition of salt is also needed for subsequent precipitation. The need for high salt concentrations to reduce the activity of endogenous ribonucleases has been obviated by the introduction of highly potent denaturants. Maximum solubility of RNA is at 0.15M Na^+. This lower ionic strength also reduces non-specific RNA aggregation.

7. Add 500µl of RNA-grade phenol saturated with water and 100´µl of a chloroform-isoamyl alcohol mixture (49:1).

7. Preparation of RNA-grade phenol: Phenol is toxic and should not be inhaled or come in contact with skin. Handling must be carried out under a fume hood, wearing gloves and goggles. RNA grade phenol is supplied by GIBCO-BRL. Since only small amounts of phenol are needed, we reconstitute 100g phenol stocks. Warm frozen phenol to room temperature, loosen bottle cap and melt crystals in a hot water bath at 65°C. Add 100mg 8-hydroxyquinoline (0.1% w/w). Saturate phenol by filling the bottle to the base of the neck with deionized water and mixing until a fine emulsion is formed. Allow the organic and aqueous phases to separate overnight at 4°C. Remove the upper aqueous phase, aliqot in practical portions and store at 4´C protected from light or at -20°C for a longer period. The aqueous phase is normally pH 3.0 - 4.5.

Procedure(cont.)   *Comments(cont.)*

8. Mix thoroughly by vortexing and set on ice for 15 min.

9. Centrifuge at 10,000g for 20 min at 4°C.

10. Carefully transfer the upper aqueous phase to a fresh Eppendorf tube paying attention not to disturb or carry over the interphase.

10. Accidental transfer of a part of the interphase - even minute amounts - leads to DNA contamination of the RNA preparation. If it is uncertain whether DNA has been carried over or not, a second phenol extraction of the aqueous phase should be performed. Our experience has shown that this is often necessary.

11. Add 1 ml cold ethanol, vortex gently and precipitate nucleic acids for at least 1 hour at -20°C.

11. Optionally, an equal amount (500µl) of isopropanol can be added.

12. Pellet RNA at 10.000g for 20 min at 4°C.

13. Thoroughly resuspend pellet in 300-400µl 4M guanidinium thiocyanate stock solution.

13. This step concentrates the RNA.

14. Reprecipate using a double volume of cold ethanol or an equal volume of isopropanol at -20°C for 1 hour or overnight.

14. Reprecipitation of the RNA pellet helps eliminate denatured ribonucleases from the nucleic acid pellet.

15. Centrifuge at 10.000g for 15 min at 4°C.

16. Discard supernatant, rinse RNA pellet with 75% cold ethanol to remove salts and centrifuge for 5 min.

17. Dissolve pellet in 50µl DEPC-treated water or in 0.5% sodium dodecyl sulfate (SDS) at 65°C for 10 min.

17. Be sure that the pellet is completely dissolved before subjecting the RNA to any further procedures. This is absolutely essential if the assay aims at quantifying mRNA transcripts. Although an RNA pellet is more readily dissolved in SDS, certain concentrations of SDS can inhibit PCR. This must be kept in mind and a pilot experiment will easily demonstrate whether SDS is diluted to a point at which it will not interfere. RNA can be stored in aqueous solution at -70°C if the sample is not going to be subjected to frequent thawing and freezing. RNA is safely stored as an ethanol precipitate at -20°C. To circumvent repeated recovery from ethanol, an aliquot of the second precipitation can be selectively precipitated.

Procedure(cont.)   Comments(cont.)

Method 2: Microadaption of the guanidinium-thiocyanate/CsCl ultracentrifugation method (Rappolee 1989 and 1990)

This protocol offers a microprocedure for isolating RNA from 1 to several thousand cells. Count the number of cells subjected to the procedure before starting.

1. Lyse cells in a minimum of 100µl 4M guanidinium thiocyanate (GuSCN) stock solution vortexing vigorously to allow for rapid homogenization.

1. Composition and preparation of 4M GuSCN stock solution is described in step 3. (Method 1). For the isolation of minute amounts of RNA it is advisable to supplement the solution with 10-20µg E.coli rRNA as carrier.

2. Layer 100µl 5.7M CsCl into the the appropriate tubes for a Beckman TL-100 tabletop ultracentrifuge or for a Beckman Airfuge.

3. Carefully overlay GuSCN cell lysate.

4. Centrifuge in the TL-100A rotor at 80,000 rpm for 2 hours or at 95,000 rpm for 1-2 hours in a Beckman Airfuge.

5. Guanidinium thiocyanate and CsCl are carefully aspirated from the transparent pellet.

6. The pellet is dissolved in 100µl DEPC-treated water.

6. Care must be taken to ensure complete resolubilization of the RNA pellet.

7. Precipitate with 10µl 2.5M ammonium acetate and a double volume of ethanol at -20°C.

8. Pellet RNA at 10.000g for 15 min at 4°C.

9. Wash pellet twice with 70% ethanol to remove residual salts.

10. The final sample is dissolved in 10-20µl DEPC-treated water and an aliquot used for OD readings at 260 and 280nm.

10. Recovery of small amounts of sample RNA with excess carrier RNA can be calculated as suggested by Rappolee:

Procedure(cont.)   *Comments(cont.)*

$$\frac{\text{recovered RNA}}{\text{input of carrier RNA} \times \text{input cell number}} = \text{recovered cell number}$$

11. RNA not exceeding 8µg total RNA in less than 9µl are directly subjected to reverse transcriptase.

Method 3: Quick RNA isolation (Ferre 1989 and J Maurer, personal communication)

1. Pellet 2×10^6 cells at 400g for 10min.

2. Wash twice in 1 x PBS.

                                                                                         2. We obtain 10 x PBS (phosphate buffered saline) from Gibco-BRL and dilute to yield a 1 x PBS solution.

3. Resuspend cell pellet in 100µl of freshly made 0.1% DEPC in double distilled water and transfer into a 1.5ml tube.

4. Boil for 5-10 min to lyse cells, degrade proteins and to remove DEPC(DEPC breaks down into CO_2 and ethanol upon boiling).

5. Centrifuge for 30 sec at 12.000g and transfer supernatant to a clean 1.5ml tube.

6. Either subject 5µl to reverse transcription immediately or continue by treating 10-20µl with 6µl of 0.1M MeHgOH in order to disrupt RNA secondary structure.

7. Incubate at room temperature for 7 min.

8. Add 3µl of 0.7M ß-mercaptoethanol and incubate 5 min at room temperature to neutralize the lysate.

9. Subject an aliquot to reverse transcription as described in section 8.3.

References

1. Berger SL. Isolation of cytoplasmic RNA: Ribonucleoside-vanadyl complexes. 1987, Methods Enzymol 152, 227-241.

2. Briscoe PR, Jorgensen TJ. Improved RNA Isolation from cells in tissue culture using a commercial nucleic acid extractor. 1991, BioTechniques 10, 594-596.

3. Chirgwin JM, Przybyla AE, MacDonald J, Rutter WJ. Isolation of biologically active ribonucleic acid from sources enriched in ribonuclease. 1979, Biochemistry 18, 5294-5299.

4. Chomczynski P, Sacchi N. Single-step method of RNA isolation by acid guanidinium thiocyanate-phenol-chloroform extraction. 1987, Anal Biochem 162, 156-159.

5. Cox RA. The use of guanidinium chloride in the isolation of nucleic acids. 1968, Methods Enzymol 12, 120-129.

6. de Martynoff G, Pays E, Vassart G. Synthesis of a full length DNA complementary to thyroglobulin 33 S messenger RNA. 1980, Biochem Biophys Res Commun 93, 645-653.

7. Ehrenberg L, Fedorcsak I, Solymosy F. Diethyl pyrocarbonate in nucleic acid research. 1974, Prog Nucleic Acid Res Mol Biol 16, 189-262.

8. Ferre F, Garduno F. Preparation of a crude cell extract suitable for amplification of RNA by the polymerase chain reaction. 1989, Nucl Acids Res 17, 2141.

9. Fuqua SAW, Fitzgerald SD, McGuire WL. A simple polymerase chain reaction method for detection and cloning of low-abundance transcripts. 1990, BioTechniques 9, 206-211.

10. Higuchi R. Simple and rapid preparation of samples for PCR. In: PCR Technology: Principles and applications for DNA amplification, Ed. Erlich HA (Stockton Press, New York, NY) 1989, 31-38.

11. Jackson DP, Quirke P, Lewis FA, Boylston AW, Sloan JM, Robertson D, Taylor GR. Detection of measles virus RNA in paraffin-embedded tissue. 1989, Lancet I, 1391.

12. Jackson DP, Lewis FA, Taylor GR, Boylston AW, Quirke P. Tissue extraction of DNA and RNA and analysis by the polymerase chain reaction. 1990, J Clin Pathol 43, 499-504.

13. Jackson DP, Haayden JD, Quirke P. Extraction of nucleic acid from fresh and archival material. in PCR: A Practical Approach. Eds.: McPherson MJ, Quirke P, Taylor GR. (Oxford University Press, Oxford, UK) 1991, 39-49.

14. Kawasaki ES. Sample preparation from blood, cells, and other fluids. In: PCR protocols: A guide to methods and applications. Eds.: Innis MA, Gelfand DH, Sninsky JJ, White TJ. (Academic Press, Inc., San Diego) 1990, 146-152.

15. Maurer J. Klinikum Steglitz, Dept. of Hematology, FU Berlin, FRG, personal communication

16. Noonan KE, Roninson IB. mRNA phenotyping by enzymatic amplification of randomly primed cDNA. 1988, Nucl Acids Res 16, 10366

17. Palmiter RD. Magnesium precipitation of ribonucleoprotein complexes. Expedient techniques for the isolation of undegraded polysomes and messenger ribonucleic acids. 1974, Biochem 13, 3606-3615.

18. Perry RP, La Torre J, Kelley DE, Greenberg JR. On the lability of poly(A) sequences during extraction of messenger RNA from polyribosomes. 1974, Biochim Biophys Acta 262, 220-226.

19. Rappolee DA, Wang A, Mark D, Werb Z. Novel method for studying mRNA phenotypes in single or small numbers of cells. 1989, J Cell Biochem 39, 1-11.

20. Rappolee DA. Optimizing the Sensitivity of RT-PCR. 1990, Amplifications A Forum for PCR Users 4, 5-7.

21. Sambrook J, Fritsch EF, Maniatis T. Molecular Cloning: A laboratory manual (Cold Spring Harbor Lab, Cold Spring Harbor, NY) 1989.

22. Wallace DM. Large and small-scale phenol extractions. 1987, Methods Enzymol 152, 33-41.

9. Reverse Transcription/PCR (RT-PCR)

Several methods have been developed for studying specific RNA molecules. These include in situ hybridization, Northern blots, dot or slot-blots, and nuclease protection assays. Of these, in situ hybridization is the most sensitive method and allows for the detection of 10-100 molecules in a single cell, while the other techniques demand at least 0.1-1.0 pg of the specific mRNA which is equal to 10^5-10^6 molecules to obtain a result (Kawasaki 1990). Except for in situ hybridization which is a rather difficult technique, the lack of sensitvity is a drawback in investigating low abundant or rare transcripts. The adaptation of PCR methodology to investigate mRNA provided a method featuring all the assets of PCR technology - speed, efficiency, specificity and sensitivity. Because RNA can not serve as a template for PCR, the successful combination of reverse transcription and PCR (Seeburg 1986) made mRNA converted into a complementary DNA (cDNA) amenable to PCR. The combined use of both techniques is colloquially referred to as RT-PCR.

The first applications of RT-PCR demonstrated a number of additional advantages other than the distinctly increased sensitivity of the method. The application of RT-PCR in investigating the BCR-ABL translocations found in 95% of CML cases finally circumvented often inefficient or sometimes even impossible amplification of genomic DNA between exons interrupted by large introns and also helped to overcome the problem posed by the amplification of a highly variable DNA in which translocations have been described at varying sites within different introns (Bernards 1987). Investigation on the mRNA level makes it possible to design an RT-PCR amplifying a cDNA fragment which spans the potential translocation junctions. In addition, the template region desired to be amplified finally possesses a length which still allows amplification with an acceptable efficieny (Kawasaki 1988). Other applications of RT-PCR will and already cover a broad field of objectives for clinical and research purposes. Applications have already been described for retroviral and viral diseases with regard to detecting the presence of RNA genomes as well as specific transcripts which can provide evidence for active infection (Hart 1988, Kawasaki unpublished results, Rowley 1991 and Schuller unpublished results). Another interesting application has shown that detection of transcripts of "multidrug resistance" genes during treatment of neoplasias may help to predict which patients will respond to a certain chemotherapeutic agent (Kashani-Sabet 1988, Goldstein 1989). Assessing the role or determining the expression cascade of low abundant growth and/or differentiation factors either in development (Rappolee 1988) or in mutagenicity has also greatly profitted from RT-PCR, especially, because of the increased sensitiviy and the possibility to screen a large number of assays in a short time. Analysis of mutated RAS proto-oncogene transcripts may also be of value to the clinician in evaluating the prognosis of certain cancers (Lacal 1988). These and many other applications all profit from the fact, that inefficient amplification of often long DNA fragments due to long introns can be circumvented and that additional information is immediately supplied with regard to phenomena such as alternative splicing.

9.1 Setting up an RT-PCR

The major advantage of ressorting to RT-PCR is, in many cases, the sensitivity of the method. Although it has been reported that the threshold can be as low as 10 transcripts using synthetic RNA (Rappolee, 1990), the threshold can vary considerably depending on the target RNA. Thus, it is important to novelly establish each RT-PCR assay considering the efficiency of each individual step required in the procedure. One must keep in mind that right from the start the total yield of RNA can vary between 20-70% making RNA preparation a crucial issue, especially, if the amount of biological material is limiting or the transcript of interest is only present in low abundancy. In addition, depending on the method selected for RNA isolation as well as the care taken to carry out the procedure, varying amounts of DNA can contaminate the RNA sample and thereby preclude a successful assay. This is discussed further on. The efficiency of reverse transcription can also vary between 10-90% (Rappolee 1990). This makes it clear that an internal standard will in many cases be necessary in order to judge the import of this step on the final result. Finally, after the mRNA has been reverse transcribed to a cDNA, the PCR assay must be designed to ensure selective amplification of the target transcript.

Reverse transcription
The necessity to reverse transcribe mRNA into a cDNA prior to subjecting the RNA template to PCR is given by the fact that the polymerase used in PCR is a DNA-dependent polymerase. Reverse transcription of mRNA requires chosing a reverse transcriptase, a means of priming the mRNA to initiate polymerisation and supplying optimal conditions for the enzymatic reaction.

Reverse transcriptases are RNA-dependent DNA polymerases which have predominantly been used to catalyze first strand synthesis (synthesis of a complementary DNA - cDNA), but also are capable of synthesizing a DNA strand complementary to a primed single stranded DNA. Two different reverse transcriptases have been commercially available over a longer period of time - the avian myeloblastosis virus (AMV) and the Moloney murine leukemia virus (MoMLV) reverse transcriptase. The avian enzyme possesses several enzymatic activities: the two stated above, namely, RNA- and DNA-dependent DNA strand synthesis, as well as an endonucleolytic activity to cleave the mRNA:cDNA hybrid: the RNase H activity processively removes rNTPs at any "nick" leading to the degradation of template RNA. This can be detrimental, if degradation of template RNA competes with DNA synthesis in the initial phase. In this case the yield of cDNA can be reduced and the length of the cDNA fragments restricted. In addition, the observation that RNase H sometimes cleaves the RNA template near the 3'-OH terminus of the newly synthesized DNA strand offers a further possibility of premature incomplete cDNA strand synthesis (Kotewicz 1988). In contrast, the murine enzyme does not exhibit such extensive endogenous degradative activity - logically, making it the more suitable choice for synthesizing longer and even full-length cDNAs. However, the fact that the murine enzyme possesses a lower optimal temperature (37°C) for maximum activity than the avian enzyme (42°C) may place the murine enzyme at a slight disadvantage, if there is extensive secondary structure in the template mRNA. As will be described in the practical section, there are several ways of effectively disrupting secondary structure. Generally, both can be used successfully - provided that optimal conditions are maintained.

Besides differences with regard to temperature requirements, the two enzymes also require different buffer systems. These differ in pH and in the molar concentration of KCl. It is important to note that even slight deviations from the optimal conditions can influence cDNA synthesis considerably. For example, the length of the cDNA synthesized by either enzyme is considerably reduced when the pH of the reaction mixture deviates from the optimum by as little as 0.2 (Sambrook 1989). The table below summarizes the factors which should be adjusted and standardized for all experiments, especially, if results are evaluated on a comparative basis.

	AMV	MoMLV
pH	8.3	7.6
KCl	145mM	72mM
Temperature	42°C	37°C

Recently, a new heat-stable DNA polymerase derived from Thermus thermophilus designated Tth pol was found to possess a very efficient reverse transcriptase activity. It has been successfully tested and compared to the activity of Taq pol (Myers 1991). The introduction of an enzyme featuring both polymerase and reverse transcriptase activity simplifies RT-PCR. In some aspects Tth pol seems to be superior to Taq pol. Tth pol is more efficient than Taq pol. The sensitivity of a coupled reverse transcription/PCR amplification using Tth pol was a 100-fold greater than that of Taq pol under similar reaction conditions. Differential evaluation of each enzymatic reaction for each enzmye suggests that increased sensitivity results from increased RT activity of Tth pol. In addition, some of the problems encountered using AMV or MoMLV can be alleviated using Tth pol. The higher optimal temperature of Tth pol activity can have an overall positive effect on reverse transcription, since secondary structure in the RNA template is disrupted. This, again, is beneficial in increasing the specificity of the primer extension reaction. Possibly the only drawback in exploiting reverse transcriptase activity of Tth pol is that increased efficiency requires Mn^{2+} as the divalent metal ion. It has been well documented for E. coli pol I that Mn^{2+} has a negative effect on the fidelity of DNA synthesis (Beckman 1985). The misincorporation rate is approximately 1 nucleotide every 500 nucleotides.

There are three approaches to priming reverse transcription: 1. oligo(dT)$_{12-18}$ binds to the endogenous poly(A)$^+$ tail at the 3' end of mammalian mRNA 2. random hexanucleotides (NNNNNN) can bind to mRNA templates at any complementary site and 3. specific oligonucleotide sequences can be used to selectively prime the mRNA of interest. Oligo(dT)$_{12-18}$ nucleotides are most frequently used to initiate first strand synthesis, if full-length cDNA synthesis is necessitated. Synthesis of non-full-length cDNAs can be achieved by either employing a specific primer or random hexamer nucleotides. The location of the specific primer - whether further upstream or downstream - will determine which region of the template RNA will be transcribed into a cDNA, either the more 5' or 3' end of the target mRNA. Since random hexanucleotides can bind to any complementary single strand nucleic acid, the synthesis of an array of cDNAs varying in size is achieved. The approach employed for priming reverse transcription will largely depend on the objectives of the assay: 1. subsequent amplification of full-length cDNAs by the PCR will probably be most successful, if oligo(dT)$_{12-18}$ is used to prime reverse transcription. 2. for diagnostic purposes, reverse transcription using a selective, specific primer has been employed successfully. If, however, the mRNA of interest is limiting, then reverse transcription using oligo(dT)$_{12-18}$ nucleotides may yield better results, since these can prime reverse transcription at several sites in the dATP-rich 3' tract, so that multiple cDNAs can be synthesized from one template. 3. As reported by Noonan et al. (1988), the use of random hexanucleotides rather than oligo(dT)$_{12-18}$ may be more superior in overcoming the difficulties encounterd by template secondary structure as well as in transcribing more 5' regions of the mRNA. It can easily be argued that the synthesis of many small cDNAs during transcription will suffice for PCR, since - at least for many diagnostic purposes - amplification of small specific regions will yield enough evidence to prove, for example, the presence of transcripts of an active agent. Random hexanucleotides can, however, bind to multiple sites on a template and thus impede extension of cDNA fragments, since any additional hexanucleotide bound to the mRNA further downstream will arrest polymerization activity. Upon denaturation for PCR the different fragments will dissociate. This may lead to the physical separation of the individual primers of a primer pair and thus preclude

PCR altogether. We believe that in many cases setting up reverse transcription or trouble-shooting should include such considerations.

9.2 Selective RT-PCR

Basically, any DNA contamination will impede assays relying on RNA quantification and second may even obscure the presence of low abundant or rare transcripts. This is determined by the fact that primer sequences chosen from two successive exons will never be able to differentiate between a cDNA and a genomic DNA template in the annealing step, if both are present in the sample. Although the cDNA template should be amplified more efficiently because of its smaller size, low abundant transcripts are always at a disadvantage when competing even against small amounts of contaminating DNA. Thus, any DNA contamination of the RNA sample will always lead to undesirable competition during PCR.

Since up- and downstream primers are usually selected from two exons spanning an intron for RT-PCR, DNA contamination of the RNA preparation can normally be judged, because the PCR products will differ in size. However, such discrimination is, not possible, if transcripts of intronless genes are being investigated. In this case, it will always be necessary to treat the RNA preparation with an RNase-free DNase prior to performing RT-PCR. This approach was chosen by Grillo and Margolis (1990) to selectively amplify transcripts of the olfactory marker protein gene - an intromless gene. Evaluation of the results requires the following PCR control assay: after DNase treatment of the RNA sample, directly subject an aliquot of the treated sample to PCR amplification (without reverse transcription) using a primer pair which permits size discrimination between PCR products originating from a cDNA and a genomic DNA template. Thus, this primer pair must be designed from a locus containing introns and span an intron. This PCR control assay permits validation of complete removal of DNA from the treated sample.

Not only intronless genes but also processed pseudogenes pose the same problem. PCR performed on a concomitant cDNA or on an aliquot of the RNA sample which was not reverse transcribed but contaminated with DNA will yield products identical in size, making it impossible to discriminate between contaminating DNA and the transcript. Unawareness of the potential of pseudogenes to mock transcripts can lead to the interpretation of false positive results. It is surprising to note, that amplification of cytoplasmic ß-actin transcripts, a locus with several known pseudogenes, has regularly been used to judge the success of RNA preparations with regard to degradation of RNA and efficacy of reverse transcription. Not only we, but also Menon et al. have observed the same hazards of relying on the amplification of the ß-actin locus to evaluate RT-PCR results. Knowledge of the misleading interpretations which can ensue if a pseudogene exists, clearly points out that successful RNA preparation as well as reverse transcription can only be judged and monitored via PCR using a primer pair from a single copy gene possessing introns and which is regularly transcribed in substantial amounts. In our laboratory, the introduction of a primer pair derived from the ß-subunit of the pyruvate dehydrogenase gene has been the solution to this problem (Rolfs et al. unpublished results). The primer pair designated "PDH1" is composed of the (+) primer (4297 -4316) 5'GGTATGGATGA GGA CCTGGA3' and the (-) primer (4481 - 4462) 5'CTTCCACAGCCCTCGACTAA3'. It is routinely used in our laboratory to monitor DNA contamination in RNA samples.

RNase-free DNase I treatment is outlined below and must be performed if transcripts of an intronless gene are being investigated.

Procedure	Comments

Method 1: RNase-free DNase treatment of RNA samples

Many commercial preparations of pancreatic DNase I are not completely free, and sometimes, even contain significant amounts of RNase. Thus, RNase must be removed from a DNase preparation prior to treatment of an RNA sample.

1. Dissolve 10mg of pancreatic DNase I in 10ml of 0.1M iodoacetic acid, 0.15M sodium acetate (pH 5.2).

2. Incubate the mixture at 55°C for 45min. Cool to 0°C, and add 1m $CaCl_2$ to a final concentration of 5mM.

3. Aliquot the treated DNase I in appropriate portions for use and store at -20°C.

4. Treat 1µg total cytoplasmic RNA with 6 units of RNase-free DNase I by incubating at 37°C for 10-60 min.

4. The RNase-free DNase from the Boehringer Co. is recommended. Nevertheless, this RNase-free DNase, too, should be tested with a control RNA beforehand to ensure that no RNase contamination remains. The integrity of the DNase-treated controlRNA should then be demonstrated in an agarose/formaldehyde gel followed by ethidium bromide staining.

Preparation of agarose/formaldehyde gels: aqueous 37% formaldehyde (12.3M) and 5x running buffer are added to the desired amount of melted agarose (50-60°C), so that a final concentration of 1 x buffer and 2.2M formaldehyde is created.

Running buffer (1x):
- 0.04M morpholinopropanosulfonic acid (MOPS), pH 7.0
- 0.01M sodium acetate
- 0.001M EDTA

Procedure(cont.)	*Comments(cont.)*

Before loading RNA samples into the gel, incubate each sample for 6min at 55°C in 2µl 5 x running buffer, 10µl deionized formamide, 3.0µl concentrated formaldehyde and 2µl loading buffer (30% FICOLL, 0.25% bromphenol blue, 0.25% xylene cyanol, 1.5mM EDTA).

5. 1µg RNA in 2µl aqua bidest. is used for DNase pretreatment.

6. Add 6U (3µl) RNase-free DNase + 28U (1µl) RNasin + 2µl 8mM $MgCl_2$ (final concentration 2mM) in a total volume of 8µl.

6. RNasin ribonuclease inhibitor (Promega #2511, 2,500U).

Preparation of an 8mM $MgCl_2$ solution: 162.4mg $MgCl_2$ x 6 H_2O to a final volume of 100ml. Autoclave to sterilize.

7. Incubate at 37°C for 1 hour.

8. Inactivate the mixture by incubating at 90°C for 5min.

9. Then put on ice immediately.

10. The cDNA synthesis can then be performed immediately, e.g., in 1 x PCR buffer or RT buffer (see page 108).

Aside from DNase treatment of an RNA sample, other approaches can be chosen to help avoid, eliminate or circumvent DNA contamination as long as no intronless gene or processed pseudogene exists for the locus to be investigated on the RNA level. Two of the suggestions address the method chosen to prepare RNA and four exquisitely demonstrate that primer design can readily help cope with DNA contamination and allow for selective amplification of the transcript:

Preparing RNA

* RNA preparation methods using a CsCl gradient yield pure RNA samples.

* If the single step GuSCN/phenol-chloroform-isoamylalcohol extraction method described by Chomczynski (1987) is used, it is crucial that acid phenol and sodium acetate, pH 4.0, are used (see chapter on the isolation of RNA). Moreover, it must be stressed that DNA contamination is promoted, if the ratio of acid phenol:chloroform (v/v) is less than 10:3. Strictly maintaining a ratio of 5:1 yields satisfactory results. This was assessed by Kedzierski (1991) in a very comprehensive study dealing with non-enzymatic DNA removal from RNA preparations

Primer design

* The standard approach has always been to choose primers that span very large introns so that the amplification of the cDNA rather than the concomitant genomic DNA sequence will be favored (Figure 9.1).

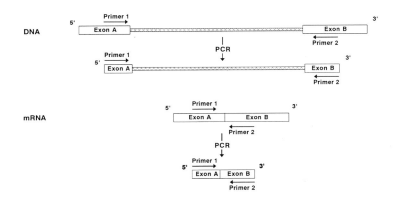

Figure 9.1: RT-PCR using a conventionally designed primer pair. PCR products are obtained on the DNA and mRNA level.

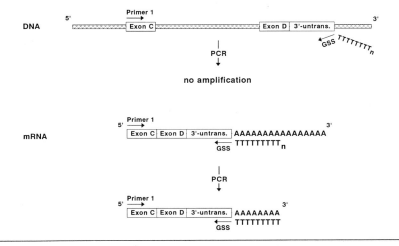

Figure 9.2: RT-PCR using the primer design proposed by Moore et al. (1990). Amplification is only possible on the mRNA level under the selected reaction conditions.

* Moore et al. (1990) have proposed an alternative approach which allows the selective detection of mRNA transcripts, even in the presence of excess DNA. A primer pair is designed in such a fashion that one of the primers binds only to the transcript, but not to the concomitant genomic DNA (fig.2). The unique composite downstream primer is designed to anneal to the 3' end of the transcript and consists of a poly(T)-tract at its 5' end (15 bases), and adjacent, a specific sequence of the 3' untranslated region of the target transcript (18-23 bases) at its 3' end. Preferential annealing of the unique composite primer only to the transcript is achieved by setting the annealing temperature slightly higher than the Tm calculated for the specific sequence of the primer, which can otherwise also bind to the DNA. The additional dTTP residues add 20°-30°C to the stability of primer annealing to the RNA transcript. This is more than enough to insure that only poly(A)$^+$-RNA is bound. The upstream primer is a specific target sequence close to the 3' end of the coding region, so that the size of the fragment to be amplified will not predominantly influence the efficiency of amplification (<500bp). This approach can be generally applied to selectively amplify mRNA under the stated conditions and has been used to amplify transcripts of the multidrug resistance gene (Moore 1990). A PCR assay using only genomic DNA as template and the primer pair designed to selectively amplify the transcript must be performed as a control to ensure that no amplification is possible on the DNA level.

* An approach which we found to work well in promoting selective transcript amplification makes use of a primer designed to span the splicing site between two exons (junction primer) and a second primer which can either be designed as described or conventionally. Which one will be the downstream or the upstream primer pair is optional, so that there are enough possibilities open in order to design a well balanced primer pair. As shown in figure 3, approximately 75% of the junction primer sequence was designed to be complementary to the 3' end of one exon - this is the 5' end of the primer - and approximately 25% was complementary to the 5' end of the following exon - this end of the primer is the 3' end. We assumed that, if the junction primer were to anneal to the concomitant genomic DNA of the transcript, then - at the given annealing temperature - the 5' end of the primer exhibiting the largest stretch of complementarity to the template would bind to the genomic template leaving the 3' end of the primer mismatched, because of the intervening intron sequence. It is definitely clear that any mismatches between the 3' end of a primer and the template can impede primer extension, and thus also amplification. In addition, the likelihood of only 5 to 7 bases at the 3' end of the junction primer annealing to any concomitant contaminating DNA template at the given annealing temperature is very low. In contrast, the junction primer can anneal to a transcript template completely over the whole sequence range, since the intron has been spliced and thus leaving no mismatched ends. The results shown in figure 4 demonstrate that, as expected, the junction primer designed for the pyruvate dehydrogenase locus (PDH2) selectively amplified the transcript despite contaminating DNA. DNA contamination in the RNA samples was demonstrated by the amplification products obtained, if a conventionally designed primer pair (PDH1) was

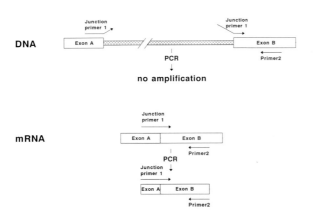

Figure 9.3: RT-PCR using a junction primer (primer1) selectively leads to the amplification of the transcript only. The junction primer together with its counterpart could not amplify the corresponding gene region on the DNA level.

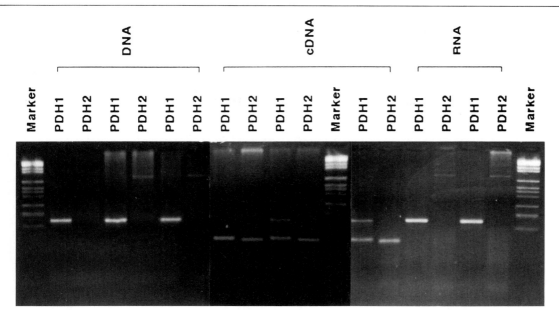

Figure 9.4: Panel "DNA": PCR was performed on three different genomic DNA samples using a conventionally designed primer pair (PDH1) and a junction primer pair (PDH2): (+) primer (4297 -4316) 5'GGTATGGATGAGGACCTGGA3' and the (-) primer spanning exons 3/4 5'CAGCCCTCGACTAACCTTGT3'. PDH1 yielded a product of the expected size (185 bp), while no amplification was possible using the junction primer pair (PDH2). Panel "cDNA": Amplification of the transcript was possible with both the PDH1 (105 bp) and the PDH2 (96 bp) primer pairs. However, PDH1 also amplified contaminating genomic DNA (185 bp). Panel "RNA": Two of the RNA samples were contaminated with genomic DNA (PDH1: 185 bp). No amplification was possible using the junction primer pair, since the RNA had not been reverse transcribed.

used in RT-PCR. In this case two products were obtained: an amplicon with the expected size on the DNA level and an amplicon with the expected size on the RNA level. Direct amplification of RNA or genomic DNA regions using PDH1 or PDH2 demonstrated that the junction primer together with its counterpart was not able to amplify the target region. This variation in primer design works generally and has also been applied to selectively amplify a defined region of the immediate early antigen transcript of human cytomegalovirus (HCMV, results not shown). In summary, the following controls ensure selective mRNA amplification: a) PCR using a DNA sample and the junction primer pair in order to prove that DNA amplification does not occur b) PCR using an RNA sample without RT and the junction primer in one assay as well as a conventionally designed primer pair (each primer sequence chosen from an individual exon) in a second assay in order to detect DNA contamination and c) RT-PCR using the two primer pairs described in b.

* A further modification of the traditional RT-PCR method, designated RNA template-specific PCR, was introduced by Shuldiner et al. (1991). Again, modified primer design promoted selective transcript amplification. A primer consisting of a gene-specific sequence (17 bases) at its 3' end was tagged with a defined sequence (30 bases) at its 5' end. This primer was used for reverse transcription. Since only novelly synthesized first strands are tagged with the defined sequence, subsequent amplification via PCR using a primer derived from the tagged sequence and a second gene-specific primer will selectively amplify reverse transcribed products only.

These examples demonstrate that simple changes in primer design can greatly influence the result of RT-PCR. It can hardly be overemphasized that great care must be taken to strictly rule out DNA contamination e.g. genomic, cDNA or DNA carry-over) or to ensure oneself that the assay established will be able to uncover as well as counteract DNA contamination. Compared to traditional RT-PCR, all three modified RT-PCR primers have greatly reduced the frequency of false positive results. Moreover, the sensitivity of the RT-PCR assay can only be maintained, if the amplification of low abundant transcripts do not have to compete with contaminating DNA.

Procedure	Comments

Method 2: Reverse Transcription using MoMLV-RT

All precautions designed to avoid RNA degradation or contamination must be strictly followed. All steps are carried out on ice unless otherwise specified. The final reaction volume is generally 20µl and for large-scale reverse transcription 50µl. The protocol described below has successfully been used to detect CMV transcripts for diagnostic purposes and the results are reproducible.

1. Dilute 1-2µg total RNA in 12µl DEPC-treated water and incubate at 65°C for 3 to 5 min on a thermal heating block. (Alternatively, 4µl 5 x RT-buffer, 1µl 10mM dNTP, 1µl Oligo(dT)$_{15}$ (40-100 pmoles) and 1-2µg total RNA adjusted to a final volume of 18µl can just as well be incubated together).

1. Regions of the RNA template that are rich in secondary structure may cause the reverse transcriptase to stop. An initial incubation at 65°C or allowing the reaction to take place in the presence of a high (e.g. 5mM) concentration of dNTPs help circumvent this problem. Treatment of the RNA with methylmercuric hydroxide should be avoided, since the substance is highly toxic. Nevertheless, initial denaturation of secondary structure remains more important if Mo-MLV reverse transcriptase (RT) is used, since the optimum temperature of this enzyme is 37°C.

2. Spin down briefly and quench on ice.

3. Add 4µl 5 x RT-buffer, 1µl 10mM dNTP and 1µl oligo(dT)$_{15}$ (40-100 pmoles), mix, spin down briefly and quench on ice.

3. 5 x RT-buffer is supplied by BRL along with the enzyme and contains: 250mM Tris-HCl (pH 8.3)
  375mM KCl
  15mM MgCl$_2$

Procedure(cont.)	*Comments(cont.)*
	* Small aliquots of 10mM dNTPs (10mM of each dNTP) should be prepared, stored preferably at -70°C and not subjected to freezing and thawing. dNTPs must be used in the millimolar range, since the K_m of reverse transcriptase is very high (Sambrook 1989).
	* If random hexanucleotides are used, add 100 pmoles to a 20µl reaction.
	* If the downstream primer is used to prime reverse transcription, then 10-50 pmoles have been tested to work well with variable amounts of RNA (Kawasaki 1989). However, limiting the amount of primer increases the specificity of the reaction, since the chance of excess primer binding to an undesirable location on the template, and then impeding extension, is decreased (Coleclough 1987). Coleclough (1987) and Frohman (1990) suggest using 10ng of gene-specific primer or 50ng of an oligo(dT)-adapter primer in a 20µl reaction. Also see section on the RACE technique.
	* For large scale reverse transcription, Sambrook et al. (1989) suggest using 2 nmoles of oligo(dT)$_{12-18}$ for 10µg of poly(A)$^+$ RNA. In our hands 40 pmoles oligo(dT)$_{15}$ (Boehringer, Mannheim) work well for 1-2µg total RNA. Fourty pmoles oligo(dT)$_{15}$ are equivalent to 0.2µg.

4. Make a master mix containing 0.1M dithiothreitol, RNasin and MoMLV-RT for all samples.	4. For each reaction include
	    0.5µl 0.1M dithiothreitol (DTT)
	    0.5µl RNAsin (40 units/µl)
	    1µl MoMLV-RT (200 units/µl)

	* RNasin is a RNase inhibitor and requires sulfhydryl reagents, e.g. dithiothreitol, for activity and denatures irreversibly, if this reagent is omitted. The minimal final concentration should be 0.5 units/µl reaction volume. Repeated freezing and thawing of the enzyme leads to denaturization.
	* 200 units MoMLV-RT (BRL) are recommended for first strand synthesis using 1µg total RNA. This is the approximate amount which can be isolated from 100,000 cells. The amount of reverse transcriptase needed for varying amounts of template RNA can be tested in a pilot assay. The combination yielding the best results should then be established.

Procedure(cont.)   *Comments(cont.)*

5. Add 2µl to each tube and incubate at 37°C for 45-60 min.

6. Heat inactivate the enzyme by incubating at 95°C for 5 min.
This also disrupts the mRNA:cDNA hybrid.

7. Spin down briefly, chill quickly and either store at -20 to -30°C or proceed to PCR.

8. For PCR either add 80µl 1 x PCR buffer containing 10-50 pmoles of each primer and 2-4 units Taq DNA polymerase

or

subject 1-2µl of the reverse transcriptase mixture to PCR in a final reaction volume of 50µl. Add 48µl 1 x PCR buffer containing 10 - 25 pmoles of each primer, dNTPs to yield a final concentration of 0.2mM each and 2 units Taq DNA polymerase.

9. After initial denaturation at 95°C for 3-5 min, use an optimized temperature profile for the thermal cycler and cycle 30 to 40 times.

10. RT-PCR products can be visualized on an ethidium bromide stained agarose gel and then subjected to further analysis.

8. No dNTPs have to be added, if the complete reverse transcriptase mixture will be used, since these are correctly diluted to yield a 0.2mM end concentration of each dNTP. dNTP loss due to first strand synthesis can be neglected.

* Primers for RT-PCR can be designed according to the suggestions given in the introduction to this chapter. As always, care should be taken to choose well balanced primers.

9. Suggested temperature profile
denature: 95°C   30 sec
anneal: 55-72°C   30-60 sec
        (set 5°C below the primer T_m)
extend: 72°C   30-60 sec

10. This procedure is extensively reported in the section dealing with analytical agarose gels.

REFERENCES

1. Beckman RA, Mildvan AS, Loeb LA. On the fidelity of DNA replication: manganese mutagenesis in vitro. 1985, Biochemistry 24, 5810-5817.

2. Bernards A, Rubin CM, Westbrook CA, Paskind M, Baltimore D. The first intron in the human c-abl gene is at least 200 kilobases long and is a target for translocations in chronic myelogenous leukemia. 1987, Mol Cell Biol 7, 3231-3236.

3. Chomczynski P, Sacchi N. Singel-step method of RNA isolationby acid guanidinium thiocyanate-phenol-chloroform extraction. 1987, Anal Biochem 162, 156-159.

4. Coleclough C. Use of primer-restriction end adapters in

cDNA cloning. 1987, Methods Enzymol 154, 64-83.

5. Frohman MA. Rapid amplification of cDNA ends (RACE): User-friendly cDNA cloning. 1990, Amplifications A Forum for PCR Users 5, 11-15.

6. Goldstein LJ, Galski H, Fojo A, Willingham M, Lai SL, Gazdar A, Pirker R, Green A, Crist W, Brodeur GM, Lieber M, Cossmann J, Gottesman MM, Pastan I. Expression of multidrug resistance gene in human cancers. 1989, J Natl Cancer Inst 81, 116-124.

7. Grillo M, Margolis FL. Use of reverse transcriptase polymerase chain reaction to monitor expression of intronless genes. 1990, BioTechniques 9, 262-268.

8. Hart C, Spira T, Moore J, Sninsky J, Schochetman G, et al. Direct detection of HIV RNA expression in seropositive subjects. 1988, Lancet II, 596-599.

9. Kashani-Sabet M, Rossi JJ, Lu W, Ma JX, Chen J, Myachi H, Scanlon KJ. Detection of drug resistance in human tumors by in vitro enzymatic amplification. 1988, Cancer Res 48, 5775-5778.

10. Kawasaki ES, Clark SS, Coyne MY, Smith SD, Champlin R et al. Diagnosis of chronic myeloid and acute lymphocytic leukemias by detection of leukemia-specific mRNA sequences amplified invitro. 1988, Proc Natl Acad Sci USA 85, 5698-5702.

11. Kawasaki ES, Wang AM. Detection of gene expression. In: PCR Technology: Principles and applications for DNA amplification. Ed.: Erlich HA. (Stockton Press, New York, NY) 1989, pp 89-97.

12. Kawasaki ES. Amplification of RNA sequences via complementary DNA (cDNA). 1989, Amplifications A Forum for PCR Users 2, 4-6.

13. Kedzierski W, Porter JC. A novel non-enzymatic procedure for removing DNA template from RNA transcription mixtures. 1991, BioTechniques 10, 210-214.

14. Kotewicz ML. Isolation of cloned Moloney murine leukemia virus reverse transcriptase lacking ribonuclease H activity. 1988, Nucl Acids Res 16, 265-277.

15. Lacal JC, Tronick SR. In: The Oncogene Handbook. Eds.: Reddy EP, Skalka AM, Curran T. (Elsevier Science Publishers B.V., Amsterdam) 1988, pp 257-304.

16. Menon RS, Chang Y, St. Clair J, Ham RG. RT-PCR artifacts from processed pseudogenes. 1991, PCR Methods and Applications 1, 70-71.

17. Moore RE, Shepherd JW, Hoskins J. Design of primers that detect only mRNA in the presence of DNA. 1990, Nucl Acids Res 18, 1921.

18. Myers TW, Gelfand DH. Reverse transcription and DNA amplification by a Thermus thermophilus DNA polymerase. 1991, Biochemistry 30, 7661-7666.

19. Myers TW, Gelfand DH. Thermostable reverse transcriptase/DNA polymerase. 1991, Amplifications A Forum for PCR Users 7, 5-6.

20. Noonan KE, Roninson IB. mRNA phenotyping by amplification of randomly primed cDNA. 1988, Nucl Acids Res 16, 10366.

21. Rappolee DA, Brenner CA, Schultz R, Mark D, Werb Z. Dvelopmental expression of PDGF, TGF-alpha and TGF-ß genes in preimplantation mouse embryos. 1988, Science 241, 1823-1825.

22. Rappolee DA. Optimizing the sensitivity of RT-PCR. 1990, Amplifications A Forum for PCR Users 4, 5-7.

23. Rowley AH, Wolsinsky SM, Sambol SP, Barkholt L et al. Rapid detection of cytomegalovirus DNA and RNA in blood of renal transplant patients by in vitro enzymatic amplification. 1991, Transplantation 51, 1028-1033.

24. Sambrook J, Fritsch EF, Maniatis T. Molecular cloning: A laboratory manual. Cold Spring Harbor Lab, Cold Spring Harbor, NY, 2nd edition, 1989.

25. Seeburg P. UCLA Symposium 1986, unpublished communication.

26. Shuldiner AR, Tanner K, Moore CA, Roth J. RNA template-specific PCR: An improved method that dramatically reduces false positives in RT-PCR. 1991, BioTechniques 11, 760-763.

10. Methods for Identification of Amplified PCR Products

10.1. Agarose gel electrophoresis

The PCR-generated fragment sizes may be estimated by gel electrophoresis, but this is usually not sufficient for checking and proving the specificity of a PCR. In cases where identity of a fragment is checked through restriction enzyme digest, however, a gel analysis may be the final step in an assay.

After gel analysis, it should be possible to see whether a PCR did work, and whether the overall experiment can be interpreted. Photographic or video documentation systems are often more sensitive than our eyes. The gel should be routinely blot-transferred for later hybridization analysis. This is usually more sensitive than ethidium bromide fluorescence and verifies the identity of the DNA fragments (or smears). The sensitivity of an agarose-gel-based detection depends, among other things, on the resolution of the DNA fragment bands and on the transparency of the gel. The maximum concentration of agarose that allows DNA migration differs between the several agarose types and makes. The procedure described below is optimized for NuSieve™ 3:1 agarose (FMC) or some self-made 6:1 mixtures with NuSieve GTG™ and normal-type agaroses (Sigma 6013 type I; Standard Low-mr, BioRad; Ultrapure™ agarose, BRL 5510). In a high-resolution gel we can detect distinct fragments containing as few as 2-4ng DNA using Polaroid photograph at long exposure times. Only freshly prepared agarose gels should be used. Fragment band resolution is sometimes reduced significantly when precast agarose gels are used after 12-24 hrs.

We routinely cast 3mm-thin agarose gels ($300\mu l/cm^2$), which allows loading of up to $11\mu l$ total sample in 5.5x1mm slots. Electrophoretic separation of DNA fragments is usually done at 3-8V/cm.

10.1.1. Electrophoresis equipment

Agarose gels may be cast into some electrophoresis apparatuses directly or into a tray that fits into the apparatus. Several models withstand gel temperatures of approx. 80°C, which allows casting of highly concentrated and TBE-buffered agarose gels. For preparative or radioactive work, UV-transparent electrophoresis equipment is available, but for maximum sensitivity the gel has to be placed directly on an ultraviolet (UV) transilluminator.

Optimum resolution of PCR-generated fragments depends on the configuration of the slot-forming comb. A good resolution is achieved with 5.5x1mm slots which are 1.5 mm apart from each other. Smaller slots result in significantly reduced resolution in our experience. For many routine applications, we use a 6.5x10 cm gel with up to three slot rows (8 slots/row), which allows 1:1 Polaroid documentation of the whole gel. We achieved satisfactory results with house-made, BIOzym/FMC, Bio-Rad, and GIBCO BRL apparatuses.

Electrophoresis buffers (stock solutions)

10 x TBE for analytical gels:
 0.9M Tris-borate, 0.01M EDTA
 108g Tris base, 55g boric acid, 20ml 0.5M EDTA, pH 8.0 (Sambrook 1989), store at RT, discard when precipitate forms.

50 x TA (Tris-acetate) buffer for preparative gels:
2M Tris-acetate
242g/l Tris base, 57.1ml/l glacial acetic acid, pH 8.0.
This buffer contains no EDTA which might interfere with enzyme activity if agarose pieces are used directly for PCR amplification. Store TA at 4°C.

10.1.2. Gel loading buffer (GLB)

Through its dye and sedimentation characteristics, the gel loading buffer (GLB) helps to load a DNA sample into the gel slots submersed under the gel running buffer in "submarine" gels. It may be helpful to use much more GLB than usual, to prevent sample eruption from the slot immediately after loading. This effect is caused by the presence of detergents or differences in salt concentration and pH between the DNA sample and the running buffer. The GLB should contain no salt (and is not a real "buffer"), because differences in salt concentration would lead to variable electrophoretic potentials, resulting in misinterpretations regarding fragment length and ethidium-bromide fluorescence intensity.

Normally, we use the specified 10xGLB in volumes 1/5 to 1/11 of the volume of the post-PCR sample. If necessary, the GLB may exceed 50% of the sample volume without interfering with pipetting or electrophoresis.

10 x GLB:
50% Glycerol in H2O
0.1% Bromphenol blue
(0.1% Xylene cyanol FF)
Store at 4°C.

Bromphenol blue migrates slightly slower in 3% agarose gels than 20mer primers, and xylene cyanol covers the 300-600bp fragment-size region with a diffuse blue color. Therefore, depending on the DNA fragment size of interest and on agarose concentration, xylene cyanol may be omitted for optimal gel transparency.

10.1.3. UV illumination and photography of stained gels

Caution: UV light is hazardous to the cornea of your eyes and causes skin burns. In addition, any UV exposure of skin affects skin lymphocytes and is mutagenic. UV irradiation creates ozone, which requires ventilation. Protection of the whole face and body surface is required. Double-stranded DNA (dsDNA) with intercalated ethidium-bromide gives a maximum fluorescence at 302nm UV transillumination, which is suitable for routine use. Sometimes, excitation with 254nm may yield higher sensitivity, but causes photo-nicking and bleaching of the visible fragments (Sealey and Southern, 1982). For preparative work, a 366nm transillumination is preferable if fragments are sufficiently visible. Preparative gels may be placed on a layer of saran wrap on the transilluminator for handling and to avoid contamination. For routine documentation, a black and white Polaroid photograph is usually sufficient. A 1:1 scale allows easy comparison to hybridization results. Otherwise, a fluorescent ruler or similar gauge should be placed beneath the gel for photography. Best sensitivity and dynamic range is achieved with negative films or slides (e.g., Fujichrome 100).

10.1.4. Molecular weight markers and semiquantitative gel analysis

Several DNA molecular weight markers are commercially available that are suitable for approximate quantitation and size analysis of PCR products. The DNA concentration of a delivered marker should be checked photometrically if the marker is used as standard for calculation of the DNA content of a visible fragment. Markers suitable for that purpose are those for which the DNA content of each fragment is known or may be calculated as a fraction of total DNA of the used marker. Sometimes, a positive control sample (fragment or plasmid) has to be quantified and diluted for optimization experiments. At least two different amounts of marker and of a DNA fragment should be analyzed in a gel to estimate the DNA concentration of the positive control sample.

Table 10.1.: Examples for molecular weight markers. In the table the following specified fragment parameters are denoted: Number of base pairs, concentration of specific fragments on a µl of whole marker basis (ng/µl), % of total marker. E.g., "587 (34ng) 13.5%" means that the marker contains a 587bp fragment and this fragment represents 34ng/µl marker which is 13.5% of the total marker.

Fragment-number	Boehringer V (# 821705) (250ng/µl) pBR322 Hae III	Boehringer VI (# 1062590) (250ng/µl) pBR322 Bgl I + pBR322 Hinf I	Clontech (# 6310-2) (1µg/µl) phi-X174 Hae III
1.	587 (34ng) *13.5%*	2176 (55ng) *22%*	1353 (250ng) *25%*
2.	540 (31ng) *12.4%*	1766 (45ng) *18%*	1078 (200ng) *20%*
3.	504 (29ng) *11.5%*	1230 (31ng) *12.5%*	872 (162ng) *16%*
4.	458, 434 (51ng) *20.5%*	1033 (26ng) *10.5%*	603 (112ng) *11%*
5.	267 (15ng) *6%*	653 (16ng) *6.5%*	310 (58ng) *6%*
6.	234 (13ng) *5%*	517 (13ng) *5%*	281, 271 (102ng) *10%*
7.	213 (12ng) *5%*	453 (11ng) *4.5%*	234 (50ng) *5%*
8.	192, 184 (21ng) *9%*	394 (10ng) *4%*	194 (36ng) *3.5%*
9.	124, 123 (14ng) *6%*	298, 298 (15ng) *6%*	118 (22ng) *2%*
10.	104 (6ng) *2.5%*	234, 234, 220 (17ng) *7%*	72 (13ng) *1,5%*
11.	89, 80 (10ng) *4%*	154, 154 (8ng) *3%*	
12.	64, 57, 51 *4%*		
13.	21, 18, 11 8 *1%*		
total	**4363bp**	**9814bp**	**5386bp**

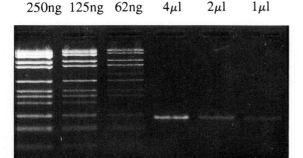

Figure 10.1: Semiquantitative gel analysis of a 282bp CMV late gene DNA fragment. Three different amounts (4μl, 2μl, 1μl) of a typical amplification product (for details, see fig. 1.13, legend) are loaded on the gel. Marker: Boehringer VI, 11 bands are visible. Estimated 282bp PCR-product concentration: 5ng/μl (see table 1). Note: Due to the dilution with dH_2O some fragments are partially denatured thus influencing migration and staining (see figure 10.3).

Procedure	Comments

Method 1: Agarose gel casting

	Caution: Wear gloves for all of the following steps. Usually, the equipment will be contaminated with ethidium bromide, which is a powerful mutagen.
1. Seal gel tray with autoclave tape and place it on a horizontal surface. The slot-forming combs should be positioned now.	1. Place the tray in a cold lab if available. This yields high transparency, and the agarose will be gelled after a few minutes. The equipment has to be free of dust and lint that might lead to interfering fluorescence under UV light.
2. Mix agarose at the desired concentration (w/v) with 1 x electrophoresis buffer in an Erlenmeyer flask, a bottle or a 50ml tube (Falcon). (Pour the agarose into the dry container first.) The gel suspension should not occupy more than 50% of the container.	2. Agarose has to be suspended completely, prior to heating. This might necessitate vigorous shaking. The buffer for gel casting and electrophoresis has to be from the same batch. Recommended gel volume: 300μl/cm² (3mm thickness).

Procedure(cont.)   *Comments(cont.)*

3. Boil in a microwave oven or in a boiling water bath. Shake from time to time, but take care: superheated gel may boil over spontaneously! Replace evaporation loss with dH_2O.

3. As long as the gel is not completely dissolved, it will boil over easily. The cap of the tube has to be loose.

4. When the gel is completely dissolved, add 1µl ethidium-bromide per 20ml gel and mix thoroughly.

4. The solution should be capped, so that no "skin" forms at the cooling surface. Ethidium bromide stock: 10mg/ml; final: 0.5µg/ml.

5. Cast the gel as hot as necessary (depending on concentration and buffer), without pause, into prepared apparatus or tray. Tilt once, so that gel flows behind the comb. Remove air bubbles with a pipet tip.

5. The gel will set with slots deeper than the overall gel thickness because of the meniscus formed at the comb surface.

6. At RT, the gel will be ready for use after 10-30 min and, when prepared in a cold lab, after approx. 5min. Submerge the gel in electrophoresis buffer before removing the combs.

Method 2: Post-PCR sample loading

Do not cross-contaminate samples during this procedure. With a nonradioactive hybridization protocol, approx. 0.1-1pg DNA can be detected, which may easily be transferred by microdroplets.

1. Preload 1µl GLB in reaction tubes or into the wells of a 96-well micro titer plate.

1. An Eppendorf combitip™ can be used.

2. Pipet 9µl sample without oil, remove oil from tip surface with a lint-free paper towel and mix the sample well with the GLB.

2. This may be done by blowing an air bubble into the water phase. The sample has to be mixed again immediately before loading into the gel.

3. Load sample slowly into slot.

3. The gel has to be submerged in electrophoresis buffer before sample loading. The slots may be filled completely. Overload may cause contamination of neighboring slot.

4. Start electrophoresis immediately.

10.2. DNA blot transfer and nonradioactive hybridization/detection

After agarose gel electrophoresis, a capillary transfer of the DNA from the agarose gel onto a nylon or nitrocellulose membrane can be performed for hybridization analysis of the PCR products. In well established, routine assays, a direct blot of the PCR products (dot blot or slot blot) may be advantageous. This procedure requires no electrophoresis, and the whole reaction product may be blotted, which might yield higher sensitivity. In addition, this method allows loading of a large number of samples with several different dilutions if desired. The drawback is that PCR by-products cannot be recognized.

In this chapter, we refer to the nonradioactive digoxigenin-11-dUTP hybridization and detection system on nylon membranes. The digoxigenin hapten can be detected with an antibody/alkaline-phosphatase conjugate. This system can be handled easily and is a robust method for assessment of post-PCR samples. The detection of DNA labelled with biotin works similarly, and digoxigenin and biotin may be detected simultaneously on one membrane.

The PCR synthesis of digoxigenin-11-dUTP-labeled probes is described in chapter 2.2 (preparative PCR). We routinely use digoxigenin-11-dUTP labeled double-stranded DNA probes. These probes hybridize to the sense and antisense target strands. For (single-stranded) oligonucleotide hybridization probes large differences in signal intensity have been observed between sense and antisense oligonucleotide probes (Skogerboe 1990). These differences may reflect asymmetric strand synthesis conditions during PCR.

After hybridization with the digoxigenin-11-dUTP-labeled probes and incubation with the antibody/alkaline-phosphatase conjugate, as few as 0.1-1pg target DNA can be detected after several hours with the dye substrates BCIP and NBT. The chemiluminescent detection of digoxigenin with the substrate AMPPD™ seems to be even more sensitive and much more rapid (Höltke 1992).

10.2.1. Capillary transfer (Southern blot)

A complete transfer of PCR-generated DNA fragments is possible without HCl treatment of the gel for depurination. Blotting without transfer buffer yields more sharpness of bands, but is usually incomplete. Many nylon blot membranes bind DNA quantitatively at medium high salt concentrations.

The following procedure was established with the nylon membranes DuralonUV™ (Stratagene) or positively charged (Boehringer) and will probably fit many other nylon membranes.

Procedure	Comments

Method 3: Southern blot from agarose gel

1. After photography, place the gel into denaturing buffer for 10 min.	1. Denaturing buffer: 1.5M NaCl (88g/l), 0.5M NaOH (20g/l)

Procedure(cont.)	*Comments(cont.)*
2. Neutralize gel for 10 min.	2. Neutralization buffer: 2M NaCl (117g/l), 1M TrisHCl (121g/l), pH 5.0
During these two incubation steps:	
3. Cut nylon membrane with a pair of scissors. The membrane should be 2mm longer and wider than the gel. Cut 3 sheets of Whatman 3MM paper with the same size as the membrane.	3. Do not touch the membrane, wear gloves, wash off the powder.
4. Place the membrane on neutralization buffer until it is completely wet, then dip it into buffer.	
5. Prepare blot apparatus, prewet Whatman 3MM paper support with transfer buffer, remove bubbles. See fig. 10.2.	5. Use neutralization buffer as transfer buffer. Several gels may be transferred simultaneously.
6. Place the gel upside down onto the wet paper support. Remove air bubbles by carefully rolling a plastic pipet over the gel. Cover the paper support surrounding the Parafilm™ or a reusable plastic frame.	6. Trim edges on gel surface with a scalpel to prevent air bubbles between the gel and the support. This prevents direct contact of paper towels with transfer buffer.
7. Overlay the gel with the wet membrane and 2-3 layers of wet Whatman 3MM paper. Remove air bubbles after each layer separately, as described in 6.	7. Prewet Whatman 3MM paper with neutralization buffer.
8. Overlay with paper towels, glass plate and 500-1000g weight. See figure 10.2. Transfer time: 2-12 hrs.	8. Use excess of paper towels so that transfer buffer does not reach glass plate.
9. After transfer, the membrane should be labeled while still lying on the gel. Label the slot positions at the edges of the membrane.	9. Make sure that the pen withstands all hybridization and detection steps. (Usually, blue pens.)
10. UV-crosslink DNA immediately after transfer while membrane is still moist.	10. Energy: 120 mJ Stratalinker (Stratagene). Alternative: Place the membrane with the DNA-side down on the UV transilluminator, 302nm, for approx. 40 sec. Note: UV-crosslinking has to be optimized for each membrane type.
11. Store dry and dustfree.	

10.2.2. Dot blot and slot blot procedures

In order to control of the blotting process, hybridization specificity and background, a blotting-buffer sample without DNA and a non-specific DNA sample, e.g. denatured salmon sperm DNA, have to be included. The array of the samples for blotting depends on the design of the hybridization assay. Usually, several hybridization probes may be mixed to detect different fragments blotted onto one membrane. Specific positive control samples are essential in diagnostics, because many patient samples are negative.

The volumes of the wells over the dots or slots depend on the type of the apparatus. Generally, it will be enough to prepare a sample volume containing the whole post-PCR sample and the blotting reagents.

Membranes have to be prepared as described above for capillary transfer of by the manufacturere´s recommendations. The filtration process (aspirator or vacuum) has to be started before sample loading and continues until each sample is blotted completely. The suction should be weak enough that it takes several minutes for the filtration to be completed. If there are some wells that are not drawn down completely, the other wells may be covered with Parafilm™ until the blot is done. Then, usually after some minutes, the blot is done. Immediately after blotting, the DNA has to be cross-linked on the blot membrane, as described for capillary transfer membranes.

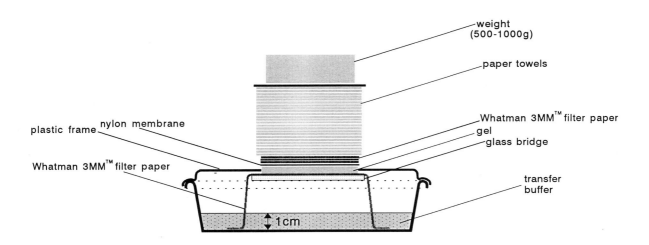

Figure 10.2.: Southern blot (for details see Method 3, chapter 10).

Procedure	Comments

Method 4: Dot blot protocol

1. Prepare membrane and blot apparatus, check function of apparatus.

2. Dilute 1 part post-PCR sample with 9 parts sample buffer.

3. Heat the diluted sample for 5-10min at 95°C. Then place on ice immediately.
4. Immediately mix the sample with an equal volume 1M NaOH and incubate at RT for 5-10min.

5. Start suction as weak as possible.

6. Load samples without any time lag. Continue suction until all the samples are blotted completely. If necessary, cover some wells with Parafilm™.

7. Lift upper part of apparatus without moving sideward.

2. Sample buffer: 1mM EDTA, 20mM TrisHCl, pH7.6.

3.&4. The DNA has to be denatured completely for maximum blotting efficiency and hybridization sensitivity.

5. Usually, a small trickle of tap water is sufficient for an aspirator.

6. Use a new pipet tip for each sample. Do not forget to blot the negative samples from PCR and a buffer-only sample.

7. Any mechanical forces applied to the membrane may lead to background hybridization.

10.2.3. Hybridization with digoxigenin-11-dUTP-labeled DNA probes

The described procedure is a modification of the protocols from the "DIG DNA Labeling and Detection Kit nonradioactive" (Boehringer Mannheim, # 1093 657) and the "DIG Luminescent Detection Kit" (Boehringer Mannheim, # 1363 514). At 62°C hybridization temperature, we were able to mix up to four different hybridization probes in a rotating hybridization tube, without any cross-hybridization or nonspecific hybridization. This is useful for many diagnostic assays, where simultaneous hybridization of different samples and targets on one membrane is desired.

Usually, a total amount of just 20ng PCR-generated hybridization probe in a 3-5ml hybridization buffer volume will be enough for high detection sensitivity, even if the blotted or dotted total amount of target DNA exceeds the probe amount significantly. If several membranes are simultaneously hybridized in one tube, more probe should be used.

Hybridization probes:

In our experience, any digoxigenin-11-dUTP-labeled PCR product synthesized according to the protocols in chapter 2 is suitable as a probe. Furthermore, we use a probe that hybridizes to the molecular weight marker DNA as a control for the hybridization and blotting system. This also allows fragment size analysis on the southern blot membrane. The probe (positive control DNA, tube #4 from the Boehringer kit) hybridizes to the molecular weight markers V and VI (Boehringer ## 821 705, 1062 590) or any pBR322 DNA-containing sample.

Stock solutions:

20 x SSC: 3M NaCl, 0.3M Na-citrate, pH 7 (20°C)
SDS: 10% (w/v)
N-Lauryl sarcosine: 10% (w/v)

Hybridization solution:

5 x SSC; 0.1% (w/v) N-lauryl sarcosine, Na-salt (Sigma); 0.02% (w/v) SDS; 2% (w/v) blocking reagent(Boehringer # 1096 176).
The blocking reagent consists of the casein fraction of nonfat, dry milk (e.g. Sigma).

Wash solution 1: 2x SSC; 0.1% (w/v) SDS

Wash solution 2: 0.1 x SSC; 0.1% (w/v) SDS

Procedure	Comments

Method 5: Membrane hybridization procedure

Procedure	Comments
1. Place the cross-linked membrane(s) into a dry hybridization tube. The DNA side of the membrane should face inside.	1. 50ml tubes (Falcon) are suitable. Do not screw the cap too tightly, and stick a syringe needle in the center of the cap. This will help to prevent the cap from bursting. All the following steps are performed in a rotating tube holder which is placed in a hybridization oven that maintains the desired temperature.
2. Prehybridize membrane(s) in 5ml hybridization solution at 62-68°C.	2. This will wash out the high salt content of the membrane from the blot procedure.

Procedure(cont.)   *Comments(cont.)*

3. Mix 10-100ng by the probe(s) with 1ml hybridization solution and heat to 95°C for 5-10min in a heat block.

3. The probes will denature.

4. Replace the hybridization solution in the hybridization tube with 2-4ml new hybridization solution prewarmed at 62-68°C. Quickly add the heat-denatured probe (1 ml), mix well, close the tube and place it immediately into the hybridization oven.

5. Hybridize for 4-16hrs.

5. The optimum hybridization temperature will be between 60 and 68°C.

6. Discard hybridization mixture and wash twice with 45ml wash solution 1 for 5min at RT.

7. Wash twice for 15min with wash solution 2 at hybridization temperature.

7. The membrane may be air-dried and stored for later detection after this step, if necessary.

10.3. Detection systems of digoxigenin labeled hybrids

Several systems exist for the visualisation of immunologically detected hybrids. The alkaline phosphatase conjugated to the anti-digoxigenin (DIG) antibody may either catalyze the turnover of the chromogen substrates NBT and BCIP or of the chemiluminescent dioxetane substrates AMPPD™ or CSPD™. The chromogen detection system seems to have fewer background problems compared to chemi-luminescence, and it fits many different membrane types. It doesn't need a darkroom, and the dye on the membrane is a permanent, membrane-bound documentation of the experiment. The protocol described in procedure 6 contains the reagent concentrations and buffers that allow NBT/BCIP or AMPPD™ detection on positively charged nylon membranes, as recommended from Boehringer Mannheim. The chemiluminescence-based detection has the potential for being more sensitive and rapid than the chromogene system. The emitted light (477nm for AMPPD™ and CSPD™ substrates) can be detected with photographic film or electronic light-detection instruments. Apparently, the combination of alkaline phosphatase, dioxetane substrate and chemiluminescent signal enhancer provides the most sensitive luminescence system, compared to other enzymes and substrates (Schaap 1989, Bronstein 1992). The sensitivity and signal-to-noise ratio of luminescence detection depends significantly on the type of membrane, blocking reagent and buffer systems. The luminescence is active for hours, which allows exposure of several films with different exposure times. After detection, the probe can easily be stripped down and the membrane can be reprobed several times, which is a major advance compared to the chromogen system.

The market for luminescence-related chemicals and instruments is rapidly growing, and it is not possible to review all the new and promising techniques in this chapter. Several companies may be contacted for further information, as, for example: Tropix; Serva; Lumigen; Amersham; Boehringer; Promega; Stratagene; BioRad.

In Method 7, an example for AMPPD™ detection is described.

Stock solutions:

Buffer 1: 0.1M maleic acid; 0.15M NaCl; pH 7.5 (20°C), adjusted with solid or concentrated NaOH.

Blocking-reagent stock solution: 10% (w/v)
The blocking reagent (Boehringer # 1096 176) consists of the casein fraction of nonfat dry milk. The reagent dissolves slowly. Use magnetic stirring rods and warm up the solution to 40-70°C. Do not boil.

Antibody conjugate: anti-digoxigenin alkaline phosphatase, (Boehringer # 1093 274)

Color solutions:
NBT 75mg/ml in 70% dimethyl formamide (v/v).
BCIP 50mg/ml in dimethyl formamide.
AMPPD™: 10mg/ml (Boehringer # 1357 328).

Working solutions:

Washing buffer: buffer 1 + Tween™ 20, 0.3% (w/v).
Buffer 2: blocking stock solution diluted 1:10 in buffer 1 (final concentration = 1% blocking reagent).
Buffer 3: 0.1M Tris-HCl; 0.1M NaCl; 50mM $MgCl_2$; pH 9.5 (20°C).
Buffer 4: 10mM Tris-HCl; 1mM EDTA; pH 8 (20°C)

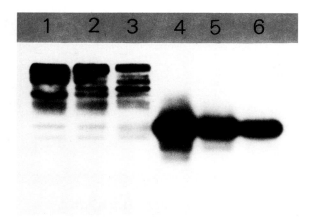

Figure 10.3: Southern blot from the gel in fig. 10.1. Membrane: Boehringer, positively charged. Hybridization with a product-internal 139bp probe (see fig 1.13, legend, for details). Chemiluminescence detection of the digoxigenin label with the substrate AMPPD™ according to method 7 of this chapter. Exposure time: 20min.

Procedure	Comments

Method 6: Chromogen detection system (NBT/BCIP)

Procedure	Comments
1. Wash membrane with washing buffer for 1-5min.	1. All steps at RT.
2. Incubate membrane in buffer 2 for 30min.	2. approx. 100ml/100cm² membrane to provide

| *Procedure(cont.)* | *Comments(cont.)* |

efficient block.

3. Incubate membrane in diluted antibody-conjugate solution for 30min.

3. Antibody-conjugate dilution: 75 mU/ml. In a plastic bag, ≤20ml will be enough.

4. Wash twice for 15min with 100 ml washing buffer.

5. Equilibrate membrane for 2-5min in buffer 3.

6. Prepare color solution by adding 45µl NBT and 35µl BCIP to 10ml buffer 3.

6. This corresponds to 3,375µg NBT and 1,750µg BCIP.

7. Incubate membrane in color solution in the dark for 30min to >12hrs. Make sure that the DNA side of the membrane is the upper side. Do not shake.

7. If placed in a plastic bag, 2-5ml solution is enough. Incubation time depends on sensitivity and background intensity.

8. Stop color reaction with buffer 4 for 5min and let the membrane air-dry.

Method 7: Chemiluminescence detection (AMPPD™)

Steps 1 to 6 as described in Procedure 6.

7. Place X-ray film cassette in 37°C oven.

7. Cut out a plastic frame with a "window" that is covered with one layer of thin saran wrap. This frame is placed in the cassette.

8. Dilute AMPPD™ 1:100 in buffer 3 and preincubate membrane in this dilution for 5min.

8. The dilution may be reused several times when stored at 4°C in the dark.

9. Place the moist membrane under the saran-wrap window in the film cassette and incubate at 37°C for 5-15min.

10. Film exposure for 5min up to 2hrs.

10. Exposure time depends on signal and background intensity. Luminescence will be present for at least 24hrs.

11. Probe stripping for rehybridization: Do not dry the membrane, wash with dH_2O; denature twice for 15min with 200mM NaOH, 0.1% SDS, 37°C; neutralize with 2 x SSC.

10.4. Polyacrylamide gel electrophoresis (PAGE)

The rapidity, flexibility and high resolution of DNA fragments over a wide range of sizes have made polyacrylamide gel electrophoresis (PAGE) an important tool in the separation and visualization of proteins and nucleic acids. Gel porosity can be varied over a wide range to meet specific separation requirements. The gel and the buffer parameters can be altered to separate the fragments on the basis of charge, size or a combination of both.
The polymerization process itself has a decisive influence on the quality of gel separation.

PAGE is based on the co-polymerization of acrylamide and bis-acrylamide (N-N'-methylene-bis-acrylamide). This vinyl addition polymerization reaction is initiated by a free-radical generating system (Sealey 1982). Polymerization is initiated by addition of TEMED (tetramethylethylenediamine) and APS (ammonium persulfate), the latter containing a persulfate-free radical which activates TEMED. TEMED serves as an electron carrier and activates the acrylamide monomer by transfer of an unpaired electron. Subsequent reaction of the activated monomer with non-activated monomers initiates the polymerization process. The elongated polymer chains are then crosslinked by bis-acrylamide in a nonselective fashion. This process finally determines the characteristic porosity of a gel.

Besides the physicochemical properties of the polymerization process, the purity of the substances, especially the acrylamide, is another important factor determining the quality of the gel. For example, acrylic acid - the deamidation product of acrylamide -, which is copolymerized with acrylamide and bis-acrylamide, may produce local pH changes, which in turn induce artifact formation, changes in the mobility of the fragments in the gel, leading to smiling effects in these areas. This can give irreproducible results and ruin experiments. Ionic contaminations can both delay and accelerate the polymerization process. In particular copper has a dramatic effect on the course of polymerization. Excessive amounts of APS and TEMED will also induce shifts in pH. Reduction of these initiators will produce longer polymer chains, decrease turbidity and increase elasticity. However, this slowing down of the polymerization reaction increases the physical solubility of oxygen in the mixture, which in turn results in gels which are too porous and mechanically weak. It is generally recommended to use equimolar amounts of APS and TEMED in concentrations of 1-10 mM. Under these conditions, the process will be completed after 90 min with visible gelling occurring after about 15 min.

In addition to the substances used, factors such as reaction temperature and oxygen concentration also have a major impact on the quality of the gel produced. Polymerization is an exothermic reaction. The initially released heat will accelerate the reaction. Gels polymerized at 4°C will be inelastic, whereas polymerization at 25°C will give transparent, less porous and more elastic gels. Thus, a polymerization temperature of 20-25°C would be ideal. Since the substances used are stored at 4°C, they have to be brought to room temperature prior to preparation of the gel.

Oxygen in the air or dissolved in the gel solution inhibits the polymerization process. It is therefore important to degas the solution in order to ensure reproducibility of the results. Degassing must be performed after heating to RT, since a 4°C solution has a higher capacity for dissolved oxygen. Prolonged degassing accelerates gel polymerization. Sufficient evacuation can thus reduce the amounts of the initiators APS and TEMED required.

The concentration of PAGE gel - like that of agarose gel - determines the fragment sizes that can be separated:

Concentration of acrylamide (%)	range of separation (bp)
3.5%	100 to 1,000
5.0%	80 to 500
8.0%	60 to 400
12.0%	40 to 200
20.0%	6 to 100

10.4.1. Separation of radioactive-labeled amplification products by denaturing PAGE and autoradiography

Despite the high amplification efficiency of the PCR, it is sometimes advisable to detect the amplified fragments by PAGE rather than on agarose gels: The greater expenditure of the former procedure compared to the latter is justified by the greater resolution of the gels and the possibility of discriminating even single base changes (e.g. in minisatellite PCR, see chapter 3). It is also possible to excise single ^{32}P- or ^{35}S-radiolabeled bands (e.g. for semiquantification of the amplified product) followed by determination of the number of radioactive decays in a scintillation counter. PAGE is required to determine whether the length of an individual amplified fragment is indicative of deletion or insertion in the area of the amplified sequence. It is also necessary to perform PAGE when only very low amounts are available for a PCR product which is to undergo cutting by restriction enzyme for specificity control.

Since the specificity of separation is determined not only by the size and charge of the PCR products but also by the presence of secondary structures, it is necessary to eliminate the differences caused by conformation. This can be achieved by electrophoresis on denaturing gels, which are produced by the

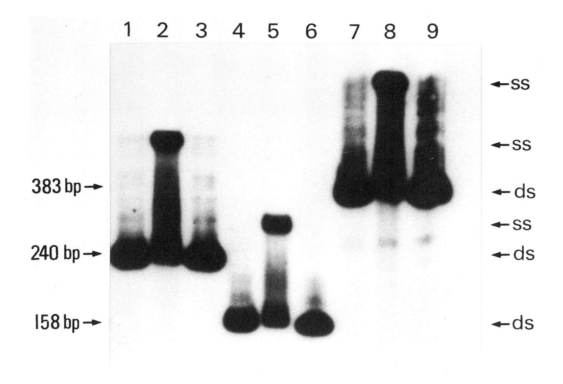

Figure 10.4: Autoradiography (2hrs) of ^{32}P-labeled PCR fragments in a 6% PAGE. Comparison of three different amplification products of M. tuberculosis (lanes **1-3** 240bp, lanes **4-6** 158bp, lanes **7-9** 383 bp) obtained under different denaturation conditions prior to loading onto a denaturing 7M urea polyacrylamide gel. All samples had a volume of 6 µl. Samples **1, 4 and 7** were admixed with 4µl of 95% formamide, samples **2, 5 and 8** additionally heated to 95°C for 5 min; samples **3, 6 and 9** stained with bromophenol blue/xylene cyanol without admixture of formamide. This image demonstrates that single-stranded DNA is formed only after admixture of formamide and heating, but not after addition of formamide alone. Note that, in this system, single-stranded DNA runs slower than double-stranded DNA. For details on the primers see chapter 12.

incorporation of denaturating agents such as sodium hydroxide, urea, formamide, methyl mercuric hydroxide, formaldehyde and sodium dodecyl sulphate (SDS). 7M urea, 98% formamide or 0.1% SDS is recommended for PAGE.

Most polyacrylamide gels can be run in a vertical gel electrophoresis apparatus; simple "homemade" devices have been described (for details see Dillon, 1985). The simplest design of a vertical apparatus consists of a square tank with an upper and a lower buffer reservoir, with the tank additionally providing the support for the front and back gel plates. The two plates are separated by spacers of any desired thickness (0.2mm - 2.0cm). Sample wells are cast in the gel, which is formed between front and back plate using a slot former. The plates are fixed on the apparatus by metal clips. One electrode is placed in the upper buffer reservoir forming the cathodic resevoir, the other in the lower buffer reservoir forming the anodic reservoir. Both reservoirs are filled with buffer and electrophoresis proceeds downward through the vertical gel.

Procedure	Comments

Method 8: Vertical denaturing polyacrylamide gel

Procedure	Comments
1. Wash the plates in distilled water, rinsed with 100% ethanol and dried. Position the spacers (typically 1.0 - 1.5 mm) between the gel plates and fix the plates with metal clips.	1. The bottom and the edges of the gel casting plates should be plugged with 2% agarose.
2. Prepare of 100 ml of 5% polyacrylamide gel solution using the quantities given in the table:	2. Use 40% acrylamide stock solution (can be stored in the dark at 4°C for several months): 380g acrylamide (DNA-sequencing grade) + 20g N-N'-methylene bis-acrylamide, distilled water to 600ml. Dissolve the chemical substances by heating to 37°C. Adjust the volume to 1.000 ml by adding distilled water. Pass the solution through a nitrocellulose filter (e.g. Nalge, 0.45 micron pore size). Store the stolution in dark bottles, since light and alkali will catalyze a deamination process gradually degrading acrylamide and bis-acrylamide to form acrylic and bis-acrylic acid. Accordingly, the solution should have a pH of approximately 7.0. **Caution:** Acrylamide is a potent neurotoxin with a cumulative toxic effect and is absorbed via the skin. It is therefore necessary to wear gloves and a mask

	Concentration of gel			
Stock solution	5%	8%	12%	18%
7 M urea (g)	42	42	42	42
40% acrylamide solution (ml)	12.5	20	30	45
twice distilled water (ml)	35.5	27	17	2
10 x TBE (ml)	10	10	10	10

| *Procedure(cont.)* | *Comments(cont.)* |

Mix all substances well. After complete dissolution, add purified water to a final volume of 98 ml.

when handling the substance.
Stock solutions:
- 10% ammonium persulfate (freshly prepared): 1.0g to 10ml H2O
- 10x TBE: 108g Tris base, 55g boric acid, 50ml 0.5M EDTA (pH 8.0), pH should be about 8.3, deionized H2O to 1 liter. Working concentrations of 1x TBE: 89mM Tris-borate, 2mM EDTA

3. Thoroughly degas the solution for about 1-2 min.

3. Sufficient evacuation is achieved when there are no longer any bubbles escaping from the solution.

4. Add 45µl TEMED and 1ml 10% APS solution. Carefully mix the solution.

5. Immediately pour the solution into the glass plates prepared as indicated under (1). Keep the glass plates in a slightly tilted position and start pouring of the liquid above one corner. Quickly insert the well forming comb. Top up with the 5% acrylamide gel.

6. Allow the gels to polymerize in a slightly tilted position at room temperature (for about 90 min).

7. When polymerization is completed, the bottom spacer between the two glass plates is removed. Fix the two plates at the upper buffer reservoir with large paper clamps.

8. Seal the space between the upper buffer reservoir and the glass plates with 1-2% agarose.

9. Add sufficient amounts of 1xTBE to both gel chambers. Make sure that the bottom of the gel is well immersed in the buffer and that the top is well covered.

10. When the chambers are filled, carefully remove the comb. Gel threads and urea crystals are removed by rinsing each slot with 1xTBE buffer.

11. Prior to loading the samples, it is important to check the functioning of the chamber. Switch on the power supply and make sure that bubbles are rising up at the platinum wire. Load 6µl of a radioactive labelled PCR sample + 4µl formamide loading buffer.

11. Formamide-dye mixture: 98% formamide, 0.025% bromophenol blue, 0.025% xylene cyanol FF. Formamide: If formamide shows a yellow color, it has to be deionized. In this case, add Dowex XG8 mixed-bed resin, stir on a magnetic stir-plate for 1 h

Procedure(cont.)	Comments(cont.)
	and passd twice through a Whatman No. 1 filter. Deionized formamide is stored in small aliquots at -70°C. For denaturation prior to transfer into the gel, PCR samples are heated to 95°C for 5 min together with the formamide loading buffer, then put on ice and immediately transferred into the gel. Note that not even formamide and heating will always achieve complete denaturation of all samples. Thus, there are often two bands in the gel. It is also important to note that in this gel system, single-stranded DNA will usually run slower than double-stranded DNA (see Figure 10.4). The simplest way of labeling the PCR fragments is to add 1μCi ^{32}P-labeled dCTP (deoxycytidine 5'tri-phosphate, α-^{32}P, NEN 013H, 3000Ci/mmol) at the start of the PCR reaction. Thus, the PCR fragments produced will be labeled by incorporation of ^{32}P-dCTP during the amplification (for details see chapter 20)
12. Start electrophoresis with 80V for 10min, followed by 140V for about 100-180min.	12. The migration of the DNA samples can be estimated from the migration of the dyes (according to Sambrook 1989)

DNA fragments (in bases) that migrate with dyes in denaturing PAGE

PAGE-conc.	Bromophenol blue	Xylene cyanol
5%	35b	130b
6%	26b	106b
8%	19b	75b
10%	12b	55b
20%	8b	28b

13. After termination of electrophoresis, remove the power cables and the buffers from both chambers (Careful! Both buffers are radioactively contaminated) and carefully remove the two glass plates.	13. Always wear gloves to avoid radioactive contamination.
14. Place the glass plates on a smooth surface and lift the upper glass plate. Spread a Whatman 3MM filter evenly on the gel avoiding bubble formation. Removal of the gel using the filter as a carrier. Insertion into an X-ray cassette with the gel on top.	

Procedure(cont.)   *Comments(cont.)*

15. All subsequent steps are to be performed in a photographic dark room. Use the safety light (red filter). Cover the radioactive gel with one layer of transparent sheeting, making sure that no bubbles are formed. Apply Kodak X-Omat RP film. Use scissors to cut an orientation mark into the film.

16. Initial exposure of the film for 2-4 hours, depending on the expected isotope activity. If required, prolonged exposition with a new X-ray film.

17. Develop the film.

15 The X-ray cassettes protect both the film and the experimenter and also ensures that the gel is tightly pressed against the film.

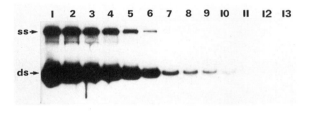

Figure 10.5.: Autoradiograph (8hrs) of ^{32}P-labeled PCR fragments in a 6% PAGE, depicting insertion of about 2,000 M. tuberculosis pathogens into approx. 0.3 ml of sputum, followed by serial dilution in 2-fold steps by addition of appropriate amounts of sputum. Subsequent purification of the DNA and amplification by PCR using the 386-bp primer is described in chapter 12. Lane **1:** approx. 2,000 pathogens (P), lane **2:** approx. 1.000 P, lane **3:** approx. 500 P, lane **4:** approx. 250 P, lane **5:** approx. 125 P, lane **6:** approx. 60 P, lane **7:** approx. 30 P, lane **8:** approx. 15 P, lane **9:** approx. 8 P, lane **10:** approx. 4 P, lane **11:** approx. 2 P, lane **12:** approx. 1 P, lane **13:** 0-1 P. The dilution steps demonstrate that the assay has a sensitivity of approx. 1 pathogen per 0.3 ml of sputum.

Radioactive detection systems can often detect 1-10 pathogens in a PCR sample (for details see chapter 12). With three published primer pairs (for details see chapter 12) and labeling of the fragments as described above, we can detect 1-5 M. tuberculosis pathogens from patient sputum. The procedure is as follows: A defined amount of M. tuberculosis (Mtb) is introduced into Mtb-negative sputum, to which more sputum is added in 2-fold serial dilution steps. The DNA isolated from the sputum samples is then used in a PCR assay. The result is given in Fig. 10.5. More recently developed immunological detection systems (AMPPD™ or CSPD™, cf. paragraph 10.3) come close to the detection limit of radioactivity (to approx. the tenth power) and can thus replace radioactive labeling in numerous experiments.

Figure 10.6 shows that, with decreasing primer concentration, the relative amount of double-stranded DNA decreases and the relative amount of single-stranded DNA increases, up to the limit where a single-stranded amplificate can no longer be detected or formed. The gel shown in figure 10.6 is conspicuous in that, on the one hand, the single-stranded DNA is retarded more than the double-stranded DNA and, on the other hand, high molecular-weight fragments are increasingly formed with increasing molar imbalance of the two primers.

Besides the detection of PCR fragments in denaturing polyacrylamide gels, it is possible to detect them using non-denaturing gel systems (without urea and without formamide). Here, the disadvantage of a possible influence on the mobilities of particular fragments by conformational differences is to be weighed against the advantage that the respective bands can be demarcated more clearly and no double bands occur as a result of single-stranded DNA and incompletely denatured double-stranded DNA (see figure 10.7). For most PCR detection systems using PAGE, non-denaturing gels meet the requirements with regard to resolution and sensitivity. However, in assays that require a separation capable of showing single-base differences (VNTR-PCR, DGGE, etc; see chapters 3 and 13), denaturing gels are indispensable. An example for a non-denaturing gel is shown in figure 10.7.

10.4.2. Detection of non-radioactive amplification products in PAGE using silver stain

The staining of DNA with ethidium-bromide is the method of choice, since this method is simple, quick, and comparatively sensitive. Other stains are also available, e.g., acridine orange, methyl green, pyronine B, toluidine blue O, etc. (Andrews 1981). In addition, DNA or RNA in PAGE may be made visible by a silver stain (Merril 1981). Silver stain is about 2-10 times more sensitive than the ethidium bromide stain (0.1ng/mm^2 [ethidium-bromide] vs. 0.03ng/mm^2 [silver stain], Allen 1989). Especially for denaturing gels, silver stain is to be recommended, since the ethidium bromide stain soon fades in these gels. Blum et al. (1987) have published a method that, based on the properties of thiosulfate (image enhancement by

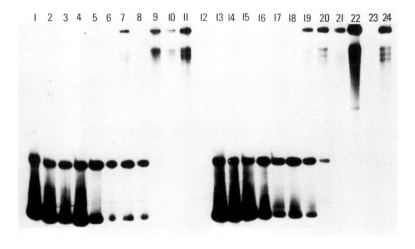

Figure 10.6.: 8% denaturing urea polyacrylamide gel. Demonstration of a 138bp fragment of the cytomegalovirus genome (Shibata 1988), where the relation of the primer concentrations to each other was altered while all other experimental conditions remained constant: 0.1µg DNA template, 200µM dNTP, 1U Taq polymerase, 50µl volume, primer 1 (5'CGT TTG GGT TGC GCA GCG GG 3'), primer 2 (5'CCG CAA CCT GGT GCC CAT GG 3'). Thermocycling: 5min 95°C for initial denaturing; 30 cycles of 20sec 95°C, 40sec 55°C, 40sec 72°C. For lanes **1-12**, primer 1 concentration constant at 100pM. Primer 2: lane **1** 100pM, lane **2** 80pM, lane **3** 40pM, lane **4** 10pM, lane **5** 8pM, lane **6** 6pM, lane **7** 4pM, lane **8** 1pM, lane **9** 0.8pM, lane **10** 0.6pM, lane **11** 0.4pM. Lane **12** negativ control. For lanes **13-24**, exactly identical experimental conditions were chosen, with the exception that, here, primer 2 remained constant at 100pM and primer 1 was diluted in the same way as primer 2 before. The experiment showed several results: 1. With increasing differences in concentration between the two primers, single-stranded DNA is preferentially formed. 2. In a denaturing PAGE, single-stranded DNA is retarded more than double-stranded DNA. 3. There are no conformational differences between the plus and minus strands of the amplificate, since both strands (single-stranded DNA) run at the same height. 4. With marked concentration differences between the two primers (e.g., lanes **9-11** and lanes **21, 22**), high-molecular fragments are formed.

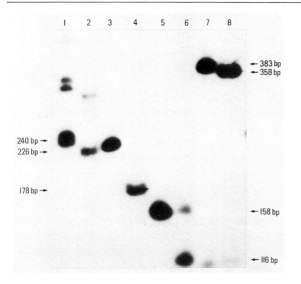

Figure 10.7: Autoradiography (2hrs) of 32P-labeled PCR fragments in a 6% non-denaturing polyacrylamide gel. Demonstrated are M. tuberculosis amplificates from blood (lanes **1 and 2**); from sputum (lanes **3 to 8**); in native condition (lanes **1, 3, 5, and 7**); and restriction-endonuclease-digested by HaeIII (lanes **2 and 4**), NlaIII (lane **6**), and HinfI (lane **8**), resp. As amplificates, a 240bp (lanes **1 and 3**), a 158bp (lane **5**), and a 383bp (lane **7**) fragment can be seen. For details of the primers used, see chapter 12. With HaeIII digestion of the 240bp amplificate, 178bp (lane **4**), 48bp, and 15bp fragments are formed with complete restriction; with incomplete digestion, a 226bp (lane **2**) and a 62bp fragment in addition. With NlaIII digestion of the 158bp fragment, a 116bp (lane **6**) and a 42bp fragment are formed. With HinfI digestion of the 383bp amplificate, a 358bp and a 25bp fragment appear. In contrast to the denaturing conditions of PAGE (see Figure 10.4), it becomes clearly visible that double-stranded DNA and the interpretation of the bands is easily possible. For most PCR applications, the results achieved with non-denaturing polyacrylamide gel are sufficient.

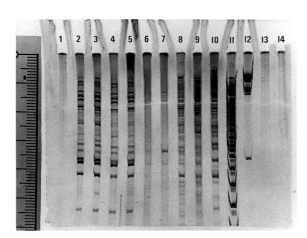

Figure 10.8.: Demonstration of amplification products of a DAF-PCR (cf. chapter 3) using the silver stain method as described under 10.4.2. As template, here, human DNA was used in different amounts in the PCR: 100ng in lanes **2 and 3**; 200ng in lanes **4 and 5**; 400ng in lanes **6 and 7**; 50pg in lanes **8 and 9**. Lane **10** negative control (contaminated with DNA). Lane **11**: 100bp marker (GibcoBRL). Lane **12**: λ-HindIII marker (Boehringer). Lane **12-13** empty lane. For amplification procedure Ampli wax™ has been used as well as the hot-start PCR method. Note that amplification efficiency decreases with increasing amount of templat. The negativ control gives a positive signal what may be due to DNA contaminated Taq polymerase with bacterial DNA. DAF seems to be extremily sensitive for the detection of DNA contamination of PCR-reagents. As primer, we used an 8mer oligonucleotide: 5´CCG TGT CG3´). 1mm polyacrylamide gel. 4µl of amplification products per lane.

pretreatment of fixed gels and formation of soluble silver complexes), makes possible improved staining of nucleic acids and detection in the sub-nanogram range, without the unspecific background increasing in intensity. Bassam et al. (1991) have described a further improvement: preexposure to formaldehyde during silver impregnation increases sensitivity, and the addition of sodium thiosulfate to the image developer reduces background staining. This improvement in background staining and sensitivity makes the silver stain the method of choice for various PCR systems that, due to the necessity of demonstrating single-base differences, require the separation of products using PAGE.

Procedure	Comments

Method 9: Silver stain of denaturing PAGE (according to modifications recommended by F Willborn/Berlin)

Separation of the PCR fragments in the denaturing PAGE is carried out as described in paragraph 10.4.1.

Procedure	Comments
1. Fix the gel overnight in 350ml of a 50% ethanol, 12% acetic acid solution.	1. Production of 350ml of 50% ethanol, 12% acetic acid solution: 175ml 100% ethanol (may be denatured), 42ml acetic acid (100%), 95µl formaldehyde (37%), 133ml purified water. The final concentrations are: 50% ethanol, 12% acetic acid, 0.01% formaldehyde. The formaldehyde serves as a stabilizer and may sometimes be omitted without quality loss. It is imperative that, for all procedures, gloves are worn and that the talcum is first removed from the gloves. The gels should always be touched at the corners only and should be totally submerged in the solutions.
2. Incubate for 90min in 250ml sodium thiosulfate/ glutaraldehyde solution.	2. 250ml of thiosulfate/glutaraldehyde solution: 75ml 100% ethanol, 5ml glutaraldehyde (25%), 0.5g sodium thiosulfate ($Na_2S_2O_3$), 17g sodium acetate, purified water to 250ml. Final concentrations: 30% ethanol, 0.5% glutaraldehyde, 0.2% sodium thiosulfate, 0.5M sodium acetate.
3. Wash twice for about 15min in 300ml purified water on a shaker.	3. If several gels are stained at the same time, care must be taken during washing to prevent them from lying on each other.
4. Impregnation with silver stain for 30min in 250ml silver solution.	4. 250ml of silver solution: 0.25g $AgNO_3$, 47µl formaldehyde (37%), purified water to 250ml. Final concentrations: 0.1% $AgNO_3$, 0.007% formaldehyde.
5. Wash the gel twice again for 2 x 1min in 300ml purified water.	
6. Develop of the stain with 350ml developer for 8-10min at 10°C.	6. 350ml of developing solution: 21g Na_2CO_3, 151µl formaldehyde (37%). Adjust pH value with a spatula tip of sodium bicarbonate. Fill up to 350ml final volume. Final concentrations: 6% Na_2CO_3, 0.016%

Procedure(cont.)   *Comments(cont.)*

formaldehyde.

7. Wash the gel twice again for about 10min in 300ml purified water.

8. Stop the reaction in 500ml 0.5M EDTA.

8. 500ml of 0.5M EDTA: 9.3g EDTA (TitriplexIII, Merck) to 500ml purified water.

9. Dry the gel on a vacuum gel dryer: 6 layers of prewatered Whatmann 3MM filter sheets are put on the grid plate of the vacuum dryer. On these filters, the gel is then dried under constant vacuum between cellophane sheets at 80°C for about 1-2h. The image of the dried stain is stable. The detection threshold of this staining method is about 1pg DNA/mm^2 band cross section.

Using this staining procedure, we have demonstrated (cf. figure 10.8) results of various experiments for the methodic evaluation of DNA amplification fingerprinting (cf. chapter 3).

References

1. Allen RC, Graves G, Budowle B. Polymerase chain reaction amplification products separated on rehydratable polyacrylamide gels and stained with silver. 1989, BioTechniques 7, 736-744

2. Andrews AT. Electrophoresis: theory, techniques and biochemical and clinical applications. 1981, Clarendon, Oxford.

3. Bassam BJ, Caetano-Anolles G, Gresshoff PM. Fast and sensitive silver staining of DNA in polyacrylamide gels. 1991, Anal Biochem 196, 80-83

4. Blum H, Beier H, Gross HJ. Improved silver staining of plant proteins, RNA and DNA in polyacrylamide gels. 1987, Electrophoresis 8, 93-99

5. Bronstein I, Fortin J, Voyta JC. Nitro-Block™ enhancement of AMPPD^R chemiluminescent signal in the detection of DNA. 1992, BioTechniques 12, 500-502.

6. Dillon JR, Bezanson GS, Yeung KH. Basic techniques. In: Recombinant DNA methodology. Eds.: JR Dillon, A Nasim, ER Nestmann. 1985, John Wiley & sons, New York, pp 13-27

7. Höltke HJ, Sagner G, Kessler C, Schmitz G. Sensitive chemiluminescent detection of digoxigenin-labeled nucleic acids: A fast and simple protocol and its applications. 1992, BioTechniques 12, 104-113.

8. Merril CR, Switzer RC, van Keuren ML. Trace polypeptides in cellular extracts and human body flu-

ids detected by two-dimensional electrophoresis and a highly sensitive silver stain. 1979, Proc Natl Acad Sci USA 76, 4335-4339

10. Sambrook J, Fritsch EF, Maniatias T. Molecular cloning. A laboratory manual. 2nd edition, CSH, 1989.

11. Schaap AP, Akhavan H, Romano LJ. Chemiluminescent substrates for alkaline phosphatase: Application to ultrasensitive enzyme-linked immunoassays and DNA probes. 1989, Clin Chem 35, 1863-1864.

12. Sealey PG, Southern EM. Electrophoresis of DNA. In: Gel electrophoresis of nucleic acids - a practical approach. Eds.: D Rickwood, BD Hames. 1982, IRL Press, Oxford, Washington, pp39-76

13. Skogerboe KJ, West SF, Murillo MD, Tait JF. PCR dot blots: large signal differences between sense and anti-sense probes. 1990, BioTechniques 9, 154-157.

11. Restriction Fragment Analysis

In molecular biology, restriction endonucleases have been exploited as a means of characterizing DNA fragments (DNA mapping) and of modifying DNA for genetic engineering (e.g. cloning). One of the most common applications of restriction endonucleases together with the PCR is validation of the specificity of the generated amplification product. Since most DNA regions amplified by PCR have been sequenced or are well characterized, the specificity of a PCR amplification product can be determined by analysing restriction fragments generated upon digest with a restriction endonuclease known to cleave the DNA fragment of interest into fragments of defined length. Knowledge of restriction endonucleases and their requirements is also very useful when the goal of the experiment necessitates cloning of the PCR product. In this case the primers used for the PCR will usually contain a restriction endonuclease recognition site sequence synthetically introduced into the 5' region of each primer. The PCR product possessing the modified 5' sequences of the primer can subsequently be cleaved with the appropriate restriction endonuclease(s) and cloned into a vector which has been subjected to identical restriction endonuclease digest(s) in order to produce compatible ends for ligation. Among the many applications in which successful restriction endonucleolytic cleavage of DNA plays a pivotal role in determining the outcome of an assay, inverse PCR is definitely one of them. Detailed information on inverse PCR is found in chapter 15.

As stated above, validation of PCR product specificity is one of the main applications of restriction fragment analysis in conjunction with PCR. Restriction fragment analysis can, however, reveal more than specificity alone. It can also be used to differentiate between closely related organisms, alleles or subtypes given that the DNA region being examined is polymorphic, such that internal sequence diversity defines a restriction site at a different position in the amplification product of each organism, allele or subtype. In this case, restriction endonuclease digestion of each polymorphic PCR amplification product will yield a distinct, unique banding pattern. Rodu et al. (1991) have very successfully employed this approach to differentiate between human papillomaviruses 6, 11, 16 and 18 which are associated with preneoplastic and cancerous lesions of the genital and digestive tracts. This approach can also be employed in the diagnosis and detection of allelic mutation associated with sickle cell anaemia and haemophilia A.

On the one hand, the combination of PCR and restriction fragment analysis offers a very simple, quick and highly sensitive detection and typing strategy. On the other hand, natural mutations leading to a change in a restriction site are very rare, thus limiting the applicability of this approach. The challenge would thus be to selectively, experimentally introduce a restriction site into one of the PCR amplicons, in other words produce a mutation. PCR-directed mutagenesis is a standard approach often exploited to introduce base changes into an amplicon. It is based on the observation that primer annealing and extension occur despite significant mismatch to the template, even if mismatches occur between the template and the 3' terminus of the primer. If a restriction site should only be introduced into one specific allele, e.g. into either the mutated or wild type (wt) allele, then certain conditions must be fulfilled: 1) The restriction site introduced into the amplicon should, if possible, not cleave the amplicon at another site. 2) The restriction site should not be introduced in the middle or at the 5' terminus of the primer, because, in this case, all alleles will carry the restriction site at the given location, thus precluding discrimination of the amplicons via restriction analysis. Therefore, the base changes necessary to introduce the restriction site into the amplicon should preferentially be placed at the 3' terminus of the primer. As stated above, mismatches between the template and the 3' terminus of the primer may still lead to the extension of the primer. This is basically determined by the fact that the Taq DNA polymerase can ignore certain base pair mismatches at the 3' terminus. These were described by Kwok et al. (1990) and are discussed in chapter 1.3. The amplicon, which should afterwards possess the "mutation", must exhibit base pair mismatching compatible with PCR. Since the Taq DNA polymerase does not possess a proof-reading activity, the mismatched 3' terminus of the primer will not be exonucleolytically removed, in which case the correct base would be extended. 3) We also find that, if the restriction site is to be selectively introduced into one of the alleles, then the first or first two bases extended at the 3' terminus of the primer should be a part of the restriction site and differ between the wt and the mutated allele. Only if this is the case, can one be fairly sure that the restriction site will only be found in one amplicon. As reported by groups using this method (e.g. Sorscher 1991), more than one allele can be amplified in most cases, despite 3' base mutation. Thus, if the first bases added to the amplicon do not differ and are not a part of the restriction site, and if the restriction site recognition sequence is exclusively contained in the 3' terminus of the primer, then the likelihood of more than one allele containing the restriction site is greatly increased. One must keep in mind, that only one successful cycle of PCR of the "wrong" target can drastically influence the outcome of the assay. The use of well defined allele-specific oligonucleotide probes can help monitor the success of the assay being established.

In the sketch below, one modified primer containing the required base changes is used to introduce PCR-directed restriction map alteration into one allele. In the example, a Cla I site (ATCGAT) is introduced at the deletion site:

wild type:
^{5}'NAACAGAAGCAATATCAT**CAGCTT**TGGTGTTN^3'
mutated allele:
^{5}'NAACAGAAGCAATATCAT..................TGGTGTTN^3'

primer: ^{5}'NAAGCAATATC*ATCGA*^{3}'

Assuming that both alleles are amplified despite mismatch at the 3' terminus, then only the mutated allele will contain the restriction site:

wild type:
^{5}'NAACAGAAGCAATATCATCGACTTTGGTGTTN^3'
mutated allele:
^{5}'NAACAGAAGCAATATC*ATCGAT*GGTGTTN^3'

11.1. Restriction Endonucleases

Restriction endonucleases actually belong to a set of enzymes enabling bacteria to protect themselves against invading foreign DNA. Such endonucleases cleave double-stranded DNA at specific sites within, adjacent or at a distance from a particular sequence known as the recognition sequence unless the specific nucleotide sequence has been modified by an appropriate enzyme - usually a methylase. Methylation of bacterial DNA at recognition site sequences renders it resistant to restriction endonuclease activity. Bacteria may protect themselves from their own restriction endonucleases by modifying their own DNA with an endogenous methylase. The restriction enzyme together with its affiliated modifying enzyme is called a restriction

Eco RI: 5' extension

5'NNNNNNNN G A A T T C NNNNNNNN 3'
3'NNNNNNNN C T T A A G NNNNNNNN 5'

5'NNNNNNNN G 3'............5'A A T T C NNNNNNNN 3'
3'NNNNNNNN C T T A A 5'............3'G NNNNNNNN 5'

Pst I: 3' extension

5'NNNNNNNN C T G C A G NNNNNNNN 3'
3'NNNNNNNN G A C G T C NNNNNNNN 5'

5'NNNNNNNN C T G C A 3'............5'G NNNNNNNN 3'
3'NNNNNNNN G 5'............3'A C G T C NNNNNNNN 5'

Dra I: blunt end

5'NNNNNNNN T T T A A A NNNNNNNN 3'
3'NNNNNNNN A A A T T T NNNNNNNN 5'

5'NNNNNNNN T T T 3'............5'A A A NNNNNNNN 3'
3'NNNNNNNN A A A 5'............3'T T T NNNNNNNN 5'

modification system.

The nomenclature of restriction enzymes was set up by Smith et al. (1973). A three letter abbreviation denotes the origin (Eco RI: Escherichia coli), while roman numerals distinguish enzymes of the same origin. A complete list of named and characterized restriction enzymes is updated annually by Roberts (1985).

Three types of restriction modification systems have been described based on subunit composition, cofactor requirements and DNA cleavage site (Yuan 1981). Type I systems contain three different types of subunits and require Mg^{2+}, ATP and S-adenosylmethionine for DNA cleavage. Cleavage occurs at a remote, non-specific site upto 7000 base pairs from the actual binding or recognition site of the enzyme. Type III systems consist of two different subunits, and require Mg^{2+} and ATP. DNA cleavage again occurs at a non specific site, but only 25-27 base pairs downstream from the enzyme recognition site. Type II systems are the least complex and most suitable for DNA analysis.

Type II endonucleases consist of only one subunit, and only require Mg^{2+} for DNA cleavage. The most favorable feature, however, is that DNA cleavage occurs at a specific site within or next to the enzyme's binding site sequence. Practically all commercially available restriction endonucleases belong to this category. Most type II recognition sites are sequences of 4-6 nucleotides (a few 7 or 8 base pairs long) and possess a dyad axis of symmetry so that cleavage on each strand is identical resulting in either a) "staggered" ends (5'-phosphate extensions or 3'-hydroxyl extensions on each strand), or b) "blunt" ends for both strands. Both 5' and 3' extensions are commonly known as cohesive ("sticky") or overhanging ends. Restriction enzymes with different recognition sequences that produce the same single-strand fragment ends form enzyme families. For example, Bam HI, Bcl I, Bgl II, Sau 3A and Xho II are members of the GATC family. This is important to note, since the nature of the ends but not the recognition sequence itself determines the suitability of the fragments for subsequent procedures such as ligation. Within an enzyme family recombinant DNA techniques should succeed. The counterpart, namely, restriction enzymes isolated from different organisms with identical recognition sequences but not necessarily with the same cleavage site - so called isoschizomers, should not be confused with enzyme families. These are not readily suitable for ligation.

11.2. Endonuclease selection

Setting up a restriction enzyme digest consists of choosing an appropriate enzyme and supplying optimal conditions for complete enzyme activity.
1. The choice of an enzyme for the validation of PCR product specificity is dictated by the product itself. For practical purposes, it is advisable to choose a restriction enzyme which will generate restriction

fragments of differing lengths, so that all generated fragments can be resolved on the same agarose gel and in addition, so that even the smallest fragment can be detected, which then will undoubtly leave no uncertainty regarding the accuracy of the assay. The minimum amount of DNA detectable by UV transillumination is approximately 10ng. This implies that a large amount of the PCR product will have to be cleaved in order to produce a detectable band of a very small restriction fragment.

2. If a restriction site sequence should be introduced into the 5' end of the primer(s) for cloning, then care should be taken to incorporate the recognition site sequence of an enzyme known to cut efficiently despite the terminal location of the cleavage site. Kaufmann et al. (1990) and Crouse et al. (1986) investigated the cleavage efficiency of a number of commonly used restriction enzymes when the recognition sequence was located at the extreme end of the DNA fragment. They found that several common enzymes, including Sal I, Hind III and Xba I, fail to cleave at the extreme ends of a DNA fragment, while others such as Sac I, Eco RI, Xho I, Acc I and Dra II generally cleave efficiently. Should the experiment require the choice of a restriction enzyme with a recognition sequence which is not easily cleaved in terminal location, then a second approach is possible. Since the 5'sequence of a primer does not play an essential role for the extension reaction during PCR, designing the primer with additional nucleotides 5' of the incorporated recognition sequence can increase the efficiency of cleavage. It is important to note that the nucleotide sequence surrounding the recognition sequence can influence cleavage efficiency. Further general helpful information is provided in the Bethesda Research Laboratories catalog.

3. If DNA is to be cleaved in an uncharacterized region prior to inverse PCR, the size of the DNA fragments as well as the type of ends generated should be considered. Whether blunt or staggered ends have been generated will decisively influence the ease or the effort with which ligation will succeed. The size of the unknown DNA fragment for amplification will influence the PCR yield (see section optimization) and this again will have an effect on any intended subsequent sequencing of the unknown region.

Although it is difficult to predict the frequency of a restriction endonuclease cleavage site, a few guidelines exist. As reported by Brooks (1987), within a perfectly random DNA sequence with a GC content of 50%, a 4-base recognition sequence would statistically occur every 256 bases, a 6 base sequence at 4kb intervals, and an 8 base sequence at 65kb intervals. Selection of a 4-base recognition sequence that does not cleave in the so-called "core" region will be most promising for initial DNA cleavage in setting up an inverse PCR protocol. If necessary, the second enzyme employed in order to linearize the DNA after ligation will then be an enzyme which seldomly cleaves genomic DNA, but in this case does cleave within the core region.

11.3. Optimal digestion conditions

All restriction enzymes require Mg^{2+} as a cofactor, and most enzymes function in a buffer system capable of adjusting the pH range to 7.2-7.6. Restriction endonucleases vary, however, in their dependence on ionic strength (Wells 1981 and Fuchs 1983). Finding out which ionic strength will allow 100% activity of the selected enzyme is facilitated by the tables supplied by the manufacturers. These also supply information on enzyme activity in different enzyme reaction buffers so that judging whether a certain buffer will be suitable for two different enzymes in one reaction is easily possible. The optimal temperature for most restriction digestions is 37°C. Only a few endonucleases such as Sma I and Taq I require different temperatures. The time as well as the units required for complete digestion of the substrate DNA can only be roughly estimated by the test digestion of lambda DNA. The base composition adjacent to the recognition sequence can affect the cleavage rate of certain enzymes up to 25 times (Thomas 1979). It is thus advisable to test selected enzymes on the target DNA substrate.

The following practical section focuses on the usage of class II restriction enzymes to evaluate PCR product specificity.

Procedure	Comments

Method : Restriction digest of PCR products

Before starting it is advisable to autoclave reaction tubes, pipet tips and reagents to reduce the likelihood of contamination with DNases.

1. After estimating the amount of DNA in µg/µl in the PCR sample, remove an aliquot containg 0.2-0.4µg DNA.

1. After PCR, the specific and sometimes also the non-specific products are visualized on an ethidium bromide gel. Appropriate DNA markers characterized by the amount in µg/µl will help judge the amount of the PCR product in the gel. The amount of DNA subsequently subjected to digestion depends on the fragment lengths which should be generated by the selected enzyme. The detection of small fragments as opposed to large fragments in an agarose gel will require the digestion of more substrate DNA. The minimum amount which can be detected by UV-transillumination is 10ng DNA.

Substances, such as EDTA, phenol, SDS and ethidium bromide, which can inhibit restriction enzyme activity, are usually not present, since these also inhibit the Taq DNA polymerase.

2. Add 2µl of the appropriate 10 x reaction buffer and autoclaved double distilled water to a final volume of 18µl.

2. An optimal reaction buffer is usually supplied by the manufacturer along with the enzyme. The buffer which works best with most commonly used enzymes contains
    100mM Tris-HCl, pH 7.5
    50mM NaCl
    10mM $MgCl_2$
    1mM dithiothreitol or 10mM 2-mercaptoethanol

Since 1 x PCR-buffer is 10mM Tris-HCl, 50mM KCl and 1.5mM $MgCl_2$, there is usually no need to precipitate the DNA prior to restriction analysis. We recommend using reaction buffers supplied by the manufacturer, since these are almost always DNase-free.

Procedure(cont.)

3. Add 5-10 units restriction enzyme in 2µl, mix and spin down briefly.

4. Incubate the mixture at 37°C for at least 2 hours.

5. Stop the reaction by heat-inactivating the enzyme at 65°C for 10 min or by adding loading buffer to yield a 1 x end concentration.

6. Visualize the cleavage products as well as an aliquot of the uncut DNA in an ethidium bromide stained agarose gel.

Comments(cont.)

3. If necessary, restriction enzymes should be diluted in storage buffer rather than reaction buffer to maintain activity.

4. This is a minimum for complete digestion. We usually perform digestions overnight. In this case, some groups suggest adding a stabilizer such as nuclease-free bovine serum albumin (Fuchs 1983).

5. Loading buffer is described in Sambrook et al. (1989). EDTA in the loading buffer will chelate Mg^{2+} ions required for enzyme activity.

6 x Loading buffer: 30% glycerol in H_2O
0.25% bromphenol blue
0.25% xylene cyanol FF

6. Refer to section agarose gel systems.

Advice: For diagnostic purposes it is crucial to ensure that the restriction enzyme selected to validate specificity of the PCR product works reliably. Pilot experiments testing a selection of enzymes should be performed to assess fidelity of individual enzymes, and then the best system established for routine analysis. In addition, we recommend introducing a "positive control" which will allow judgement of enzyme activity. Without this information an uncut PCR product may be falsely interpreted as a non-specific product.

REFERENCES

1. Arber W. DNA modification and restriction. 1974, Prog Nucleic Acid Res Mol Biol 14, 1-37.

2. Brooks JE. Properties and uses of restriction endonucleases. 1987, Methods Enzymol 152, 113-129.

3. Crouse J, Amorese D. Double digestions of the multiple cloning site. 1986, Focus (Bethesda Research Laboratories) 8, 9.

4. Fuchs R, Blakesly R. Guide to the use of type II reatriction endonucleases. 1983, Methods Enzymol 100, 1-38.

5. Kaufmann DL, Evans GA. Restriction endonuclease cleavage at the termini of PCR products. 1990, BioTechniques 9, 304-306.

6. Kwok S, Kellog DE, McKinney N, Spasic D, Goda L, Levenson C, Sninsky JJ. Effects of primer-template mismatches on the polymerase chain reaction: human immunodeficiency virus type I model studies. 1990, Nucl Acids Res 18, 999-1005.

7. Roberts RJ. Restriction and modification enzymes and their recognition sequences. 1985, Nucl Acids Res 13, r165-200.

8. Rodu B, Christian C, Snyder RC, Ray R, Miller DM. Simplified PCR-based detection and typing strategy for human papillomaviruses utilizing a single oligonucleotide primer set. 1991, BioTechniques 10, 632-636.

9. Sambrook J, Fritsch EF, Maniatis T. Molecular cloning: A laboratory manual (Cold Spring Harbor Lab, Cold Spring Harbor, NY) 1989.

10. Sorscher EJ, Huang Z. Diagnosis of genetic disease by primer-spacified restriction map modification, with application to cystic fibrosis and retinitis pigmentosa. 1991, Lancet 337, 1115-1118.

11. Smith HO, Nathans D. A suggested nomenclature for bacterial host modification and restriction systems and their enzymes. 1973, J Mol Biol 81, 419-425.

12. Smith HO. Nucleotide sequence specificity of restriction endonucleases. 1979, Science 205, 455-462.

13. Thomas M, Davis RW. Studies on the cleavage of bacteriophage lambda DNA with EcoRI Restriction endonuclease. 1979, J Mol Biol 91, 315-328.

14. Wells RD, Neuendorf SK. Cleavage of "single-stranded" viral DNAs by certain restriction endonucleases. 1981, Gene Amplif Anal, 101-111.

15. Yuan R. Structure and mechanism of multifunctional restriction endonucleases. 1981, Ann Rev Biochem 50, 285-319.

12. Multiplex PCR

Multiplex PCR is the use of several primer pairs in one PCR assay. Simultaneous amplification of more than one DNA region of interest in one reaction mixture (cf. Figure 12.1) reduces twork, time, cost, and the risk of cross contamination, since sample handling is minimal.

Chamberlain and co-workers (1990, 1988) have succesfully employed multiplex PCR to diagnose Duchenne muscular dystrophy (DMD). Genetically, although certain point mutations are believed to be associated with DMD, single different deletion patterns spanning several hundred kilobases in the DMD locus

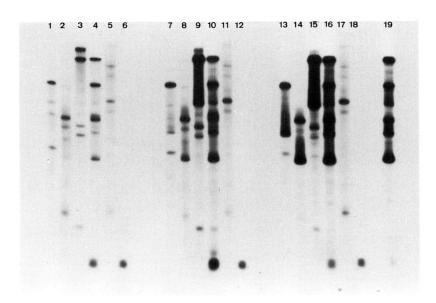

Figure 12.1: Amplification results using single primer pairs and multiple primer pairs in single PCR assays. Demonstration of *Mycobacterium tuberculosis* amplicons for different gene regions (383bp, 240bp, 158bp; for details, see text) with variation of number of bacteria initially used. Lanes **1-5, 100** bacteria; lanes **7-11**, 1,000 bacteria; lanes **13-17**, 10,000 bacteria. Lanes **6, 12, 18**: negative control without DNA, but with multiprimer use. Lane **19**: positive control (PC) with 10ng M. tuberculosis H37Rv DNA. Lanes **1, 7, 13**: 240bp fragment. Lanes **2, 8, 15**: 158bp fragment. Lanes **3, 9, 16**: 383bp fragment. Lanes **4, 11, 17**: multiprimer PCR mixture with all three primers at optimized quantitative ratio. Lane **3, 9, 18**: internal control with ß-actin primer (196bp fragment: (+) primer 5'acg gct ccg gca tgt gca ag 3', (-) primer 5'tga cga tgc cgt gct gca tg 3'). The experiment proves that the multiprimer assay with optimized primer ratio can clearly detect 100 mycobacteria for all three gene regions. However, further reduction of number of bacteria, lowers sensitivity by a factor of 10-20 as compared to the use of single primer pairs.

are detected in approximately 60% of the patients. The multiplex PCR assay developed by Chamberlain et al. (1988) using six different primer pairs enables the detection of six deletion-prone exons of the DMD gene and thereby the diagnosis of 70% of all DMD cases.

Since the introduction of multiplex PCR, the method has been widely applied. For example, Rodriguez et al. (1991) described the simultaneous detection of the myosin heavy-chain gene and the human immunodeficiency virus type I (HIV-1) in endomyocardial biopsy specimens, while Bej and co-workers (1990) described the use of multiplex PCR for the detection of infectious agents. They point out, however, that the application of multiplex PCR in diagnostics (e.g. viral agents) is mostly associated with a lower sensitivity of the assay. In contrast, the detection of mutations, deletions, rearrangements or insertions in single-copy genes is a more suitable application of multiplex PCR. According to Bej et al. (1990) reproducible results can only be obtained if the optimized ratio of the respective primers to each other are stringently used. In one case, it was even crucial to perform a preamplification (mip sequence). Thus, practical experience with multiplex PCR clearly emphasizes the importance of primer design and of the optimization of the amounts of primers used. Even more than in a PCR assay using only one primer pair, care must be taken to avoid any 3' complementarity between any of the primers (see chapter 20.1). Hot start set-up strategy will probably significantly improve multiplex PCR.

The following recommendations for the optimization or standardization of multiplex PCR assays can be formulated:

1. Thermocyclers: only devices exhibiting constant physical properties should be used. Minute changes in the thermoprofile can lead to complete failure of the assay.

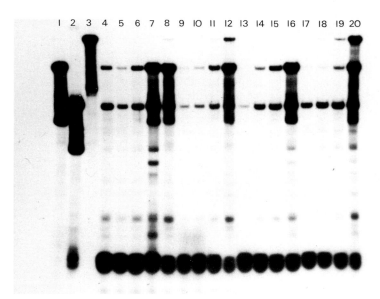

Figure 12.2: Denaturing polyacrylamide gel demonstrates the results obtained using different ratios of the three primer pairs in separate multiplex PCR assays. A prerequisite for multiplex PCR are optimal primer concentrations so that equal numbers of cycles will result in strong signals from the different target regions. The amplicons for the detection of the *Mycobacterium tuberculosis* genes are demonstrated one by one in the first three lanes (383bp, 240bp, 158bp). All three primer pairs were used in amounts of 80pmol. The best results are those of the multiplex PCR in lane **19**, in which all three amplicons yield equally strong signals. For the description of test details, see text and method.

2. The length of the primers should be between 22bp and 30bp - i.e. somewhat longer than in standard PCR assays. Primers with short sequences strictly must be avoided.

3. Multiplex PCR assays may require the addition of a cosolvent. Additions such as dimethyl sulfoxide (DMSO) at a final concentration of 10% have proved to be advantegous in certain systems requiring high sensitivity (Kogan 1987).

4. Prolongation of the annealing time to approximately 1min in the first five cycles, followed by a short annealing time (not longer than 30sec), at the highest possible temperatures, can increase the stringency of the assay.

5. Every additional new primer pair must be evaluated anew in the context of the whole assay.

6. Increasing the Taq polymerase amount up to 4-6U/100µl in the reaction mixture will in some systems improve sensitivity.

Procedure	Comments

Method: Detection of three different mycobacterial genome regions in a single PCR tube

Procedure	Comments
1. Prepare bacterial DNA as described in chapter 6.1.3. Suspend bacteria from the culture plate in 1ml 10mM Tris-HCl/1mM EDTA buffer and incubate for 90min at 37°C after adding 10mg lysozyme (30mg/ml).	1. Preparation of 100ml of a 10mM Tris/1mM EDTA buffer: Store 1ml of a 1M stock solution of Tris, pH 7.4, plus 40µl of a 0.25M EDTA solution, pH 8.0, 99.3ml double destilled water, at room temperature. Lysozyme solution: 30mg lysozyme (Sigma) per 1ml double destilled water, always prepare solution fresh.
2. Add 9ml proteinase-K solution for lysis. Incubate at 65°C for 90min.	2. Proteinase-K solution: 2mg/ml proteinase K in 10mM Tris (pH 7.4), 10mM EDTA, 150mM NaCl. Supplement with SDS to yield a final concentration of 0.8%.
3. Sonicate the mycobacterial DNA for 15min at 80Hz in a 50°C water bath.	3. For details of the DNA preparation, see chapter 7.
4. Add an equal volume of phenol/chloroform (1:1). Mix vigorously for about 10min.	

Procedure(cont.) *Comments(cont.)*

5. Separate the phases by centrifuging at 10,000 rpm for 10min at 4°C.

6. Remove the upper aqueous phase. Repeat steps 4 and 5 twice.

7. Transfer the aqueous phase into a new tube.

8. Add 1/10 volume of 3M sodium acetate and 2.5ml volumes of ice-cold 100% ethanol. Precipitate DNA at -70°C for 20min.

9. Centrifuge for 10-15min at 13,000rpm. Then wash the pellet with 80% ethanol and again with 70% ethanol.

10. Resuspend the pellet in 500µl of 50mM Tris-HCl/ 5mM EDTA buffer. Measure the DNA concentration (OD_{260}). In all subsequent PCR mixtures, about 5ng M. tuberculosis DNA was used per 50µl PCR mixture.

11. Label 20 tubes from 1 to 20. Pipet the PCR: 5µl of 10x PCR buffer each, 8µl of a dNTP stock solution each.

11. All additions are pipetted on ice. For details of the PCR mixture, see chapters 1 and 2.
10 x PCR buffer: 500mM KCl, 100mM Tris-HCl (pH 8.3), 15mM $MgCl_2$, 0.01% gelatin.
dNTP stock solutions (Boehringer) dATP, dCTP, dGTP, dTTP 100mM each. Premixed stocks: 0.125mM.

12. Add the M. tuberculosis primers according to the following scheme:

a) In each of tubes 3-20, 4µl (corresponding to 80pmol) of the primer pair for the 65kD region (hereafter called 383bp primer) is added.
b) 4µl of the primer pair for the MPB 64 protein (hereafter called 240bp primer) are added in tubes 1 and 3-7; 3µl, in tubes 9-12; 2µl, in tubes 13-16; 1µl, in tubes 17-20.
c) 4µl of the primer pair for the 2.4kB insert (hereafter called 158bp primer) are added in tubes 2, 4, 5, 9, 13, 17; 3µl, in tubes 6, 10, 14, 18; 2µl, in tubes 7, 11, 15, 19; 1µl, in tubes 8, 12, 16, 20.

12. In this assay, the following published primers are used:

1. MPB 64 protein: 240bp fragment (Shankar 1990)
(+) primer: 5'tcc gct gcc agt cgt ctt cc 3'
(-) primer: 5'tgg cct aga ctc gcg agg ac 3'

2. 2.4kB DNA insert, pPH7301 clone: 158bp fragment (Hermans 1990)
(+) primer: 5'ggt cct gac ggt aat ggg gt 3'
(-) primer: 5'cgc cca tcc aca tcc cgc cc 3'

3. 65kD antigen: 383bp fragment (Hance 1989)
(+) primer: 5'gag atc gag ctg gag gat cc 3'
(-) primer: 5'agc tgc agc cca aag gtg tt 3'

Procedure(cont.)	Comments(cont.)
	After synthesis and OD_{260} measurement: 1. dilute primers to 40µM stock solutions using double destilled water. 2. For reducing the set-up pipetting steps the stock solution may be premixed to 20µM primer pair stock solution by mixing equal amounts/volumes. 1µl of such a 20µM stock contains 20pmol of each primer. (thus, 4µl = 2 x 80pmol).
13. Add water to fill up to the final volume of 50µl, taking into account the subsequent addition of DNA, enzyme, and ^{32}P-dCTP.	
14. Cover the mixtures with a layer of 75µl light mineral oil.	
15. Below the oil, add 10ng M. tuberculosis DNA plus 1µl ^{32}P-dCTP (10mCi/ml) each to label the amplicons.	15. Make sure that, before adding it to the PCR mixture, the DNA is heated at 95°C for 5min to denature any protease that may still be present. However, this denaturing step should not be performed immediately before addition to the PCR mixture, since the DNA needs some time to renature completely. If incompletely renatured DNA is added to the PCR mixture, it will increase the risk of unspecific annealing of primers followed by elongation.
	From this step on, the use of radioactive material is involved, so that special care must be taken when handling the material.
16. Preheat the thermocycler to the desired denaturing temperature of 92°C.	
17. Add 4U diluted Taq polymerase.	
18. Place all tubes in the preheated thermocycler as soon as possible.	
19. Start the amplification cycles: Cycles 1- 5: 60sec 95°C, 60sec 56°C, 45sec 72°C Cycles 6-35: 60sec 95°C, 30sec 56°C, 45sec 72°C	
The elongation time is prolonged by 3sec in each cycle. After the last cycle, a final extension step, 10min at 72°C, is carried out and the samples then cooled to 4°C.	

Procedure(cont.)

20. 10µl each of the radioactively labeled crude PCR product are separated by electrophoresis under denaturing conditions in a 6% polyacrylamide gel (see chapter 10.4). Expose a Kodak X-ray film (see chapter 10.4) for 2-4 hours.

References

1. Bej AK, Mahbubani MH, Miller R, DiCesare JL, Haff L, Atlas RM. Multiplex PCR amplification and immobilized capture probes for detection of bacterial pathogens and indicators in water. 1990, Molecul Cell Probes 4, 353-365

2. Chamberlain JS, Gibbs RA, Ranier JE, Caskey CT. Multiplex PCR for the diagnosis of Duchenne muscular dystrophy. In: PCR protocols. A guide to methods and applications. Eds.: MA Innis, DH Gelfand, JJ Sninsky, TJ White. 1990, Academic Press, San Diego, pp272-281

3. Chamberlain JS, Gibbs RA, Ranier JE, Ngyen PN, Caskey CT. Deletion screening of the Duchenne muscular dystrophy locus via multiplex DNA amplification. 1988, Nucl Acids Res 16, 11141-11156

4. Hance AJ, Grandchamp B, Lévy-Frébault V, Lecossier D, Rauzier J, Bocart D, Gicquel B. Detection and identification of mycobacteria by amplification of mycobacterial DNA. 1989, Molecul Microbiol 3, 843-849

5. Hermans PWM, Schuitema ARJ, van Soolingen D, Verstynen CPHJ, Bik EM, Thole JER, Kolk AH, van Embden JDA. Specific detection of Mycobacterium tuberculosis complex strains by polymerase chain reaction. 1990, J Clin Microbiol 28, 1204-1213

6. Kogan SC, Doherty M, Gitschier J. An improved method for prenatal diagnosis of genetic diseases by analysis of amplified DNA sequences. 1987, N Engl J Med 317, 985-990

7. Rodriguez ER, Nasim S, Hsia J, Sandin RL, Ferreira A, Hilliard BA, Ross AM, Garrett CT. Cardiac myocytes and dendritic cells harbor human immunodeficiency virus in infected patients with and without cardiac dysfunction: detection by multiplex, nested, polymerase chain reaction in individually microdissected cells from right ventricular endomyocardial biopsy tissue. 1991, Am J Cardiol 68, 1511-1520

8. Shankar P, Manjunath N, Lakshmi R, Aditi B, Seth P, Shriniwas. Identification of Mycobacterium tuberculosis by polymerase chain reaction. 1990, Lancet I, 423

13. Detection of Single Base Changes Using PCR

Numerous methods are now available for the detection of single base changes in a given DNA fragment (for a reviwe, see Caskey 1987, Landegren 1988, Myers 1988, Cotton 1989). With all methods, it has to be considered what requirements the detection system should meet: (1) Is the point mutation known and should it now be detected in a preamplified fragment? (2) Should the given DNA product be screened for the presence of DNA point mutations? (3) Should a possibly present point mutation be pinpointed in the fragment or does the statement that a mutation is present suffice? (4) Should all possibly present mutations be detected? (5) Should the used method represent a routine screening procedure? The method of choice for the detection of single base changes depends on the purpose.

The reasons why today point mutations are searched for in the DNA sequence are manyfold: (1) explanation of the mechanism of a disease, (2) elucidation of evolutionary relationships between species, (3) investigation and understanding of the mechanism of mutagenic substances, (4) detection of disease-related genes for the diagnosis of certain diseases, (5) investigation of certain pathogenicity traits of various causative agents, (6) comprehension of the basis of resistance development against chemotherapeutic substances by microorganisms, (7) genetic linkage studies.

The PCR technique has brought considerable experimental simplifications into many methods for the detection of point mutations. As examples, the most important procedures will be introduced in this chapter. However, reference can be made once more to the excellent review article by Richard Cotton (1989), which can serve as a complement.

13.1. Allele-specific amplification (ASA, PASA, ASP, ARMS)

A brief survey of the methodology of allele-specific amplification (ASA) - also called PCR amplification of specific alleles (PASA), allele-specific PCR (ASP), or amplification refractory mutation system (ARMS) - has already been given in chapter 3.2. The basis of this procedure is the hypothesis that a mismatch at the 3' end of one or both of the used oligonucleotides - with high probability - prevents the 3' elongation of the primer by Taq polymerase. Of course, only DNA polymerases that do not exhibit proofreading activity must be used for such an assay (cf. chapter 21). Figure 13.1 demonstrates the basic principle of the method. In each of two separate PCR mixtures, a specific primer (here, primer 1 and primer 2) is used as well as an unspecific one. Primer 1 (with a C residue at the 3' end) only detects the G allele; primer 2 (with a G residue at the 3' end), only the C allele. If a patient is heterozygous, amplicons of identical length will result in both mixtures. If he is homozygous for the G allele, an amplicon can only be produced with primer 1 (see figure 13.1, panel A); if he is homozygous for the C allele, an amplification product will only result with primer 2 (figure 13.1, panel B). Therefore, it must be possible to detect a band in at least one reaction mixture.

Allele-specific amplification

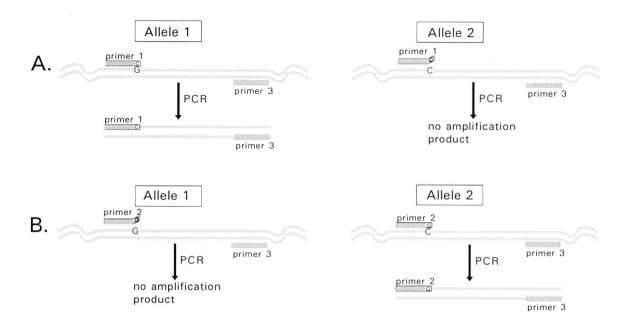

Figure 13.1: Basic principle of the allele-specific amplification (ASA), for details see the text above

In 1989, Wu et al. published the first results regarding the allele-specific PCR. The authors used the ASA for the detection of the normal or sickle-cell ¨-globin allele in genomic DNA. The primers they used showed an A-A or T-T mismatch. To optimize their systems, they employed 14bp-long primers, at an annealing temperature of 55°C. A discrimination between the two alleles was not possible at lower annealing temperatures. Several articles on the methodology of the ASA were published by the group surrounding Steve S. Sommer (Dutton 1991, Sarkar 1990, Sarkar 1991, Sommer 1992). The authors make the following recommendations for the optimization of the ASA:

(1) A mismatch directly at the 3' end or within the first 3-5 bases of the 3' end yields the highest specificity.
(2) Primer lengths of between 14 and 17bp yield better results, due to increased relative influence of the mismatch on the annealing behavior.
(3) The DNA concentration should be chosen as low as possible, since concentrations that are too high reduce the specificity. Proposed were amounts of 1ng/1µl PCR assay.
(4) The primer concentrations should be reduced to 0.05µM.
(5) Lowering of the magnesium concentration to approximately 1.5mM, and of the dNTP concentration to 25-50µM.
(6) Reduction of the Taq polymerase amount to 0.2-0.3U/25µl PCR mixture.
(7) The addition of 2-5% formamide may improve the

specificity of the assay, esp. if G-C-rich regions are present.
(8) The number of cycles should be kept as low as possible. Interestingly, the authors report that they were successful with all combinations of mismatched primer and template pairs.

This is in contrast to the data from Kwok et al. (1990), who showed that only the C-C, G-A, A-G and (to a lesser degree) A-A mismatches prevent, with high certainty, an elongation of the 3' end by Taq polymerase (cf. Table 13.1). The specificity of an allele-specific amplification is determined by two kinetic variables: the rate at which the annealed primer dissociates from the template before the primer is elongated (P_{off}) and the rate at which the annealed primer is elongated by the DNA polymerase (P_{elong}). From this, it can be deduced that, for the optimally matched primer, $P_{elong} \gg P_{off}$ should be true and, for the mismatched primer, $P_{elong} \ll P_{off}$. If, due to less than optimal reaction conditions or physicochemical properties of the enzyme, these proportions are not kept to during amplification, no allele-specific amplifications can be performed.

Table 13.1: Efficiency of elongation of primer-target mismatches by Taq polymerase (according to Kwok 1990)

	T	C	G	A
T	1.0	1.0	1.0	/
C	1.0	<0.01	/	1.0
G	1.0	/	1.0	<0.01
A	/	1.0	<0.01	0.05

The presence of haplotypes - the combination of closely linked alleles that cosegregate - makes it possible to perform a double ASA, as an extension of the simple ASA. Here, the presence of an allele is no longer tested by only two specific primers and one unspecific primer in two separate mixtures; instead, altogether four specific primers (5' primers #1 and #2, 3' primers #3 and #4) are used in four possible permutations (1+3, 2+3, 1+4, 2+4) to detect the four possible haplotypes. Sarkar and Sommer (1991) have shown this using two biallelic polymorphic sites of the human dopamine D2 receptor as an example. The four primers used had lengths of 14bp and 15bp, resp. 5% formamide was added to the reaction mixture. Conspicuously long, 120sec, was the chosen annealing time. One difficulty of this system resulted from the fact that a missing specific amplicon has the same significance as the presence of a specific PCR band in the gel. For, the investigated sample may well be negative for the allelity tested by the primer used in this reaction. To have at least an internal amplification control, the authors coamplified a 551bp fragment of the human factor IX from a cloned template. Even more than the simple ASA, the double ASA involves the risk that, by "erroneous" elongation of a mismatched primer, a false-positive result may be simulated. All the more carefully, all factors cited above for optimization purposes must be taken into account. Apparently, the number of cycles especially is a problem. An experiment exactly following the data from the publication by Sarkar and Sommer (1991), performed by us on three subjects for the detection of the different alleles of the dopamin D2 receptor (figure 13.2), shows that, for all three, plausible results are obtained after 30 cycles. In contrast, after 40 cycles, one subject (#3, lane 3 in panel A, B, C and D) is found to allegedly have three alleles. This is a result that should not occur and cannot be explained biologically, so that a false-positive result of the ASA is to be assumed. This small experiment does not question previous ASA achievements, but it shows that both implementation and interpretation must be done with great care.

Greater reliability regarding the specificity of ASA might be achieved if the allele-specific primer is destabilized by additional deliberate mismatches near the 3' end in such a way that the probability of elongation, in spite of the mismatch, is even more reduced (Newton 1989).

The method of ASA, as hitherto described, requires at least two PCRs per tested allele. Several ideas exist as to how the presence of one or more alleles in a reaction tube might be investigated. Dutton and Sommer (1991) distinguish two amplicons that could occur when heterozygosity is present, due to the fact that the allele-1-specific amplicon is longer by 31bp than the one for allele 2 because the corresponding primer was

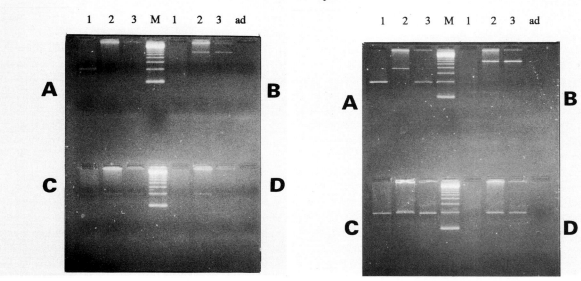

Figure 13.2: Results of a allele-specific amplification using primers published by Sarkar and Sommer (1991). The experiments demonstrates the unplausible constellation that patient #3 reveals after 40 cycles - in contrast to 30 cycles - three alleles [A, C, D] (for details see p151). This gives a hint for the fact that ASA has obtained a false-positive result and highlights the problems of this method.

synthesized with an additional 31 bases at the 5' end. This makes it possible to safely distinguish between the two alleles simply through their difference in size. Even though, purely by way of calculation, the Tm value for the two differently sized primers may be the same, different Pelong and Poff values must nevertheless be assumed for the two oligonucleotides, which will have a critical impact on the specificity of the reaction. An alternative and methodologically somewhat safer way was chosen by Ye et al. (1992). Their ASA assay, modifying the one-tube nested PCR (see chapter 3.3), uses two primer pairs in one tube, where the outer primers (#1 and #2) have a Tm value higher by 10°C (cf. figure 13.3). With these outer oligonucleotides, a pre-amplification is performed over 10 cycles at a correspondingly higher annealing temperature (63°C). The two inner primers (#3 and #4) are, at the same location of the gene, designed in such a way that #3 is completely complementary to the sense strand of allele 1 and #4, to the antisense strand of allele 2. However, primers #3 and #4 are asymmetrically located on the pre-amplicon, so that the products formed in the second part of the PCR (lower annealing temperature, 46°C) with involvement of primers #3 and #4 have different sizes. The amplicon from primers #1 and #3 is approximately 30-50% larger than the amplicon from primers #2 and #4 (unfortunately, the authors do not state exact fragment sizes). This procedure makes it possible that the corresponding primers (here, #1 and #2, and #3 and #4, resp.) are designed identical with regard to size, Tm value, mismatches, etc.; that the gene locus is pre-amplified through the first 10 cycles and thereby has a clear quantitative advantage in relation to the background DNA; and that, in any case, a specific amplicon must be formed in each reaction tube.

All in all, the method of ASA can be looked upon as an extremely helpful and interesting enrichment of the PCR technique. However, the problems inherent in this method are not yet solved, esp. if the method is to be applied in diagnostic assays. By far the main problem is how the specificity of a single primer can be increased with regard to the detection of a single point mutation.

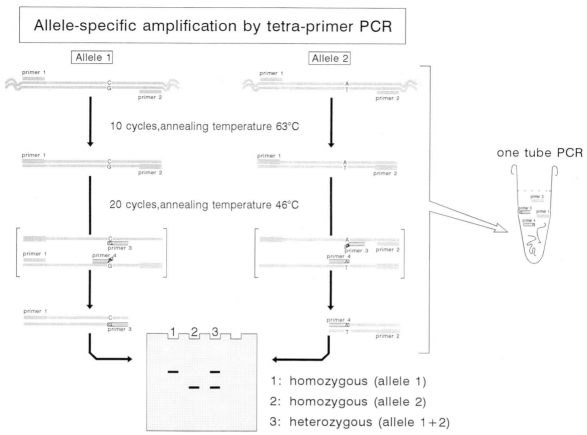

Figure 13.3: Schematic course of an allele-specific amplification by tetra-primer PCR modified according to Ye at al. (1992). For details of the reaction course, see description in the text.

13.2 Allele-specific oligonucleotide (ASO) hybridization

Allele-specific oligonucleotide hybridization (ASO) is the method of choice for all PCR assays that are to be performed - mostly with one primer pair - within a greater framework and for which no specific restriction sites are available for the subsequent discrimination of allelity. Above all, there are no expensive optimization experiments for primers, as they have been described for the ASA in the previous chapter. A further advantage of ASO is the presence of the specific PCR product in high concentration and with low complexity. For the detection of single point mutations in the amplicon, short probes (oligonucleotide length, usually 18-30 bases long) therefore offer themselves. Saiki et al. (1986) describe the system using as example the detection of normal (ß^A), sickle-cell (ß^S), and hemoglobin C (ß^C) sequences. ß^A, ß^C, and ß^S globin differ by the presence of a specific base mutation in the region of codon 4-17 (A vs. T). In addition, the mutations of the ras oncogen were extensively investigated using the method of ASO (e.g., Farr 1988). The only prerequisite for the method is that the hybridization conditions are chosen in such a way that the presence of a single base difference in the different targets is sufficient for discrimination. The decrease in stability of the primer-target hybrid is about 1.5°C for every percentage of mismatched bases. From this results that the melting temperature of a 20-nucleotide hybrid is reduced by 5-7.5°C when an internal mismatch is present. This difference is, as a rule, sufficient to distinguish between perfectly matched and internally mismatched oligonucleotides. With increasing length of the detecting oligonucleotide, the relative impact of a mismatch decreases. When choosing the length of an oligonucleotide, the gain in specificity associated with the use of a longer oligonucleotide must be weighed against increasing problems in the detection system. Furthermore, it must be noted that, apparently, clear differences in the sensitivity of the detection system occur again and again, depending on whether the detection is done with the sense probe or the corresponding anti-sense probe (Skogerboe 1990). This difference may be caused by the sense and anti-sense strands of the PCR product having different affinities to the carrier (blot membrane), by asymmetrical formation of (+) strand and (-) strand in the PCR, or by different secondary structures of the two strands. Therefore, it is always to be recommended to test both sense and anti-sense oligonucleotide probes during the optimization of the ASO test. As detection system, the slot- or dot-blot method recommends itself, since here the various necessary hybridizations can be performed with manageable expenditure. Two variants come into consideration here: in one test system, the PCR product is blotted on the membrane; in the other one, the detecting probe is spotted on the membrane through a homopolymer tail and covalently bound by UV irradiation (Saiki 1989). For the hybridization of oligonucleotides larger than 16 bases, the use of tetramethyl ammonium chloride (TMACl) is recommended instead of sodium chloride if probes of identical length are used. TMACl is available from the Aldrich Co. In this solution, the T_m value of the hybrid is largely independent of base composition and depends primarily on its length (Wozney 1989, Wood 1985). The recommended hybridization temperatures in 3M TMACl solution for oligonucleotides of different lengths are as follows: 17mer 48-50°C, 19mer 55-57°C, 20mer 58-66°C.

Procedure	Comments

Method 1: Oligonucleotide hybridization using TMACl buffer

The dot-blot procedure is described in detail in chapter 10.2.2.

1. After UV-linking of the blotted DNA on the nylon membrane, the filter is pre-hybridized for 1 hour at the temperature determined by the choice of length of the oligonucleotide. For this, we recommend a buffer of 3M TMACl/50mM Tris-HCl (pH 7.8), 2mM EDTA/	1. 10x Denhardt's reagent: 1g Ficoll (Type 400, Pharmacia), 1g polyvinyl pyrrolidone, 1g bovine serum albumin (Sigma) and aqua bidest. to 500ml. Preparation of the 3M TMACl solution: TMACl can be obtained in 500g packages from the Aldrich Co.

Procedure(cont.) | *Comments(cont.)*

0.3% SDS/denatured sonicated salmon sperm DNA 80µg/ml/5x Denhardt's solution.

To this amount, 400ml aqua bidest. are added. This will result in an approx. 5M solution. Mild heating of the solution to about 50°C. Filtration through a Whatman No.1 filter, then renewed filtration through a Nalge (0.45µ pore-size) filter. To determine the exact molarity, the concentration must be measured in the refractometer and can then be calculated using the formula $C = (n-1.33)/0.018$, where C is the molar concentration of the quaternary alkyl ammonium salt and n is the refractive index.

2. Approximately 1-5pmol of the probe are subsequently introduced into the mixture and the hybridization continued for another one hour.

3. Wash the filter twice with 2x SSPE/0.2% SDS at 20°C for 10min each.

3. 2x SSPE: 17.5g NaCl, 2.8g NaH2PO4 x H2O and 0.74g EDTA in 800ml aqua bidest., adjust pH to 7.6 with NaOH, adjust the volume to 1,000ml. Sterilize by autoclaving.

4. Wash again in the 3M TMACl/50mM Tris-HCl (pH 7.8), 2mM EDTA/0.3% SDS buffer for 60min at the appropriate temperature (see above).

5. Exposure of the blot or development in the colorimetric detection procedure (see chapter 10.3).

13.3. Chemical mismatch cleavage method

Various methods for the detection of point mutations require the preparation of heteroduplex hybrids from wild-type DNA and mutant DNA. For this, wild-type DNA and mutant DNA are mixed, heated together and thereby melted; with subsequent lowering of the temperature, they re-anneal, forming heteroduplices. If single base-pair changes are present in the mutant DNA, base-pair mismatches are formed within the heteroduplices that can subsequently be detected by various methods (ribonuclease A, ABC nuclease, chemical cleavage of mismatches [CCM]). The stability of DNA is, over long stretches, determined by the complementarity of the G-C and A-T pairings, G-C being much more stable than A-T. Due to the different distribution of base pairings, DNA doamins with different melting behavior inone DNA fragment result.

Heteroduplex investigations are always to be recommended where the gene to be investigated is too long for routine sequencing and when point mutations can occur at different locations, so that they cannot be detected by a specific primer.

When investigating heteroduplices with the chemical cleavage method, it is important to note that the formation of these hybrids preferentially takes place when the amount of wild-type DNA is limited. One of the wild-type DNA strands is labeled radioactively. In contrast to incorporation by [^{32}P]dCTP, the labeling of the wild-type DNA by a radioactively labeled primer makes it possible to choose between labeling the plus strand and the minus strand of the wild-type DNA. Treatment of the heteroduplex with hydroxylamine (H) leads to a modification of mismatched C bases, and with osmium tetroxide (OT), to a modification of mismatched T bases (Cotton 1988). If the heteroduplices pretreated in that way are subsequently incubated with piperidine, a cleavage of the modified residue will result. The resulting radioactive fragments can then be made visible in a high-resolution polyacrylamide gel with subsequent autoradiography. Thereby, all possible mismatches can be demonstrated in four reaction mixtures - one mixture with radioactively labeled (+)-strand of wild-type DNA, one with radioactively labeled (-)-strand of wild-type DNA, both treated with hydroxylamine and with osmium tetroxide, respectively. Besides DNA-DNA hybrids, the chemical cleavage mismatch method can also be applied to RNA-DNA hybrids. Thus, Cotton and Wright (1989), using CCM, have demonstrated mutations in a DNA-mRNA hybrid in an RNA virus. An important advantage of CCM is the fact that all reactions have the same kinetics and efficiency, in contrast to enzymatic reactions using RNaseA. The following method for CCM is mainly based on the data published by Belinda Rossiter et al.

Procedure	Comments

Method 2: Chemical cleavage of mismatches in PCR products

1. The end labeling with [^{32}P]dATP of the 5' and 3' primers for the labeling of the PCR-generated wild-type DNA is done according to the method given in chapter 10.	
2. The two PCR mixtures - one reaction for the labeled 5' primer and one reaction for the labeled 3' primer - are carried out in a 100µl volume as described in chapters 1 and 2. The purification of the two radioactive end products is done using a low-melting agarose from which the two probes are cut out.	2. The determination of specific activity is necessary for the more precise planning of the experiment as follows. In our experience, it should be around 5×10^7-10^9cpm/µg primer. Because of possible radiolysis, the probes can be stored at -70°C for about 4-5 weeks.
3. 20ng wild-type DNA probe (about 1×10^6cpm) are united with about 200ng unlabeled mutant DNA in 20µl mixing buffer and heated for 5min to 95°C.	3. 5x mixing buffer: 1.5M NaCl, 15mM MgCl$_2$, 15mM Tris-HCl (pH 7.8).

Procedure(cont.)   *Comments(cont.)*

---

4. After heating, put the whole mixture on ice immediately for 10min and heat for 100min to 40°C.

5. Subsequent precipitation of the DNA hybrids by addition of 60µl ice-cold ethanol and incubation at -70°C for 20min. Centrifuge the hybrid DNA at maximum rotation in a desk centrifuge. Wash the mixture with 70% ethanol and subsequently resuspend in 15µl aqua bidest.

5. Altogether two hybrid mixtures are carried out, where in one case the (+) strand is labeled and in the other case the (-) strand is labeled. In the following, two chemicals are employed for the cleavage and therefore 2 x 2 reaction mixtures are needed. With all mixtures, one should be aware that radioactivity is being handled; therefore, gloves must be worn and all contaminated articles must be disposed of properly.

6. Pipet 7µl of the two 15µl hybrid mixtures from paragraph 5 into each of four Eppendorf tubes (1-4). Thus, the mixture containing the labeled (+) strand is in tubes 1 and 2, and the mixture containing the labeled (-) strand is in tubes 3 and 4. In tubes 1 and 3, the hydroxylamine reaction is performed; in tubes 2 and 4, the osmium tetroxide reaction.

7. Add 24µl hydroxylamine solution to tubes 1 and 3, mix well and incubate for 30min at 37°C. Then add 240µl stop buffer and 750µl ice-cold 100% ethanol. Chill at -70°C for 30min and spin in a microcentrifuge for 15min at 13,000rpm. Rinse the pellet twice with 80% ethanol, then dry in a vacuum-speed centrifuge.

7. Hydroxylamine solution: Dissolve 1.39g hydroxylamine in 1.6ml aqua bidest. while slightly heating. Add approximately 1ml diethylamine to adjust the pH value to 6.0. The solution can be stored for about 10 days at 4°C.
Stop buffer: 0.3M sodium acetate (pH 5.4), 0.5mM Na_2-EDTA, 30µg/ml tRNA. The solution should always be freshly prepared, or the tRNA carrier should be freshly added to the sodium acetate/Na_2-EDTA stock solution.

8. Add 2.5µl 10x osmium tetroxide buffer and 15µl 2% osmium tetroxide in tubes 2 and 4 on ice. Mix well (the solutions will turn yellow) and, while constantly shaking, incubate at 37°C for 7.5min. Then incubate again on ice and add 240µl stop buffer as well as ice-cold absolute ethanol. Chill at -70°C for 30min and spin in a microcentrifuge for 15min at 13,000rpm. Rinse the mixture twice with 80% ethanol, then dry in a vacuum-speed centrifuge.

9. Add 50µl 1M piperidine in tubes 1-4, mix vigorously. Incubate at 90°C for 30min. Chill on ice, add 50µl 0.6M sodium acetate (pH 5.4) and 300µl ice-cold 100% ethanol. Chill at -70°C for 30min and

Procedure(cont.) *Comments(cont.)*

spin in a microcentrifuge for 15min at 13,000rpm. Rinse the mixture twice with 80% ethanol, then dry in a vacuum-speed centrige.

10. Completely dissolve the pellet in 10µl 100% formamide. Heat the sample for 5min to 90°C and immediately cool in ice to prevent renaturation.

10. Approximately 50-60% at least of the initial radioactivity should be in the tube.

11. The samples are loaded on a 5% denaturing polyacrylamide gel. Bromphenol-blue buffer added to the samples gives a help to check the position of the samples in the gel.

11. For the polyacryamide-gel technique, see chapter 10.

12. For autoradiography expose the gel for about 2-6 hours, as described in chapter 10.

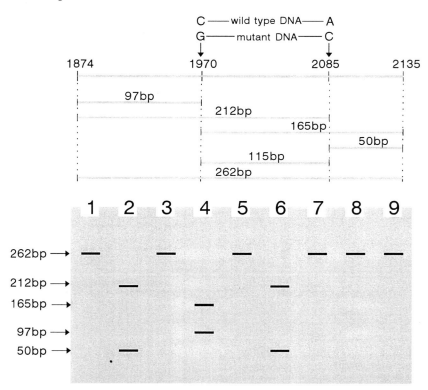

Figure 13.4: Chemical cleavage of the HIV-I nucleocapsid gene (BH10 nomenclature). Schematic representation of the gene region, the loci of possible base changes and the gene fragments resulting from cleavage. In the schematic gel picture, the anti-sense probe [(-) strand] was used for labeling in lanes **1, 2, 5 and 6**; the sense probe [(+) strand], in lanes **3, 4, 7 and 8**. Lanes **1, 3, 5, 7**, reaction with hydroxylamine; lanes **2, 4, 6, 8, 9**, reaction with osmium tetroxide. Lane **9** wild-type DNA. Lanes 1-4, HIV-I isolate 34B; lanes **5-8**, HIV-I isolate 12IK. Results: Lane **2** detects the point mutation "C" in the (+) strand of the 34B isolate; lane **4**, the point mutation "C" in the (-) strand of the same isolate. Isolate 12IK only shows the point mutation "C" at locus 2085 (lane **6**).

13.4. Denaturing gradient gel electrophoresis (DGGE)

Due to their different melting temperatures, two double-stranded DNA fragments differing in single bases can be physically separated from each other through a standard polyacrylamide gel with a linear ascending gradient of DNA denaturants - as, e.g., formamide and urea or temperature. A single DNA fragment does not have a uniform melting temperature, but can be divided, according to its sequence, into melting domains of mostly 50-200bp. These melting domains are regions that melt at the same temperature (T_m for a given domain). The T_m value of the melting domains is mostly between 65°C and 80°C. If a single base is altered within a melting domain, the T_m value of that domain may change by more than 1°C. The domain having the lowest melting temperature (low-melting domain) is the first one to melt open in the gel (branched DNA fragment). The melting point of this low-melting domain must, of course, still be above the temperature at which the plates are heated in the gel apparatus. If, in the course of electrophoresis, the first domain melts open, the running behavior of the fragment in the gel changes - its mobility is retarded. Simply stated, the extent of mobility retardation is a function of the length of the low-melting domain melted open - the longer this region the greater the gel retardation. If two DNA fragments with an altered sequence in the low-melting domain are separated in a gradient gel, the one domain of the wild-type DNA fragment melts, e.g., at 65°C, while the corresponding domain of the mutant DNA altered by the mutation only melts at 68°C. Thereby, the two fragments are demonstrated in the gel at different heights. Base changes in the region having the highest melting temperature (high-melting domain) cannot be detected anymore, since the melting open of this region leads directly to the single-stranded state of the DNA fragment, resulting in a loss of sequence-dependent mobility. This problem can partly be solved by introducing, through a modified primer, a G-C clamp at the end of the PCR-generated fragment, resulting in a very high-melting domain (Myers 1985a, 1985b). With this modification, it becomes possible to detect about 90% of all DNA polymorphisms. The resolution and sensitivity of the system can be further improved if, beforehand, - similar to the cleavage system - the mutant DNA is hybridized with the wild-type DNA and a heteroduplex is thus formed (see Figure 13.3). // Einheitlich "Figure/Table" oder "figure/table"!// The reason why a mismatch in a heteroduplex contributes to improved resolution is that a single base mismatch contributes to a destabilization of the system, thereby increasing the differences in melting temperature.

The method of DGGE can, understandably, only be employed for the screening of DNA fragments, since the exact locus of the mutation cannot be determined by it. Velleman (1992) describes how the DGGE can be optimized for the detection of DNA polymorphisms. It is important to note that the range of the gradient must at first be chosen quite wide (e.g., 20-80% linear-gradient polyacrylamide gel). Once a gradient region has been identified, the separation by fragment mobilities can be intensified by narrowing the gradient to ±15% around the point of strand separation. After completed separation, the fragments can also be detected using a probe after performance of a southern blot, instead of by the radioactive hybrid complex (see Figure 13.3). This technique circumvents the procedure of heteroduplex preparation. The separation of the DNA fragments, which usually takes about 16 hours, is very much accelerated by the technique published by Raja et al. (1991). The authors employ the Phast system, about 8x5cm, for electrophoresis, use a 0.2mm acetate sheet between a 0.6mm spacer and the glass plates - which simplifies the handling of the 6% polyacrylamide gel - and detect the DNA heteroduplices with silver stain (see chapter 10.4). According to the authors, the whole procedure shortens the 16-hour electrophoresis run time to 20min.

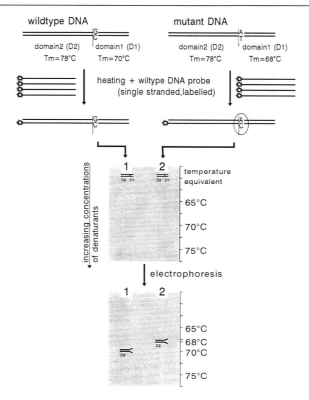

Figure 13.5: Schematic representation of the detection of point mutations by DGGE (based on R.M. Myers et al. 1988). After heating to 95°C, a single-stranded radioactively labeled DNA probe is added in excess to the mutant DNA and the wild-type DNA (as internal control). After cooling down of the reaction mixtures, heteroduplices form, contributing to a destabilization of domain 1. From the start, domains 1 and 2 differ in their T_m values, due to a point mutation (G-C vs. A-T). Both heteroduplices are loaded on the gel as double-stranded DNA (gel on the left). The gel system is characterized by a rising gradient of a denaturant equivalent to 65°C at the top and 75°C at the bottom. Domain 1 of the wild-type DNA heteroduplex melts at 70°C (lane **1**), while domain 1 of the mutant DNA already melts open at 68°C. The usual length of fragments that can be investigated in this way is between 100 and 1,200bp.

Procedure	Comments

Method 3: Denaturing gradient gel electrophoresis

The essential data for the polyacrylamide gel have already been given in chapter 10.4. It is important to be aware that we are here dealing with a constant-temperature gradient gel requiring special equipment. To be recommended are the heated carrier plates usually employed for DNA sequencing (water-jacketed

Procedure(cont.)   *Comments(cont.)*

electrophoretic apparatus). As a rule, the temperature of the plates is kept at 60°C. The usual acrylamide concentration of the gels is between 6% and 7%. Only where DNA fragments are smaller than 300bp, higher acrylamide concentrations of between 10 and 14% may be used. For the casting of the linearly increasing gradient gel, a gradient maker is needed.

1. Assemble the plates and seal the edges with agarose as described in chapter 10.4. The thinner the gels can be casted the better the resolution is. Therefore, spacers with approximately 0.2mm thickness should be used.

2. Preparation of the 40% acrylamide stock solution, 20x gel running buffer, 0% denaturing and 80% denaturing stock solutions.

2. Acrylamide stock solution: 100g acrylamide, 2.7g bisacrylamide, fill up with aqua bidest. to 250ml. In this stock solution, bisacrylamide is present at only half its usual concentration. The reduction in crosslinking thereby achieved (see also chapter 10.4) results in a better separation of the DNA fragments (see also Maxam and Gilbert 1980).

Caution: Acrylamide is neurotoxic. Therefore, only handle (weigh, etc.) this substance under a vent with gloves and oral protective mask.

20x gel running buffer: 800mM Tris base, 400mM sodium acetate, 30mM EDTA, pH 7.6.
For this, the following gram amounts must be used: 190g Tris base, 110g sodium acetate, 22.5g Na2EDTA. Fill up with aqua bidest. to about 1.95 liters, adjust the pH value to 7.6 with acetic acid and then complement to exactly 2 liters.

0% denaturing stock solution / 7% acrylamide:
44ml of the acrylamide stock solution, 12.5ml 20x gel running buffer. Fill up with aqua bidest. to a volume of 250ml.

80% denaturing stock solution / 7% acrylamide:
44ml of the acrylamide stock solution, 80ml deionized formamide (final concentration 32%), 85g ultrapure urea (5.6M), 12.5ml 20x gel running buffer.

3. Add 5µl TEMED and 80µl of a 10% ammonium persulfate stock solution to 8ml of the 80% denaturing stock solution, mix well and store on ice until the solution from paragraph 4 is also ready.

Procedure(cont.) *Comments(cont.)*

4. Add 5µl TEMED and 80µl of a 10% ammonium persulfate stock solution to 8ml of the 0% denaturing stock solution, mix well.

5. Put the solution from paragraph 3 into the left cylinder of the gradient maker, and the solution from paragraph 4, in the right cylinder.

5. Depending on the gel size, approximately 30-60ml solution are needed altogether. It is important that all air bubbles are removed from the gradient maker system.

6. Continual thorough mixing of the solutions in the cylinders of the gradient marker with a magnetic stirrer.

7. Slowly fill up the space between the two gel plates, the highest concentration (80%) of the denaturing solution being at the bottom of the gel.

8. Let the gel polymerize as described in chapter 10.4.

9. For the preparation of the heteroduplices, the following steps are performed: Approximately 0.1pmol of a labeled single-stranded DNA probe are thoroughly mixed with about 50ng of a PCR-generated DNA fragment (about 1/10 of a 100µl standard PCR reaction mixture), and the volume is filled up with aqua bidest. to 20µl.

10. Heat the mixture to 85°C for about 10min to separate the DNA strands.

11. Then incubate the mixture immediately at 50°C for 30min to anneal the probe (wild-type DNA probe).

12. After that, the reaction mixture is put on ice, 70µl aqua bidest. and 5µg carrier tRNA are added, and the whole mixture is precipitated with 100% ethanol (see Method 1 in this chapter).

13. Wash the pellets and dry in a vacuum centrifuge. Resuspend the mixture in 20µl loading buffer.

13. Loading buffer: 2g Ficoll 400 (final conc. 20%), 100µl 1.0M Tris-HCl (pH 8.0) (final conc. 10mM), 20µl 0.5M EDTA (pH 8.0), 10mg bromphenol blue (final conc. 0.1%). Fill up with aqua bidest. to 10ml.

14. Load 10µl each of the resuspended sample. Electrophoretic separation in the gel, with about 60V being applied for 16 hours.

14. It makes sense to electrophorese, as a control, the probe as well as wild-type DNA hybridized with the wild-type probe in a separate lane.

Procedure(cont.)   *Comments(cont.)*

15. Subsequent exposition of the gel as described in chapter 10.4. Analysis of the autoradiogram.

13.5. PCR single-strand conformation polymorphism (PCR-SSCP)

Single-strand conformation polymorphism relies on the principle that single-stranded DNA or RNA strands of different sequences exhibit different mobilities during electrophoresis in non-denaturing polyacrylamide gels. The strategy of the method is to amplify the segment of interest of a gene by PCR and then to compare the mobility of the denatured DNA with that of a reference segment of known sequence. Since single point mutations within a sequence already lead to a changed running behavior in the gel, this method is very well suited for detecting the presence of mutations in a segment of DNA. Under non-denaturing conditions, single-stranded DNA exhibits a folded structure, which is determined essentially by intramolecular interactions and thus by the sequence. The occurrence of mutational changes in the DNA sequence causes a changed folded structure. Thus, in

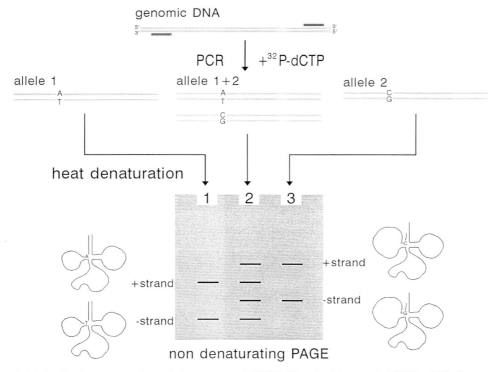

Figure 13.6: Methodical representation of the course of SSCP. The double-stranded-DNA PCR fragment is heat-denatured and the resulting single-stranded fragments are separated in a non-denaturing polyacrylamide gel. Fragments of equal length that, however, differ in sequence migrate in different positions, according to their conformational changes. It is important to note that complementary strands show altered mobility. The appearance of a point mutation (allele 2) causes an altered secondary structure and therefore a different migration pattern in the gel.

the SSCP analysis, the detection of a mutated sequence is determined by the changed mobility in the polyacrylamide gel electrophoresis. Length and sequence of the PCR fragment determine quite decisively the informativeness of the method. The demonstration of the different mobilities of individual PCR fragments is achieved either through incorporation of 32P-dCTP in the PCR fragment and autoradiography (Shuldiner 1992), ethidium bromide staining (Yap 1992), silver staining (Lo 1992) or with fluorescent PCR primers (5'carboxyfluorescein [FAM]-labeled or 6-carboxy-X-rhodanine [ROX]-labeled) followed by visualization on a UV transilluminator (Lo 1992). Orita et al. (1989a, 1989b) report that, using SSCP, they were able to demonstrate all mutations (12 of 12) in various human RAS gene PCR fragments (103 and 162bp fragment length, resp.). In addition, the method has hitherto been used for the detection of a polymorphism in Alu repeats (Orita 1990), in the human dopamine D2 receptor gene (Bolos 1990) and in the human p53 gene (Murakami 1991). Sarkar and co-workers (1992) have shown in a systematic study that, under optimized conditions and depending on the size of the PCR fragment, the SSCP method detects 92% (183bp fragment) and 59% (307bp fragment) of all mutations, resp.

Critical for the reproducibility of the method is, however, the electrophoresis procedure. Above all, heating of the gel during electrophoresis must be avoided under all circumstances, since this would alter decisively the running behavior of the samples. Favorable is a cooling of the gel plates to 5-7°C with the use of a water-jacketed electrophoretic apparatus (Danenberg 1992). Therefore, little ohmic heating, efficient cooling and the use of thin gels are essential. In addition, the composition of the gel matrix has considerable influence on the running behavior. In this respect, according to our own observations and to that of other authors (Sarkar 1992), a percentage of N,N'-methylene bisacrylamide of 5% of total acrylamide, a total acrylamide concentration of 5% (Hayashi 1991) and the addition of 5-10% glycerol has proved advantageous. Interpreting the results of SSCP gels may prove difficult if, on the one hand, in spite of point mutations being present in the DNA sequence, the migration pattern remains unchanged or if, on the other hand, in spite of the sequences being identical, one DNA strand is separated into two or more bands in the gel (Murakami 1991). This phenomenon can have several causes: 1. Slight differences in temperature between the region near the glass plate and the middle of the gel. 2. The strands are in a transitional state of two conformations (Hayashi 1991). 3. Incomplete denaturation of the double-stranded DNA fragment.

In order to solve such problems, esp. to increase the informativeness of the method, two working groups (Danenberg 1992, Sarkar 1992) have established the method of RNA-SSCP. The conversion of PCR-amplified DNA fragments to complementary RNA can be achieved easily through amplification primers of which one or two are modified by the addition of a T7 (5'TAA TAC GAC TCA CTA TA 3') or SP6 (5'CAT ACA CAT ACG ATT TAG GTG ACA CTA TA 3') polymerase promoter sequence. If only one primer is modified in this fashion, single-stranded RNA will be present after completed transcription, so that the usually necessary denaturation of double-stranded DNA can be dropped for the performance of the SSCP gel analysis. Further important differences between RNA- and DNA-SSCP are: 1. the larger repertoire of RNA secondary structures because of shorter hairpins from stable duplexes and because the 2'hydroxyl group is available for sugar-base bonds; 2. RNA can assume elaborate tertiary structures; 3. conformations of RNA molecules seem to be more sensitive to single-base substitutions. From this, a greater probability results for the RNA-SSCP being able to demonstrate single-base substitutions by electrophoretic differences. The first experimental results of the two working groups confirm this theoretically deduced hypothesis. Sarkar et al. (1992) showed that, in a 307bp fragment in which they were only able to detect an average of 58% of all mutations with DNA-SSCP, they found 77% of all mutations using RNA-SSCP. A similar superiority became obvious when examining a 2.6kb fragment of factor IX genomic sequence separated into nine PCR fragments (180bp-497bp). Only 35% of all 20 different sites could altogether be detected using DNA-SSCP, whereas RNA-SSCP indicated a considerable 70% of all mutations. Interestingly, Danenberg et al. (1992)

show that sense and anti-sense RNA strands of the same DNA segment of the p53 gene exhibit different conformational patterns, providing an additional opportunity for the detection of mutations. Both RNA strands can be produced easily by synthesizing the T7 sequence to one PCR primer and the SP6 sequence to the other primer and then transcribing the DNA amplicon once with T7 polymerase and again with SP6 polymerase in two separate reactions.

Procedure	Comments

Method 4: Single-stranded conformation polymorphism (SSCP)

1. The PCR is carried out essentially as described in the standard recommendations in chapters 2.1 and 10.4. Since, however, only small volumes are required for the gel analysis, PCR reactions can be carried out with a total volume of 5-10µl. For the performance of the SSCP gel analysis, the PCR fragment lengths should be between 120bp and a maximum of 220bp.

1. 70µM deoxynucleoside triphosphates (dNTPs), 0.1µl 32P-dCTP (3,000 Ci/mmol), 1µl 10x PCR buffer (100mM tris-HCl, 500mM KCl, 15mM MgCl2, 0.01% gelatin), 1U Taq polymerase, 100ng DNA, total volume 10µl. The reduction of the usual dNTP concentration to one-third improves the incorporation of the radioactively labeled dCTP.

2. 2µl of the original PCR reaction are mixed with 48µl of 95% formamide, 20mM EDTA, 0.05% bromphenol blue and 0.05% xylene cyanol. The mixture is heated to 95°C for 5min, followed by quick chilling on ice for 10min.

2. With DNA fragments, it is necessary to dilute the samples with stop solution before applying them to the gel, since otherwise reannealing of the denatured double-stranded DNA molecules often occurs. When performing an RNA-SSCP analysis, this is not necessary, since the RNA can already be present single-stranded. Danenberg et al. (1992) recommend two types of loading buffer for RNA-SSCP samples: (i) 4µl of the transcription reaction mixed with 1µl 50% glycerol or (ii) 8µl of the transcription reaction mixed with 1.8µl of 40% sucrose, both containing 0.05% bromphenol blue.

3. Casting of a 40cm 5% acrylamide/bis-acrylamide (19:1) gel (0.8mm) (Pharmacia LKB) containing 45mM tris-borate (pH 8.5), 3mM EDTA, 10% glycerol.

3. The quality of the DNA-SSCP analysis depends crucially on the electrophoresis conditions. Resolution and the number of conformations seen in the gel depend on the electrophoresis temperature, salt concentration, presence or absence of glycerol, and the ratio of acrylamide and bis-acrylamide. The necessity of the glycerol additive will be discussed controversially. Some authors report better results with adding 7% sucrose (Danenberg 1992).

Procedure(cont.)

4. After the samples have been loaded onto the gel, they are focussed by setting the power at 200 volts for 10min. The gel is then run at 30 watts at a constant 6°C for 6 hours.

5. After electrophoresis, the gel is dried and exposed to XAR film (Kodak).

Comments(cont.)

4. It is important to always remember loading a control fragment of known sequence (wild-type) every 5 lanes. This will later simplify evaluation.

References

1. Bolos AM, Dean M, Lucas-Derse S, Ramsburg M, Brown Gl, Goldman D. Population and pedigree studies reveal a lack of association between the dopamine D2 receptor gene and alcoholism. 1990, JAMA 264, 3156-3160

2. Caskey CT. Disease diagnosis by recombinant DNA methods. 1987, Science 236, 1223-1229

3. Cotton RGH. Detection of single base changes in nucleic acids. 1989, Biochem J 263, 1-10

4. Danenberg PV, Horikoshi T, Volkenandt M, Danenberg K, Lenz H-J, Shea LCC, Dicker AP, Simoneau A, Jones PA, Bertino JR. Detection of point mutations in human DNA by analysis of RNA conformation polymorphism(s). 1992, Nucl Acids Res 20, 573-579

5. Dutton Ch, Sommer SS. Simultaneous detection of multiples single-base alleles at a polymorphic site. BioTechniques 11, 700-702

6. Farr ChJ, Saiki RK, Erlich HA, McCormick F, Marshall Ch J. Analysis of RAS gene mutations inacute myeloid leukemia by polymerase chain reaction and oligonucleotide probes. 1988, Proc Natl Acad Sci USA 85, 1629-1633

7. Hayashi K. PCR-SSCP: A simple and sensitive method for detection of mutations in the genomic DNA. 1991, PCR Methods Applicat 1, 34-38

8. Kwok S, Kellog DE, McKinney N, Spasic D, Goda L, Levenson C, Sninsky JJ. Effects of primer-template mismatches on the polymerase chain reaction: human immunodeficiency virus type 1 model studies. 1990, Nucl Acids Res 18, 999-1005

9. Landegren U, Kaiser R, Caskey CT, Hood L. DNA diagnostics - molecular techniques and automation. 1988, Science 229-237

10. Lo Y-MD, Mehal WZ, Fleming KA, Bell JI, Wainscoat JS. Analysis of complex genetic systems by ARMS-SSCP: application to HLA genotyping. 1992, Nucl Acids Res 20, 1005-1009

11. Murakami Y, Hayashi K, Sekiya T. Detection of abberations of the p53 alleles and the gene transcript in human tumor cell lines by single-strand conformation polymorphism analysis. 1991, Cancer Res 51, 3356-3361

12. Murakami Y, Katahira M, Makino R, Hayashi K, Hirohashi S, Sekiya T. Inactivation of the retinoblastoma gene in a human lung carcinoma cell line detected by single-strand conformation polymorphism analysis of the polymerase chain reaction product of cDNA. 1991, Oncogene 6, 37-42

13. Myers RM, Fisher SG, Maniatis T, Lerman LS. Modification of the melting properties of duplex DNA by attachment of a GC-rich sequence as determined by

denaturing gradient gel electrophoresis. 1985a, Nucl Acids Res 13, 3111-3129

14. Myers RM, Fisher SG, Lerman LS, Maniatis T. Nearly all single base substitutions in DNA fragments joined to GC-clamp can be detected by denaturing gradient gel electrophoresis. 1985b, Nucl Acids Res 13, 3131-3145

15. Myers RM, Sheffiled VC, Cox DR. Detection of singel base changes in DNA: ribonuclease cleavage and denaturing gradient gel electrophoresis. In: Genome analysis - a practical approach. Ed.: KE Davies. 1988, IRL Press, Oxford - Washington, pp95-140

16. Newton CR, Graham A, Heptinstall LE, Powell SJ, Summers C, Kalsheker N, Smith JC, Markham AF. Analysis of any point mutation in DNA. The amplification refractory mutation system (ARMS). 1989, Nucl Acids Res 17, 2503-2516

17. Orita M, Suzuki Y, Sekiya T, Hayashi K. A rapid and sensitive detection of point mutations and genetic polymorphisms using polymerase chain reaction. 1989a, Genomics 5, 874-879

18. Orita M, Iwahana H, Kanazawa H, Hayashi K, Sekiya T. Detection of polymorphisms of human DNA by gel electrophoresis as single strand conformation polymorphisms. 1989b, Proc Natl Acad Sci USA 86, 2766-2770

19. Orita M, Sekiya T, Hayashi K. DNA sequence polymorphisms in Alu repeats. 1990, Genomics 8, 271-278

20. Saiki RK, Bugawan TL, Horn GT, Mullis KB, Erlich HA. Analysis of enzymatically amplified ß-globin and HLA-DQ_ DNA with allele-specific oligonucleotide probes. 1986, Nature 324, 163-166

21. Saiki RK, Walsh PS, Levenson CH, Erlich HA. Genetic analysis of amplified DNA with immobilized sequence-specific oligonucleotide probes. 1989, Proc Natl Acad Sci USA 86, 6230-6234

22. Sarkar G, Cassady J, Bottema CDK, Sommer SS. Characterization of polymerase chain reaction amplification of specific alleles. 1990, Anal Biochem 186, 64-68

23. Sarkar G, Sommer SS. Haplotyping by double PCR amplification of specific alleles. 1991, BioTechniques 10, 436-440

24. Sarkar G, Yoon H-S, Sommer SS. Screening for mutations by RNA single-stranded conformation polymorphism (rSSCP): comparison with DNA-SSCP. 1992, Nucl Acids Res 20, 871-878

25. Shuldiner AR, Tanner K. Detection of point mutations by SSCP of PCR-amplified DNA after endonuclease digestion. 1992, BioTechniques 12, 64-66

26. Sommer SS, Groszbach AR, Bottema CDK. PCR amplification of specific alleles (PASA) is a general method for rapidly detecting known singel-base changes. 1992, BioTechniques 12, 82-87

27. Velleman SG. A method for empirically optimizing the detection of DNA polymorphisms in genomic DNA by denaturing gradient gel electrophoresis. 1992, BioTechniques 12, 521-524

28. Wood WI, Gitschier J, Lasky LA, Lawn RM. Base composition-independent hybridization in tetramethylammonium chloride: a method for oligonucleotide screening of highly complex gene libraries. 1985, Proc Natl Acad Sci USA 82, 1585-1588

29. Wozney JM. Using a purified protein to clone its gene. 1990, Methods Enzymol 182, 738-751

30. Wu DY, Ugozzoli L, Pal BK, Wallace RB. Allele-specific enzymatic amplification of ß-globin genomic DNA for diagnosis of sickle cell anemia. 1989, Proc Natl Acad Sci USA 86, 2757-2760

31. Yap EPH, O'D.McGee J. Nonisotopic SSCP and competitive PCR for DNA quantification: p53 in breast cancer cells. 1992, Nucl Acids Res 20, 145

32. Ye S, Humphries St, Green F. Allele specific amplification by tetra-primer PCR. 1992, Nucl Acds Res 20, 1152

14. Non-Radioactive, Direct, Solid-Phase Sequencing of Genomic DNA Obtained from Polymerase Chain Reaction

In the last few years DNA sequencing has become increasingly important to molecular biology and biotechnology. There is an effort to determine the sequence of the complete genome of different species, and this requires technically easy, automated procedures which are reproducible and give the best results.

Here, we describe a solid-phase protocol for automated direct sequencing of genomic PCR products, using magnetic beads coated with streptavidin as solid support. This solid-phase method is very useful for template purification and strand separation of DNA obtained from polymerase chain reaction, as well as for high quality sequencing. The method can easily be automated as well.

The two most widely used methods for the sequence analysis of DNA fragments are the enzymatic synthesis of DNA fragments (Sanger 1977) and the base-specific cleavage of DNA (Maxam 1980). Although these methods are relatively simple and provide reliable results, radioactive detection (^{32}P or ^{35}S isotopes) presents some serious disadvantages: 1. Contact with radioactive material is not harmless and therefore entail relaively high investment costs (isotope laboratory, safety devices). 2. The costs incurred when disposing of radioactive waste are now very great. 3. Radioactive samples have relatively short half-lives and, because of this, cannot be stored very long before they are used. 4. The interpretation and execution of radioactive experiments is time consuming.

Leroy Hood (1986) brought new vigor to the search for alternatives to sequencing with radioisotopes. He used four different fluorescent markers, one for each nucleotide (A, C, G, T), to develop a non-radioactive method of sequencing.

Until recently, sequencing methods have required an electrophoretic separation in the polyacrylamide slab gel format. In spite of some simplification and standardization, these gels are prone to variability due to differences among commerical sources of reagents and differences induced during the polymerization process (for details see also chapter 10.4). The development of methods using capillaries filled with polyacrylamide gel (Cohen 1988) has provided an alternative to conventional sequencing gels. These new methods offer a number of advantages, including: faster runs, higher sensitivity, improved electrophoretic separation, more sensitive fluorescence detection and a potential for automation (Karger 1991, Zagursky 1990). Capillary gel electrophoresis has some problems, but it seems to have the highest potentil for a complete automation of the process of nucleic acid sequencing. For instance, the development of a stable separation phase would allow much more automation of sample delivery. Complete automation would make capillary slab gel electrophoresis a very attractive alternative to the slab gel systems currently, particularly if this reduces costs.

So far, several automated sequencing systems have been designed using different fluorescent-dye-labeled primers or terminators (Knight 1988). The principle of this sequencing method is based on Sanger's enzymatic sequencing method employing chain-terminating dideoxynucleotides (Sanger 1977). Four primers were used, each one labelled with a different fluorescent dye. Each primer is used in a separate reaction, which include one of the four dideoxynucleotides. Because each of the four dyes fluoresces at a different wavelength it is possible to perform the electrophoresis on a single lane of a polyacrylamide gel. During gel migration, the fluorescently labelled DNA fragments are excited by an argon ion laser at a fixed position. Detectors register the fluorescent-dye-specific signal and give the user the analyzed sequencing data in the form of chromatograms.

Although the electrophoresis is performed on a denaturing gel and at high temperatures, to avoid secondary structures and the consequent anomalies in electrophoretic mobility, there are still problems in determining DNA sequences with high GC contents. The difficulty lies in so-called "band compressions". To reduce this phenomenon, it is best a) to substitute ITP for GTP (Mills 1979) and b) to replace dGTP by c^{7}dGTP if a particularly high GC content is present (Mizusawa 1986). It might also be possible that A residues cause such "band compressions". In this case, an improvement is achieved by the use of c^{7}dATP instead of ATP (Jensen 1991).

Several enzymes are useful for dideoxy chain-terminating sequencing (Sambrook 1989). The bacteriophage T7 DNA polymerase Sequenase™, particulary *Sequenase™* version 2.0, appears to be the preferable enzyme because of its high processivity (processivity is an important factor in reducing background phenomena in sequencing gels) and its high rate of polymerization. In addition, it tolerates nucleotide analogs such as dITP and 7-deaza-dGTP. *Sequenase™* version 2.0 completely lacks 3'-5'exonuclease activity. The sequencing data produced by *Sequenase™* show a high uniformity of signal intensity for several hundred nucleotides (the data are even more uniform when manganese [Mn^{2+}] is present [Tabor 1989]). Taq DNA polymerase produces signals which vary in intensity much more than those of *Sequenase™*. The advantage of using the thermostable Taq DNA polymerase, however, is that we can perform sequencing reactions at elevated temperatures. This leads to a more stringent primer-to-template association and to a reduction of secondary DNA structures (for example, GC-rich regions). Using *Sequenase™*, a long elongation run, 30 minutes or longer, can lead to unusually weak signals. This phenomenon is caused by a sequence specific pyrophosphorolysis (reverse reaction of polymerization) catalyzed by the polymerase. However, with the addition of sufficient inorganic pyrophosphatase to the termination reaction this effect can, fortunately, be eliminated (Tabor 1990).

14.1. Generation of single-stranded DNA fragments

To perform DNA sequencing under optimal conditions it is necessary to obtain a well purified and single-stranded DNA template. Additional primers and dNTP's have to be removed from the amplified DNA, because they will disturb the sequencing reaction; furthermore, a single-stranded DNA template is necessary to avoid the reassociation of the two amplified strands.

A number of methods for generating single-stranded DNA have been described:
1. Generation of single-stranded DNA by asymmetric polymerase chain reaction (Gyllensten 1988,

Gyllensten 1989, Wilson 1990, ABI 1989).
2. Generation of single-stranded DNA by blocking-primer PCR (Gyllenstein 1989).
3. Separation of single-stranded DNA from a denaturing polyacrylamide gel (Gyllensten 1989).
4. Production of single-stranded DNA by addition of complementary single-stranded DNA following polymerase chain reaction (Gal 1989).
5. Exonuclease digestion of the phosphorylated strand of the double-stranded PCR product (Higuchi 1989).
6. Immobilization of amplified biotinylated double-stranded DNA by avidin and strand-specific elution using alkali:
   a) Affinity agarose gel (Stahl 1988, Mitchell 1988),
   b) Capturing biotinylated PCR product using streptavidin-coated magnetic beads (Syvänen 1991, Hultman 1991, Jones 1991, Kaneoka 1991).

There are two major advantages to single-stranded DNA sequencing:
1. The required amount of DNA template is less than that for double-stranded DNA sequencing; therefore, a smaller amount of starting DNA is sufficient.
2. Single-stranded DNA template does not present the problem of rapid reassociation of the amplified strands, so the complementary strand will not compete with the annealing of the sequencing primer. Consequently, the "length of read" and the accuracy in base assignment are improved.

The disadvantage of single-stranded DNA sequencing is that the generation of single-stranded DNA is associated with additional steps prior to the sequencing reaction and is, consequently, more time-consuming. Also, most procedures lead to a loss in the yield of the amplified DNA template. Furthermore, the isolation of single-stranded DNA from a strand-separating gel involves the risk of cross-contamination with other PCR products.

Considering the advantages and disadvantages described above, we decided to perform DNA sequencing with the solid-phase method using streptavidin-coated magnetic beads. Another reason for this decision was that we have developed a fully automated method for the biotin-streptavidin-mediated template preparation and sequencing reaction in a 96-well microtiter plate.

The biotinylated PCR product is produced using a 5' biotin-labeled (for biotinylation see chapter 20) amplification primer (forward primer, P1) containing the specific sequence and a 5'sequence identical to that of the M13 universal fluorescent sequencing primer (ABI), and a non-biotin-labeled amplification primer (reverse primer, P2) containing the specific sequence of the 3'primer and a 5'sequence identical to that of the reverse M13 fluorescent sequencing primer (ABI). For PCR, the primers are used in an equimolar ratio. After PCR, the specific biotinylated amplification product is bound to streptavidin-coated paramagnetic beads, followed by alkaline elution of the non-biotinylated strand. Both amplified strands present suitable templates for (manual and automated) fluorescent single-stranded sequencing. The beads with

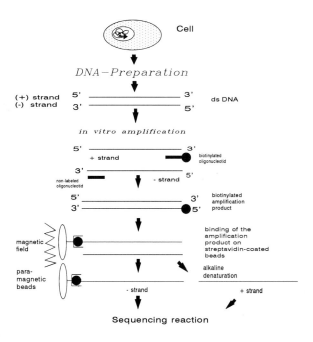

Figure 14.1: Schematic flow-sheet demonstrating the procedure of the biotinylation of PCR fragments followed by the strand separation with streptavidin coated paramagnetic beads.

the immobilized single-stranded DNA are used for solid-phase sequencing performed with the reverse M13 sequencing primer, because this strand contains its complementary sequence; likewise, sequencing of the eluted non-biotinylated strand is performed with the M13 universal sequencing primer.

For some complex DNA samples we recommend a nested amplification method. The first PCR reaction uses two primers containing the specific sequence only. The mean size of the amplification products designed for outer PCR is about 1 kb. We don't run these amplification products in an agarose gel. We take an aliquot (usually 1µl of a 25µl PCR reaction) and put it directly into the inner, or secondary, PCR. The amplification products of the second PCR reaction, which have a length of between 400 and 500 bp, are detected in an agarose gel to demonstrate the expected amplification product and its approximate amount (see Figure A, A73).

Here, we describe a solid-phase sequencing protocol performed with Sequenase™ and a sequencing protocol for the eluted strand performed with Taq polymerase. Why do we use two different DNA polymerases? Looking for single point mutations requires sequencing data of high accuracy. Therefore, both single strands need to be sequenced. Sequenase™ is not always able to determine all bases - in some cases we find two to five bases which are unreadable because of a high background or false termination events. For this reason, we perform sequencing reactions of the eluted strand with Taq polymerase. This usually leads to good sequencing data from those regions which are problematic for Sequenase™ (see Figure B, A74).

We perform sequencing reactions with reagents from Applied Biosystems, Foster City, USA. The automated sequence analysis is carried out on a 373A sequencer. Streptavidin-coated magnetic beads, Dynabeads M280-Streptavidin, are obtained from Dynal AS, Norway. A neodymium-iron-boron permanent magnet, MPC-96, is used to sediment beads in the microtiter plate during the removal of the supernatant and washing procedures. Apart from some modifications, we use reagents and amounts recommended by the manufacturers.

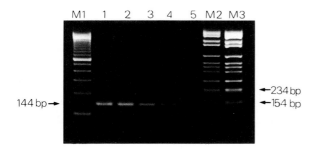

Figure 14.2: Agarose gel analysis of a 144bp PCR fragment (5SrRNA) from Legionella pneumophila (ATCC 43110 Oxford). 10µl, 7.5µl, 5µl, 2.5µl and 1.25µl (lane **1 to** 5) of a 100µl PCR sample were separated in a 3% agarose/Nusieve™ gel in 1xTBE buffer. Molecular weight markers: M1: 1µl 100bp-ladder (Gibco BRL), M2 and M3: 1µl and 2µl, respectively of the Boehringer VI marker (Boehringer Mannheim. PCR products and markers were visualized by ethidium bromide staining (for more details see also Fig. A, pp   ).

14.2. Sequencing of Biotinylated PCR Products

Procedure	Comment

Method 1: Manual sequencing procedure

Dynabeads, M280 Streptavidin (Dynal AS, #112.05) are paramagnetic polystyrene beads with a diameter of 2.8μm, a specific gravity of 1.3g/cm^3 and a surface area of 3-8m^2/gram. Commercially available Dynabeads M280 Streptavidin suspension contains 6-7 x 10^8 beads per ml dissolved in PBS (0.1% BSA, 0.02% NaN$_3$, pH 7.4).

Binding capacity: minimum of 300pmol biotin per mg beads. The amount of biotinylated DNA produced is essentially dependent upon the quality grade of the biotin. 1mg Dynabeads (ca. 100μl) bind about 200pmol oligonucleotides or 25pmol of a 300bp double-stranded fragment, respectively.

A. Preparation of Dynabeads:

Procedure	Comment
1. Pipette 40μl Dynabeads into a 96-well microtiter plate.	1. Store Dynabeads at 4°C and, on opening, take care to guard against bacterial contamination. Extract with sterilized equipment only and, before handling the beads mix the stock solution well in a flexible assay plate (Falcon™, Becton Dickinson Lab., #3911).
2. Add 40μl of binding buffer, shake briefly, place the microtiter plate on the MPC-96 until the beads are completely separated (usually about 20 sec), remove and discard the supernatant.	2. Binding buffer: 10mM TrisHCl, pH 7.5, 100mM NaCl, 1mM EDTA, 0.15% Triton X 100. Subsequently filter sterilize. If the buffer is autoclaved, salt complexes develop. Magnetic Particle Concentrator MPC-96 for microtiter

Procedure(cont.)   *Comments(cont.)*

	plate (Dynal AS, Norway, #120.05).
3. Remove the microtiter plate from the MPC, resuspend the beads in 40µl binding buffer.	
4. Restore the microtiter plate to the MPC, separate the beads, remove and discard the supernatant.	
5. Remove the microtiter plate from the MPC, resuspend the beads in 40µl binding buffer, add 27µl of 20x SSPE buffer plus 40µl biotinylated PCR product, shake well	5. 20x SSPE buffer: 3M NaCl, 2mM $NaH_2PO_4 \cdot xH_2O$, 2mM EDTA. Subsequently filter sterilization.
6. Tape up the microtiter plate, incubate the reaction components for 30 min at 37°C in a waterbath, if possible with gentle rotation.	6. During incubation, biotinylated PCR product is bound to the beads by using the streptavidin bridges.
7. Separate the beads, now coated with the biotinylated DNA fragment, by placing the microtiter plate on the MPC, remove and discard the supernatant.	
8. Remove the microtiter plate from the MPC, resuspend the beads in 100µl binding buffer, shake well.	
9. Restore the microtiter plate to the MPC, separate the beads, remove and discard the supernatant.	
10. Remove the microtiter plate from the MPC, add 50µl of denaturation buffer, resuspend the beads thoroughly, incubate the reaction components for 3 min at room temperature.	10. Denaturation buffer: 0.1M NaOH, 0.04mM EDTA.
11. Restore the microtiter plate to the MPC, separate the beads completely, remove the supernatant, but do not discard; rather, place the supernatant in a new reaction tube and quickly neutralize with 5µl 1M HCl (for further instructions, see "Sequencing of the non-biotinylated strand").	11. The supernatant contains the non-biotinylated strand that must be kept for further sequencing.
12. After removing the microtiter plate from the MPC, resuspend the beads in 200µl binding buffer.	
13. Place the microtiter plate on the MPC, separate the beads, remove and discard the supernatant.	

Procedure(cont.)   *Comments(cont.)*

14. Remove the microtiter plate from the MPC, resuspend the beads in 16µl doubly distilled water.

B. Solid-Phase Sequencing:

1. Distribute the resuspended beads into four different tubes ("A"-, "C"-, "G"- and "T"-reaction) as follows:

Pipetting scheme :

Reagents	A	C	G	T
Dynabeads	2µl	2µl	6µl	6µl
5x buffer	1µl	1µl	3µl	3µl
M13 rev.primer	1µl (JOE)	1µl (FAM)	2µl (TAMRA)	2µl (ROX)
total volume	4µl	4µl	11µl	11µl

Pipette together the reaction components as described, centrifuge briefly, resuspend the beads carefully.

2. Incubate for 5 min at 65°C in a heating block. Switch off the Thermoblock, leave the reaction tubes in the Thermoblock for further 5 min, let the reaction tubes stand for a further 5 min at room temperature. Then place on ice for 5 min. Centrifuge briefly to collect any condensat.

3. Prepare the enzyme dilution before starting the termination reactions. Dilute the Sequenase DNA polymerase 1:6 with ice-cold dilution buffer.

1. Except for the M13 reverse primer, the sequencing reagents for solid-phase sequencing are from the Sequenase™ Dye-Primer Sequencing Kit, Applied Biosystems, # 401117 (the kit must be stored at -20°C). M13 Reverse Primer Kit, Applied Biosystems, #400929. The kit contains 80pmol of the "A"- and "C"-specific primers, JOE and FAM, plus 160pmol of the "G"- and "T"-specific primers, TAMRA and ROX. For this protocol, the concentration of each primer is 0.4µM (0.4pmol/µl). M13 reverse primer sequence: 5'-[JOE, FAM, TAMRA, ROX]-CAG GAA ACA GCT ATG ACC-3'.
Dye-labeled primers must be stored at -20°C in the dark. Before handling the primers, they must be thawed in the dark, vortexed and centrifuged briefly. During the pipetting steps, the primers should be kept on ice and in the dark as much as possible. It is recommended to aliquot the stock solutions. The 5x buffer is mixed by pipetting together equal volumes of 10x MOPS buffer (400mM MOPS, pH 7.5, 500 mM NaCl, 100mM $MgCl_2$) and 10x Mn solution (50mM $MnCl_2$, 150mM isocitrate); fresh 5x buffer should be prepared daily. The pipetting steps should be carried out on ice.

2. Annealing reactions

3. Sequenase™ Version 2.0 (USB)T7 DNA Polymerase (13U/µl) containing pyrophosphatase (12U/ml); enzyme dilution buffer (10mM Tris, pH 7.5, 0.1mM EDTA). The diluted enzyme must be stored on ice for no more than 60 min.

Procedure(cont.) *Comments(cont.)*

4. Add the different d/ddNTP termination mixes and the enzyme dilution to the annealed template reactions as follows:

Pipetting Scheme:

4. d/ddATP termination mix (1mM each of dATP, dCTP, dTTP, c⁷dGTP, 3.3µM ddATP); d/ddCTP termination mix (1mM each of dATP, dCTP, dTTP, c⁷dGTP, 3.3µM ddCTP); d/ddGTP termination mix (1mM each of dATP, dCTP, dTTP, c⁷dGTP, 3.3µM ddGTP); d/ddTTP termination mix (1mM each of dATP, dCTP, dTTP, c⁷dGTP, 3.3µM ddTTP)

Reagent	A	C	G	T
d/ddNTP Mix	d/ddATP 1µl	d/ddCTP 1µl	d/ddGTP 2µ	d/ddTTP 2µl
Diluted Enzyme	1µl	1µl	2µl	2µl
Total Volume including volume of annealing reaction	6µl	6µl	15µl	15µl

When adding the diluted enzyme, it is recommended that the reaction components be thoroughly mixed- incomplete mixing may cause "stops" in the sequence.

5. Incubate the reaction components for 30 min at 37°C in a heating block.

5. Termination reactions: Incubation time can vary between 5 and 40 minutes. An incubation time of about 30 min seems to give the best results.

6. Place on ice for 5min and centrifuge briefly.

6. Place on ice to stop the reactions, centrifuge briefly to collect any condensate.

7. Add the contents of the "A"-, "C"- and "G"-tubes to the "T"-tube for each template

8. Place the reaction tube on the MPC, separate the beads completely, remove and discard the supernatant.

9. Resuspend the beads in 5µl of formamide/EDTA (6:1).

9. Gel-loading mixture containing deionized formamide and 50mM EDTA at a ratio of 6:1.

10. Heat the samples for 2 min at 72°C, restore the reaction tubes to the MPC, separate the beads, remove the supernatant and load it directly on a sequencing gel.

10. Denaturation.

Procedure(cont.)

11. Resuspend the beads in 40µl binding buffer and store them at 4°C

Comments(cont.)

11. The resuspended beads, still coated with the "original" biotinylated single-stranded PCR fragment, present a suitable template for further solid-phase sequencing reactions. It is possible to perform 3 to 4 further sequencing reactions with this template.

Only the supernatant which contains the newly synthesized dye-labeled strands is loaded on the sequencing gel for electrophoresis and automated sequence analysis. The electrophoresis is carried out on a 6% polyacrylamide sequencing gel.

Gel components (per 100 ml):
50g urea (BRL, #540-5505),
15 ml 40% acrylamide stock solution [acrylamide (BIO-RAD Lab., #161-0107) and bis-acrylamide (BIO-RAD Lab., #161-0201) diluted 19:1 in deionized, distilled water stored at 4°C in the dark for up to 1 month],
1-2g mixed-bed, ion-exchange resin (Amberlite, Serva Corp., #40711).
Adjust the volume to 90 ml with dH_2O.

Stir the solution while gently heating (not more than 50°C) until all urea crystals have dissolved completely. Add 10 ml of 10x TBE buffer. (10x TBE stock solution (per liter): Tris base 108.0g (BIO-RAD Lab., #161-0719), Boric acid 55.0g (Merck Corp., #165.1000), EDTA 8.3g (Sigma Corp., #ED4SS). Vacuum-filter the solution through a 0.2µm filter for 2 min, transfer it to a beaker, add 500µl of 10% ammonium persulfate (BIO-RAD Lab., #161-0700, make fresh solution daily or store at 4°C for up to 1 week; avoid water "contamination" of solid APS, which would result in a loss of activity. Add 45µl TEMED (BIO-RAD Lab., #161-0800). Swirl gently for a few seconds and immediately pour he solution between prepared glass plates. To avoid air bubbles it is important not to interrupt the flow of the solution while pouring. Let the gel polymerize in a horizontal position at room temperature for at least 2 hours. The gel should be used within 48 hours after polymerization. For electrophoresis, prepare a fresh 1x TBE buffer, the stock solution described from above.

Procedure(cont.)   *Comments(cont.)*

C. Sequencing of the non-biotinylated strand

1. For precipitation of the non-biotinylated strand, add to the neutralized supernatant 5µl of 3M sodium acetate, pH 5.2 and 120µl of 95% ethanol. Vortex and store at -20°C for about 30 min.

2. Centrifuge in a microcentrifuge for 15 min at about 13.000 rpm.

3. Remove supernatant as much as possible

4. Wash the pellet by adding 300µl of 70% ethanol, vortex and centrifuge again for about 15 min at 13,000 upm.

5. Remove the supernatant and vacuum-dry the pellets in a vacuum centrifuge for 3-5 min.

         5. Do not overdry

6. Resuspend the pellet in 6µl deionized, distilled water.

7. Prepare four microcentrifuge tubes according to the four base-specific reactions "A", "C", "G" and "T"

8. Pipette the sequencing reagents and template as follows:

         8. Taq Dye Primer Cycle Sequencing Kit, -21M13, Applied Biosystems, # 401119, containing 5x cycle sequencing buffer (400mM Tris-HCl, pH 8.9, 100mM ammonium sulfate, 25mM magnesium chloride) AmpliTaq™ DNA Polymerase (Perkin Elmer Cetus).

40pmol of the "A"- and "C"-specific -21M13 dye primer JOE and FAM, plus 80pmol of the "G"- and "T"-specific -21M13 dye primers, TAMRA and ROX. For this protocol, the concentration of each primer (resuspended in TE buffer: 10mM Tris-HCl, pH 8.0, 1mM EDTA) is 0.4µM (0.4pmol/µl). -21M13 primer sequence: 5'-[JOE, FAM, TAMRA, ROX]-TAA AAC GAC GGC CAG TGC CA-3'.
d/ddATP termination mix (1.5mM ddATP, 62.5µM dATP, 250µM dCTP, 375µM c^{7}dGTP, 250µM dTTP);

Procedure(cont.)   *Comments(cont.)*

Pipetting Scheme

Reagents	A	C	G	T
5x Buffer	1µl	1µl	2µl	2µl
-21M13 primer	JOE 1µl	FAM 1µl	TAMRA 2µl	ROX 2µl
d/ddNTP Mix	d/ddATP 1µl	d/ddCTP 1µl	d/ddGTP 2µl	d/ddTTP 2µl
Template DNA	1µl	1µl	2µl	2µl
Diluted Taq	1µl	1µl	2µl	2µl
Total Volume	5µl	5µl	10µl	10µl

d/ddCTP termination mix (0.75mM ddCTP, 250µM dATP, 62.5µM dCTP, 375µM c^{7}dGTP, 250µM dTTP); d/ddGTP termination mix (0.125mM ddGTP, 250µM dATP, 250µM dCTP, 94µM c^{7}dGTP, 250µM dTTP); d/ddTTP termination mix (1.25mM ddTTP, 250µM dATP, 250µM dCTP, 375µM c^{7}dGTP, 62.5µM dTTP)

Storage and handling conditions see comments above (B) Solid-phase sequencing).

The pipetting steps should be carried out on ice.

Enzyme dilution:
     0.5µl AmpliTaq™ DNA Polymerase (8U/µl)
     1.0µl 5x cycle sequencing buffer
     5.5µl dH$_2$O
Mix well and centrifuge briefly.

9. Centrifuge briefly and overlay the sequencing reactions with 20µl light mineral oil.

9. Light mineral oil (Sigma Corp., #M-5904).

10. Place the tubes in a thermal cycler and perform the termination reactions using temperatures as follows:

10. Polychain™ thermal cycler (Polygen Corp., Germany).
Cycle sequencing is used to amplify sequencing signals in case only a small DNA template amount is available. The important element of cycle sequencing is the incorporation of label into the sequencing products, e.g., dye primers.

15 cycles	97°C	30 sec
	55°C	30 sec
	70°C	1 min
20 cycles	97°C	30 sec
	70°C	1 min

followed by cooling to 4°C

11. Add the contents of the "C"-, "G"- and "T"-tubes to the "A"-tube for each template, centrifuge briefly, pipette the reaction volume to a fresh tube. Be careful not to transfer any oil.

12. In order to precipitate the reaction, add 3µl of 3M sodium acetate, pH 5.2, and 60µl of 95% ethanol to each pooled sample. Vortex and place at -20°C for about 30 min.

13. Centrifuge in a microcentrifuge for 15 min at about 13,000 rpm.

14. Aspirate carefully and discard the supernatant.

15. Add 250µl of 70% ethanol to wash the pellet, vortex and centrifuge again for about 15 min at 13,000 rpm.

16. Remove the supernatant and vacuum-dry the pellet in a vacuum centrifuge for 2-5 min.

16. Do not overdry

17. Resuspend the pellet in 5µl of formamide/EDTA (6:1).

17. Gel loading mixture containing deionized formamide and 50mM EDTA at a ratio of 6:1
For complete resuspension of the pellet, mix well and heat the sample at 50°C for a few minutes if necessary.

18. Heat the sample for 2 min at 90°C and load it directly on a sequencing gel (for details see pp   )

18. Denaturation.

Procedure(cont.)   *Comments(cont.)*

Method 2: Automatic sequencing procedure

Several methods for fully automated DNA sequencing procedures have already been described (Zimmermann 1988, D'Cunha 1990, Koop 1990).

We have developed a fully automated method for generating single-stranded DNA using magnetic beads followed by a fluorescent sequencing procedure.

In the following, we describe the instrument we have developed with heating, magnetic and mixing functions (PolySeq™). The procedure (reagents, - amounts, pipetting steps, incubation times and temperatures) is, except slight modifications, similar to the procedure described above (Method 1: Manual sequencing procedure); the reactions are also performed in a 96-well microtiter plate.

The following design for automation is postulated:
1. Strong, simultaneously homogenic magnetic field in all 96 wells of the microtiter plate.
2. Agitation function
3. Temperature control up to 90°C
4. Simple adaptation to an existing pipetting robot

A further factor which is important is that the 96-well microtiter plate is immersed directly in the heating/magnet block, so that we have a satisfactory heat transfer between the block and the sample (we don't use any liquid interphase) and the ramp-time (the time required to heat the sample from temperature 1 to temperature 2) is short enough. (The polymerase does not work at non-optimal temperatures).

PolySeq™, which we conceived of, was constructed by Polygen Corp. (Frankfurt, FRG); the robotic workstation (Biomek 1000) which carries out the pipetting steps is from Beckman Instruments (USA).

The current version of PolySeq™ consists of a block with integrated temperature, magnet and agitation unit as well as a controller. Those have been constructed for the approach of a complete working station which can also linked to a pipetting robot, in our case the Biomek 1000. The heating block can accommodate a 96-well microtiter plate with a U-bottom (the mictrotiter plates we use are flexible plates from Falcon™ Becton-Dickinson, Lab. #3911) and has a regulation precision of ± 0.2°C from the temperature

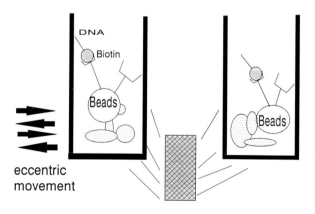

Figure 14.3: Schematic drawing of the principles of automated separation of paramagnetic beads in 96-well plate using the PolySeq™.

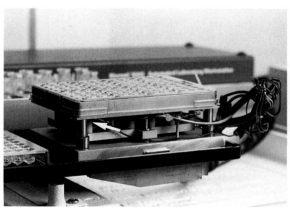

Figure 14.4: The prototype of PolySeq™ with heating block, agitation unit and the magnets at the top of the pins (arrow) - 1 per 4 wells - integrated in the robotic workstation Biomek 1000.

Procedure(cont.)

range from 30°C to 98°C. Regarding the whole block, the uniformity of the temperature achieves a tolerance of ± 0.4°C. The heating performance is 1°C/sec. The cooling is done by an inbuilt ventilator and the cooling performance is about 0.8°C. The heating block is easily agitated with a stroke of ± 1mm. Length and frequency of agitation can be regulated by the controller. The movement of agitation allows the uniform redistribution of magnetic beads after separation has taken place. The maximum volume which can be agitated without spilling of any liquid is about 200µl. In addition, PolySeq™ contains a magnet hoist supplied with neodymium-iron-boron magnets (Neo-Delta, IBS Magnet, FRG). Each individual magnet is located in the middle of a four-well group within the matrix of the microtiter plate. Such location of magnets affords an excentric separation of magnetic beads on the sidewall of each well. The hoist allows the magnets to enter the heating block. Height position as well as the delay time of the magnets inside the heating block is freely controlled through the controller. Depending on the total volume of material being processed, the complete separation of magnetic beads is achieved over 5-15 seconds.

The problem of evaporation occuring during the reaction in the uncovered microtiter plates and particularly during the heating steps is solved by adding dH_2O (usually 2µl) after the annealing step. This is necessary because evaporation increases the concentrations of the reagents and this is detrimental to the polymerase. Moreover, during the heating steps, we cover the microtiter plate with a flexible lid

Comments(cont.)

(Falcon™, Becton Dickinson Lab., #3913). When sequencing the non-biotinylated strand with Taq polymerase, we currently do not perform cycle sequencing. The termination reactions are performed at a temperature of 70°C for 15 min. The annealing step is similar to the procedure with Sequenase™: 5 min at 65°C followed by slow cooling to room temperature within 10 min. Although the pipetting steps are not performed at 4°C and cooling after the execution of the annealing and termination steps (4°C) is not possible with the current version of PolySeq™, no significant variation in sequencing quality has been observed.

In short, when comparing the quality of sequencing data obtained in manually performed sequencing reactions with that obtained with the robot and Polyseq™, both procedures give good results (see Figure C, p A75).

Advantages of the fully automated method we use are:

1. Standardization of sample handling and manufacturing
2. Pipetting errors all but eliminated
3. Greater sample security
4. Time saved compared with manual procedures (manual sequencing procedure including generation of single-stranded DNA and sequencing reaction for 24 samples takes about 12-18 hrs, fully automated sequencing procedures take about half the time)
5. Saves energy ("man power")
6. Standard range of sequenced base pairs about 15,000 per week.

References

1. Applied Biosystems. Fluorescence-based sequencing of templates amplified by asymmetric PCR. 1989, User Bulletin Number 13.

2. Cohen AS, Najarian DR, Paulus A, Guttman A, Smith JA, Karger BL. Rapid separation and purification of oligonucleotides by high-performance capillary gel electrophoresis. 1988, Proc Natl Acad Sci USA 85, 9660-63.

3. D'Cunha J, Berson BJ, Brumley RL Jr, Wagner PR, Smith LM. An automated instrument for the performance of enzymatic DNA sequencing reactions. 1990, BioTechniques 9, 80-90.

4. Gal S, Hohn B. Direct sequencing of double-stranded DNA PCR products via removing the complementary

strand with single-stranded DNA of an M13 clone. 1989, Nucl Acids Res 18, 1076.

5. Gyllensten UB, Erlich HA. Generation of single-stranded DNA by the polymerase chain reaction and its application to direct sequencing of the HLA-DQA locus. 1988, Proc Natl Acad Sci USA 85, 7652-56.

6. Gyllensten UB. PCR and DNA sequencing. 1989, BioTechniques 7, 700-708.

7. Higuchi RG, Ochman H. Production of single-stranded DNA templates by exonuclease digestion following the polymerase chain reaction. 1989, Nucl Acids Res 17, 5865.

8. Hultman T, Bergh S, Moks T, Uhlen M. Bidirectional solid-phase sequencing of in vitro-amplified plasmid DNA. 1991, BioTechniques 10, 84-93.

9. Jensen MA, Zagursky RJ, Trainor GL, Cocuzza AJ, Lee A, Chen EY. Improvements in the chain-termination method of DNA sequencing through the use of 7-deaza-2'-deoxyadenosine. 1991, DNA-Sequence-J DNA Sequencing and Mapping, 233-239.

10. Jones DSC, Schofield JP, Vaudin M. Fluorescent and radioactive solid phase dideoxy sequencing of PCR products in microtitre plates. 1991, DNA-Sequence-J DNA Sequenc Mapp 279-283.

11. Kaneoka H, Lee DR, Hsu K-C, Sharp GC, Hoffman RW. Solid-phase direct DNA sequencing of allele-specific polymerase chain reaction-amplified HLA-DR genes. 1991, BioTechniques 10, 30-34.

12. Karger AE, Harris JM, Gesteland RF. Multiwavelength fluorescence detection for DNA sequencing using capillary electrophoresis. 1991, Nucl Acids Res 19, 4955-62.

13. Knight P. Automated DNA sequencers. 1988, BioTechnology 6, 1095-96.

14. Koop BF, Wilson RK, Chen C, Halloran N, Sciammis R, Hood L. Sequencing reactions in microtiter plates. 1990, BioTechniques 9, 32-36.

15. Maxam AM, Gilbert W. 1980. Methods Enzymol 65, 499-559.

16. Mills DR, Kramer FR. Structure-independent nucleotide sequence analysis. 1979, Proc Natl Acad Sci USA 76, 2232-35.

17. Mitchell LG, Merril CR. Affinity generation of single-stranded DNA for dideoxy sequencing following the polymerase chain reaction. 1989, Anal Biochem 178, 239-242.

18. Mizusawa S, Nishimura S, Seela F. Improvement of the dideoxy chain termination method of DNA sequencing by use of deoxy-7-deazaguanosine triphosphate in place of dGTP. 1986, Nucl Acids Res 14, 1319-1324.

19. Sambrook J, Fritsch EF, Maniatis T. Sequencing techniques and stratagies, DNA polymerases. 1989, Molecular Cloning, A Laboratory Manual, 2nd edition, CSH, chapter 13.7.

20. Sanger F, Nicklen S, Coulson AR. DNA sequencing with chain-terminating inhibitors. 1977, Proc Natl Acad Sci USA 74, 5463-67.

21. Smith L, Sanders J, Kaiser R, Hughes P, Dodd C, Connell CR, Heiner C, Kent S, Hood LE. Fluorescence detection in automated DNA sequence analysis. 1986, Nature 321, 674-89

22. Stahl S, Hultman T, Olsson A, Moks T, Uhlen M. Solid phase DNA sequencing using the biotin-avidin system. 1988, Nucl Acids Res 16, 3025-38.

23. Syvänen A-C, Hultman T, Aalto-Setälä K, Söderlund H, Uhlen M. Genetic analysis of the polymorphism of the human apolipoprotein E using automated solid-phase sequencing. 1991, GATA 8, 117-123.

24. Tabor S, Richardson CC. DNA sequence analysis with a modified bacteriophage T7 DNA polymerase. Effect of pyrophosphorolysis and metal ions. 1990, J Biol Chem 265, 8322-28.

25. Tabor S, Richardson CC. Effect of manganese ions on the incorporation of dideoxynucleotides by bacteriophage T7 DNA polymerase and Escherichia coli DNA polymerase I. 1989, Proc Natl Acad Sci USA 86, 4076-80.

26. Wilson RK, Chen C, Hood L. Optimization of asymmetric polymerase chain reaction for rapid fluorescent

DNA sequencing. 1990, BioTechniques 8, 184-189.

27. Zagursky RJ, McCormick RM. DNA sequencing separations in capillary gels on a modified commercial DNA sequencing instrument. 1990, BioTechniques 9, 74-79

28. Zimmermann J, Voss H, Schwager C, Stegemann J, Ansorge W. Automated Sanger dideoxy sequencing reaction protocol. 1988, FEBS Letters 233, 432-436.

15. Application of PCR to Analyze Unknown Sequences

15.1. Inverse PCR

The polymerase chain reaction exhibits per se a method for readily amplifying characterized DNA regions whose borders are defined by the two primers employed in the PCR which are directed towards each other and encompass the target region. In each PCR cycle, primer extension yields a newly synthesized DNA strand containing a binding site for the opposite primer. Thus, repeated cycles lead to an exponential amplification of the target region. However, if the DNA sequence of interest lies outside of the characterized DNA region, then the requirement for primers complementary to both ends of the generated target DNA segment cannot readily be fulfilled and only a linear amplification into the unknown region can be performed using one primer during PCR. Three groups independently developed a method for overcoming this problem (Triglia 1988, Ochman 1988 and Silver 1989).

The method now known as the inverse polymerase chain reaction (IPCR) relies on initial digestion of the source DNA using restriction enzymes, circularization of the cleaved products (ligation), linearization of the circularized DNA with a restriction enzyme cutting within the characterized region (optional), and amplification of the circularized or linearized fragments employing primers which lie within the "core" DNA (characterized region) and are oriented in opposite directions. Due to the orientation of the primers, extension proceeds into the unknown flanking region,

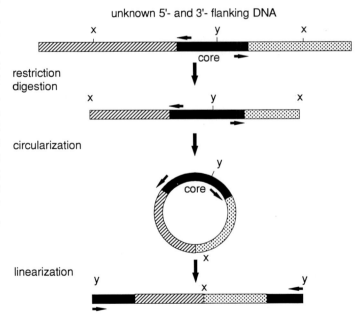

Figure 15.1. Scheme of the IPCR procedure for amplifying unknown 5'- and 3'-flanking sequences employing restriction enzyme "x" for initial genomic DNA template digestion, circularization (ligation) and linearization of the circularized DNA using the restriction enzyme "y".

crosses the junction formed by ligation of the compatible ends, and continues through to the opposite primer. Primer extension again yields DNA strands containing the complementary sequence of the opposite primer and exponential amplification ensues. Figure 15.1 schematically shows the steps outlined above.

The application of this technique can in many cases help circumvent cumbersome construction and screening of DNA libraries in order to walk hundreds or even thousands of base pairs into flanking DNA regions by repeating IPCR on each novelly characterized DNA sequence. Inverse PCR can also assist in the characterization of insertion sites of transposable elements or retroviruses or offer a method for establishing end specific probes to be used in further hybridization assays (Ochman 1988 and Silver 1989).

Digesting Source DNA and Circularization

Selection of a restriction enzyme for initial cleavage of source DNA depends on the known restriction map of the core region and should take into account the probable size of the resulting DNA fragment so that monomeric circularization is favored. Choice of a restriction enzyme in context with the known restriction map of the core region will determine whether the application of inverse PCR will unravel unknown flanking sequences to both sides or to only one side of the known sequence. In the first case the enzyme should not cut within the core region, while in the latter case the enzyme must cut within the core region close to the 3'-end of one of the primers. Figure 15.2 demonstrates the localization of the cleavage sites in order to pursue either one-sided amplification.

The size of the resulting DNA fragments to be circularized can be estimated by conventional Southern blot hybridization using a probe from the core region prior to attempting ligation. Fragments shorter than 200-300 base pairs are difficult to circularize (Shore 1981), while fragments larger than 3 kilo bases are not easily amplified during the PCR, especially, in a complex mixture. The restriction enzymes used should also, if possible, generate staggered ends as opposed to blunt ends, since these are ligated more efficiently (see section Restriction Endonucleases). A good choice for initial cleavage is an enzyme with a four-base recognition sequence. This will help avoid the generation of very large fragments and simultaneously allow manipulation of which unknown flanking sequence will be amplified in the PCR depending on the absence or the convenient location of a cleavage site in the core region (see figure 15.2).

Linearization

The need for this step is controversial. Silver *et al.* (1989) assert that linearization increases the efficiency of the PCR a 100-fold. They argue that covalently closed circular double-stranded DNA is a poor template for the first round of primer extension due to "snap-back" reannealing of the denatured DNA strands. Although inverse PCR can be carried out omitting this step (Ochman 1988), in cases in which the template is limiting, linearization will tend to enhance success. Should linearization be performed, then the selection of a six-base recognition sequence cutting between the 5'-ends of the primers will best assure that cleavage will not also occur in the unknown circularized segment in which case amplification would be precluded. An alternative to enzymatic linearization is random nicking by heating (Frohman 1988) or by mild DNAse treatment. Both approaches help to overcome the initial difficulties of amplifying circular DNA template in the first cycles but may adversely lead to extensive destruction of many templates.

Amplification

Amplification is carried out with the strategies in mind which were suggested in the section "PCR Optimization" (chapter 2).

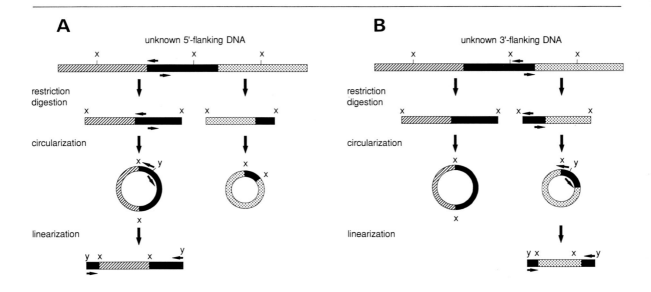

Figure 15.2. Selective amplification of either A. the unknown 5'-flanking sequence or B. the unknown 3'-flanking sequence. The relative position of the restriction enzyme "x" to the primer pair determines whether the 5'- or 3'-flanking sequence will be amplified selectively.

Procedure	Comments

Method 1: Inverse PCR

1. Digest 2-5µg of source DNA diluted in the 1 x restriction enzyme buffer supplied by the manufacturer with 10-40 units of the selected enzyme at the optimum temperature (37°C) for at least 2 hours. Suggested reaction volume: 50µl.	1. An excess of enzyme is necessary for complete digestion of genomic DNA. In this case, digestion should be performed overnight.

2. Confirm digestion by subjecting an aliquot to gel electrophoresis. Use a 1% (w/v) agarose gel (SeaKem) in 1 x TBE buffer.

2. 10 x TBE buffer: 0.89M Tris-base
　　　　　　　　　　0.89M boric acid
　　　　　　　　　　0.002M EDTA (pH 8.0)

If only a certain fragment length is required for circularization in the following procedure, then excise the appropriate fragments from the gel and elute using a method established in the laboratory.

3. Extract once with an equal volume phenol/chloroform and once with an equal volume of choroform. Ethanol precipitate (standard protocol) and resuspend in 50-100µl 1 x TE buffer.

3. Residual phenol must be removed in order to avoid denaturation of enzymes in subsequent steps.
If incompatible ends have been generated, then the following steps must be carried out prior to circularization: A. 3'-OH recessed ends can be filled in to form blunt ends by the addition of the Klenow enzyme and deoxynucleotides. B. 5' or 3' protruding ends can be removed by treating the DNA with S_1 or mung bean nucleases generating blunt ends (Cobianchi 1987).

4. For circularization, dilute 0.1 µg DNA (2-5µl) in ligase buffer to a final volume of 20µl, add 1 unit T4 DNA ligase (Boehringer, Mannheim) and incubate overnight at 15°C.

4. Ligase buffer:
　　50mM Tris-HCl pH 7.6
　　10mM $MgCl_2$
　　0.7mM ATP
　　10mM dithiothreitol (DTT)
　　1mM spermidin
　　1mg/ml bovine serum albumin

- Low DNA concentrations favor the formation of monomeric circularized molecules. The relative likelihood of one end of a molecule ligating with its other end, as opposed to the end of another molecule, is expressed in the equation

$$1900 / c \cdot (bp)^{1/2}$$

where c is the DNA concentration in µg/ml and bp the length in base pairs. For ratios greater than 1 almost all molecules will theoretically circularize (Sambrook 1989).
- T4 DNA ligase is the preferable enzyme, since either staggered complementary or blunt ends can be ligated to one another. In the latter case, more enzyme is needed for ligation. Optimal conditions for ligating DNA have been described by Dugaiczyk et al. (1975). Although the extent of circularization can be monitored

in an ethidium bromide agarose gel (ethidium bromide increases the mobility of covalently closed circles and decreases the mobility of linear DNA), this is rather difficult if the DNA fragments form a heterogenous population as is the case in this assay. Nevertheless, a mock ligation assay using the same reagents and an appropriate template will aid in determining whether components of the assay were faulty.

5. Phenol extract and ethanol precipitate the ligation reaction as described above. Resuspend in 50µl 1 x TE buffer.

6. Subject 10-20µl to restriction digestion for linearization. Add the appropriate amount of the concentrated restriction buffer to yield a 1 x concentration and 10-20 units of the selected enzyme. Incubate for the recommended time or overnight at 37°C.

7. Phenol extract, ethanol precipitate and resuspend in 20-40µl 1 x TE buffer.

8. Perform a standard PCR using approximately 1µg template, 10-30pmol of each primer, 0.2mM dNTPs and 1-2 units Taq polymerase in 50µl PCR reaction volume.

8. After initial denaturation at 95°C for 5 min, the standard PCR cycle programm we employ is composed of 35 cycles: denature at 95°C for 30 sec, anneal at 55-65°C (depending on Tm of the primer pair) for 30 sec, and extend at 72°C for 30 sec. Variations: If the DNA template is limiting, lengthen the annealing time to allow for screening of the right complementary sequence. Since the length of the novel flanking sequence which will be amplified is not known, it might be advisable to start with an extension time of 1 min or to lengthen the extension step in each cycle.

Evaluation:

One of the main difficulties in performing successful IPCR resides in the fact that individual steps cannot be easily monitored. Initial digestion of genomic template DNA can be visualized on a gel and satisfactorily judged whether complete or incomplete digestion has occurred. Restriction enzyme activity can be checked by digesting a known DNA substrate. As asserted by Silver (1991), circularization is probably the most crucial and difficult step in IPCR. Because of the complex nature of the genomic template DNA, the approach suggested to monitor circularization in IPCR can only yield circumstantial evidence regarding circularization of the target DNA. The second enzyme employed to relinearize circularized DNA can also have its drawbacks, if by chance this enzyme cleaves the circularized DNA at a position which leads to the physical separation of the two primers. However, if the assay was not jeopardized in one of these three essential steps, then IPCR still remains more powerful than approaches relying on a hemi-specific primer for amplification. The likelihood of two specific primers or nested specific primers leading to specific amplification and thus increasing the sensitivity of the assay is greater than in an approach employing hemi-specific primers.

15.2. Alternative methods to inverse PCR

15.2.1. "Alu-PCR"

It is known that all mammalian genomes contain short interspersed DNA sequences which are found up to 10^6 times in a haploid genome. These short interspersed repeated DNA sequences are referred to as SINES (Singer 1982). The major short repeated DNA sequence in the human genome is the Alu repeat sequence. Since the estimated copy number in the human genome is approximately 900,000 and repeated sequences are found ubiquitiously, the average distance between two Alu repeat sequences would be about 4 kilo bases (Britten 1968). A closer analysis of the distribution of repetitive sequences in the human genome, however, clearly demonstrated that SINES are more freqently found as clusters in distinct regions on a chromosome (Korenberg 1988). Because this holds true, it is possible to attempt establishing a new PCR method in order to unravel unknown sequences by designing primers with sequences from highly conserved Alu repeat regions and then performing PCR to amplify the intervening unknown DNA sequence. This approach was established by Nelson et al. (1989) and designated Alu polymerase chain reaction (Alu PCR).

Alu PCR was developed as a technique that could possibly circumvent the construction of libraries of somatic cell hybrids - rodent cells containing human chromosomes or subchromosomal fragments - in an endeavor to map the human genome. There are several factors which will influence the sensitivity, specificity and/or efficiency of the Alu PCR assay: 1. When attempting to perform an Alu PCR, it is initially not known just how Alu repeats are arranged on the target DNA. This may preclude any amplification at all, if no Alu repeats exist in a certain region or two Alu repeats are separated from each other by a long intervening sequence. The detection of unknown genomic DNA sequences or of cloned subchromosomal DNA fragments is thus biased. 2. If different mammalian genomes have been genetically engineered and exist combined, then pilot experiments are necessary to verify that the Alu-specific primers are only detecting Alu-specific sequences in one of the species but not in both. Highly conserved Alu repeat sequences in one species can also be highly conserved in another species, thus, allowing no discrimination between the two (Nelson 1989). 3. Depending on the orientation of the Alu repeat in the genome, it is either possible to perform Alu PCR using only one primer if

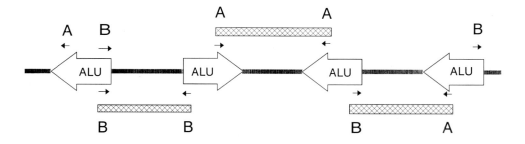

Figure 15.3. Fictive integration of Alu repeats (bars marked with "Alu") in genomic DNA and possible amplification products (hatched bars) when Alu repeats are in close proximity to one another using the selected primers A and B reflecting sequences from highly conserved regions of the repeat.

the Alu repeats are directed towards each other or it may be necessary to employ two Alu-specific primers oriented in opposite directions, if pairs of Alu repeats occur in the same orientation on the target DNA. Figure 3 schematically shows possible Alu PCR amplification of unknown DNA regions considering these facts.

Although this approach is biased by the distribution of Alu repeats, it has been reported to yield satisfactory results and has been employed to create probes for unknown sequences. A major advantage of this approach is the minimal handling of the sample which reduces the risk of contamination as well as the loss of valuable material otherwise promoted by additional steps demanding several reprecipitations throughout the procedure.

15.2.2. Targeted gene walking PCR

Targeted gene walking PCR is based upon the observation that a primer with only partial homology at its 3' end to a known or unknown DNA sequence may initiate Taq-mediated polymerisation. The combination of a "target" primer annealing to a known region of DNA and a "walking" primer exhibiting sufficient base pair annealing to an uncharacterized preexisting sequence either downstream or upstream of the targeted primer has been used in designing a modified PCR capable of amplifying a contiguous unknown DNA sequence (Parker 1991). Amplification of the target region occurs, if the "walking" primer is extended toward the "target" primer and the distance between the two primers is preferably under one kilobase, so that the PCR is still fairly efficient. To overcome some of the problems which might arise, if a walking primer binds at an undesirable distance or in the wrong orientation, a number of individual PCR reactions are performed parallel, employing an array of different "walking" primers. Even if this approach is chosen, it is clear that any "walking" primer can also anneal to multiple sites of the complex genomic DNA template and generate a large number of non-specific products. In order to differentiate between specific and non-specific products, Parker et al. (1991) included a second single cycle PCR using a kinased "internal" detection primer downstream of the target primer with no overlapping sequence. Figure 15.4 displays the basic set-up.

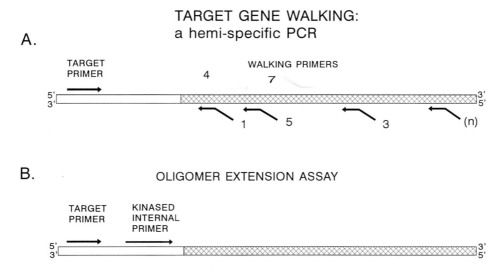

Figure 15.4: Targeted gene walking: A. PCR using a target primer and different walking primers in individual tube assays. B. Oligomer extension assay to detect specific amplification products using a kinased nested primer in a single cycle PCR. Unfilled region designates known DNA region, hatched area unknown DNA region.

The oligomer-extension products are then resolved on a gel, transferred to a nylon membrane and exposed to X-ray film. Positive bands are excised from the gel, eluted and an aliquot of each eluted DNA subjected to asymmetric reamplification using the "target" and appropriate "walking" primer in a ratio of 1:20. The "target" or "internal" primer was subsequently used for direct sequencing of the PCR product.

Employing "targeted gene walking" as an alternative method for resolving unknown flanking DNA sequences circumvents molecular modification of the template DNA. First, it is not necessary to cleave the DNA with a restriction enzyme or to purify the generated restriction fragments for subsequent enzymatic steps. No ligation step nor linearization of circularized DNA is involved. This definitely reduces the risk of contamination as well as the loss of valuable material more readily introduced by extensive manipulation and incomplete recovery. In addition, little time is needed to obtain preliminary results, because the isolated DNA is directly subjected to PCR. However, the method requires screening of a number of "walking" primers in order to detect which ones will lead to the amplification of the unknown region of interest. This can be somewhat tedious, since each "walking" primer can anneal at many different sites in the complex DNA mixture. Thus, some of the "walking" primers may never lead to sufficient amplification of the region of interest. If there is enough evidence that the PCR is yielding a sensible array of products, then detection of specific sequences using an "internal" kinased primer in a one cycled "nested" PCR as suggested by the authors (Parker 1991) can readily be managed technically.

15.2.3. "Panhandle PCR"

One of the limitations of setting up an efficient PCR assay to unravel unknown flanking DNA sequences is the use of one non-specific primer in the reaction as is the case in targeted gene walking. A very ingenious method for appending a known sequence to the end of the unknown sequence was devised by Jones et al. (1992). The method named the "panhandle PCR" is briefly described and illustrated in figure 15.5. As in

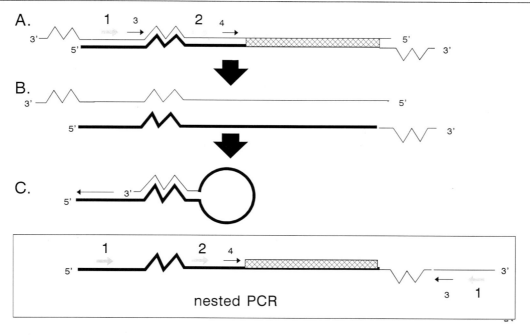

Figure 15. 5. Abridged illustration of panhandle PCR as described by Jones et al. (1992). A. Genomic template DNA is cleaved using a restriction enzyme to create 5' overhanging ends. A synthetic single-stranded oligonucleotide with a 3' sequence complementary to the 5' overhang, and a 5' sequence complementary to a sequence in the known region is ligated to genomic DNA restriction fragments: known double-stranded DNA sequence (thin and thick lines), unknown DNA sequence (hatched area), single-stranded appended oligonucleotides and region of complementarity (staggered lines). Primer pairs are depicted by identical arrows with diferent numbers. B. Denaturation of the construct. C. Panhandle formation of only the single-strand depicted by the thick line by allowing the complementary regions to hybridize to one another followed by a 3' extension. Nested PCR on the denatured panhandle DNA template is illustrated in the box.

most protocols, genomic DNA is first digested with a restriction enzyme to create 5'-overhangs at the ends of the generated restriction fragments. Subsequent treatment with calf intestinal alkaline phosphatase or partial fill-in using less than 4 dNTPs helps prevent self ligation and circularization of the restriction fragments. Synthetic single-stranded oligonucleotides containing 5' ends complementary to the 5'-overhang and an additional sequence complementary to a part of the known sequence (staggered sequence region) are then ligated to the genomic restriction fragments using T4 DNA ligase (figure 15.5A). These modified double-stranded restriction fragments with 3'-overhangs are denatured to yield single-strand DNA (figure 15.5B). Since denaturation and subsequent annealing occur under dilute conditions, intra-strand annealing is favored leading to annealing of the 3' appended sequence to the complementary region in the known portion of DNA. This produces a recessed 3' end which can prime extension, so that the sequence added is complementary to the sequence of the known 5' end of the original single strand transformed into the "panhandle"(figure 15.5C). The unknown sequence is now flanked by a known sequence at both ends. Since the "new" sequence at the 3' end is complementary to the sequence at the 5' end, one primer can anneal to one strand in the first PCR cycle and then prime the newly synthesized strand backin the second cycle. In the first PCR two primers are employed of which one functions as stated above (primer 1) and the other primes unidirectionally (primer2). The sensitivity and specificity of the assay other methods employing ligation of a specific sequence to the ends of restriction fragments, this method circumvents the problems that arise when the appended sequence is used in order to walk back to the sequence of the specific primer. The difficulty which resides in this approach is simply the fact that all restriction fragments with ligated specific sequence can be primed equally well, thus making it difficult for the specific polymerase chain reaction to take place between the ligated primer sequence. It can thus be difficult to optimize primer concentration, if the is increased by performing a nested PCR (primer pair 3 and 4). The PCR product can then be sequenced.

This approach to detecting unknown flanking sequences is superior to other methods. In contrast to ligated primer sequence is sacrificed for unspecific amplification. However, the method proposed by Jones et al. (1992) never uses the ligated sequence to prime strand synthesis in PCR.

This sequence is solely used to append a known sequence to the opposite end of single-strand DNA so that specific primer sequences can be used exclusively to prime one specific PCR - thus avoiding the amplification of a large number of unwanted products. Although the method presupposes knowledge of diverse basic techniques in molecular biology and many steps are needed in the procedure (endonucleolytic cleavage, dephosphorylation, ligation and DNA purification using glass beads - Geneclean), it remains an intriguing approach waiting to be explored.

13.5 "Rapid amplification of cDNA ends" (RACE)

Opposed to the methods described above which deal with the amplification of unknown DNA sequences, the method designated "RACE" offers an efficient method for amplifying and unravelling unknown 5' and 3' mRNA sequences provided that a short sequence of an exon is known so that primers oriented in the 3' and 5' direction can be designed (Frohman 1988). In order to amplify the unknown 3' end of a mRNA, mRNA is first reverse transcribed using a primer with 17 dTTP residues at its 3' end which will anneal to the natural poly(A)-tract of a mRNA and an adapter sequence at its 5' end which can be designed to contain a rare restriction enzyme recognition sequence for cloning purposes and also be used as a primer on its own for PCR. Second, a specific primer sequence from the known region complementary to the synthesized (-) strand and directed toward the 3' end is used to prime (+) strand synthesis. Cyclic amplification is then carried out using the adapter primer sequence and the specific primer (3'-RACE). The unknown 5' sequence of a mRNA is amplified by first reverse transcribing using a specific primer sequence from the known region complementary to the mRNA and heading upstream. In order to prime (+) strand synthesis of the 5' cDNA end, poly(A)-tailing is carried out using the terminal deoxynucleotidyl transferase prior to (+)strand synthesis using the same $(dT)_{17}$-adapter primer as in 3'-RACE. Amplification is carried out using the adapter primer and the same specific primer or a nested specific primer, in which case specificity is increased (5'-RACE). The basic procedure is outlined in figure 15.6.

The benefits that ensue using the RACE technique are largely those generally endowed by PCR: speed, a high sensitivity and specificity. The RACE technique has successfully been employed to obtain and characterize full length cDNA sequences even of low abundant mRNA. It has been more powerful in tackling the difficult task of obtaining the 5' end sequence of a mRNA than conventional approaches since it relies on two reverse transcription steps producing two shorter, more readily synthesized overlapping cDNA fragments. In some instances, however, the mRNA may be so large that one attempt with the 5'- and 3'-RACE technique might not yield complete sequence information. An interesting alternative suggested by Fritz et al. (1991) with regard to primer design extends

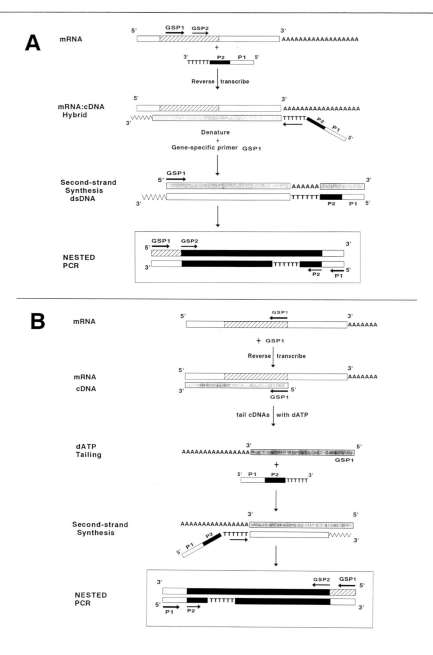

Figure 15.6 : Scheme of the 3' RACE protocol (Panel A) and of the 5' RACE protocol (Panel B). A hatched bar symbolizes the region of known RNA template sequence. In 3' RACE the oligo(dT)-adapter primer is used to initiate first strand synthesis and the gene-specific primer (GSP1 in bold letters) to synthesize the (+) strand. First strand synthesis in 5' RACE is initiated by the gene-specific primer and followed by dATP tailing and (+) strand synthesis using the same oligo(dT)-adapter primer as in 3' RACE. In both protocls, nested PCR is carried out using GSP1/p1 for the outer PCR and GSP2/p2 for the inner PCR.

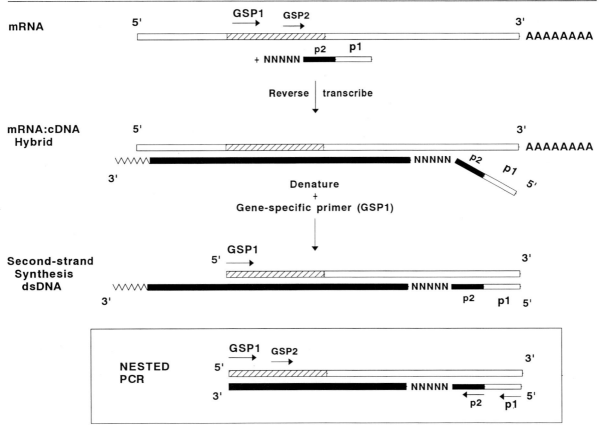

Figure. 15.7: Scheme of the novel 3' extension technique described by Fritz et al. (1991). A hatched bar symbolizes a region of known RNA template sequence. The procedure illustrated is nearly identical to the conventional 3' RACE protocol, except that the oligo(dT)-adapter primer has been substituted by a NNNNNN-adapter primer.

the applicabilty of the RACE technique, so that the complete sequence of a mRNA can be determined despite its length. The approach is outlined in figure 7. The primer used in their novel 3' extension technique was designed to contain a random hexamer sequence at its 3' end and an additional 5' sequence which could serve as a sequence for an adapter primer. Reverse transcription was carried out using 100ng of the "hybrid" primer. Second strand synthesis was achieved with a primer designed from a known exon sequence. Cyclic amplification was performed with the gene-specific primer and an adapter primer. An array of products between 100 and 1000bp were purified by Geneclean (Bio 101) and reamplified using nested primers. This highly increased specificity, so that direct PCR product sequencing was possible. As asserted for some of the other approaches described above, each novel sequence information can be used to unravel more of the unknown sequence in a step by step fashion. Finally, whether in this case or very generally, the use of nested primers greatly increases the specificity of the RACE technique.

Procedure	Comments

Method 2: Rapid amplification of 3' cDNA ends (3'-RACE) according to Frohman et al. (1988, 1990)

1. Incubate 5µg total or 1µg poly(A)⁺ RNA in 11µl DEPC-treated water at 65°C for 3min and then immediately place reaction tubes on ice.

1. 5µg total RNA is equivalent to the amount of RNA which can be extracted from 5×10^5 cells (10pg/cell). Fictitiously, this would mean that if there were only one mRNA copy/cell, then the starting number would figure 5×10^5 copies.

2. Place all reverse transcription components on ice.

3. Add 4µl of 5 x RT buffer, 50ng of $d(T)_{17}$-adapter primer in 2µl, 1µl of a 10mM (each) dNTP stock solution, 20 units RNasin (0.5µl), 0.5µl of 0.1M DTT and 200 units of Mo-MLV reverse transcriptase (1µl).

3. 5 x RT buffer and Mo-MLV reverse transcriptase were purchased from Bethesda Research Laboratories (BRL).

    5 x RT buffer:
    250mM Tris-HCl (pH 8.3)
    375mM KCl
    15mM $MgCl_2$

Using a limiting amount of primer for reverse transcription decreases the probability of transcription being blocked by primers incompletely binding to an unpredicted internal site.

4. Incubate at 37°C for 1 hour and dilute the reaction mixture to 1ml with 1 x TE (10mM Tris-HCl, pH 7.5-8.0 and 1mM EDTA) and store at 4°C.

5. Use 1-10µl of the "cDNA pool" for amplification. Add 5µl 10 x PCR reaction buffer, 25pmol of each primer (3' specific primer and adapter primer), 200-400µl each dNTP and 2.5 units Taq DNA polymerase.

5. Keep all reaction components and reaction tubes on ice.

6. Overlay with oil and place reaction tubes into a preheated (95°C) thermal cycler and denature for 5min.

7. Anneal at 50-55°C for 2min and extend for 2-4min in the first cycle. Then amplify as follows for 30 to 40 cycles: 94°C for 45sec, 50-58°C for 30-45sec, 72°C for 2-3min and a final extension at 72°C for 5-10min.

7. It is important to optimize the PCR for the gene-specific and adapter primer used. Be sure that the primer pair is well balanced (see section Synthesis of Oligonucleotides). Since the adapter primer has the same orientation as the $(dT)_{17}$-adapter primer, the adapter primer alone should only be able to anneal to a newly synthesized (+) strand.

8. PCR products can be visualized on an ethidium bromide stained agarose gels or an aliquot subjected to a nested PCR in order to increase specificity or sensitivity.

Method 3: Rapid Amplification of 5' cDNA ends (5'-RACE) according to Frohman et al (1990)

1. Incubate 5µg total or 1µg poly(A)$^+$ RNA in 11µl DEPC-treated water at 65°C for 3min and then immediately place reaction tubes on ice.

2. Place all reverse transcription components on ice.

3. Add 4µl of 5 x RT buffer, 1-20 pmole of a gene-specific primer in 2µl, 1µl of a 10mM (each) dNTP stock solution, 20 units RNasin (0.5µl), 0.5µl of 0.1M DTT and 200 units of Mo-MLV reverse transcriptase (1µl).

4. Incubate at 37°C for 1 hour and dilute the reaction mixture to 1ml with 1 x TE (10mM Tris-HCl, pH 7.5-8.0 and 1mM EDTA).

5. Remove excess primer from the newly synthesized 5' cDNA ends using Centricon 100 columns (Amicon Corp.) for spin filtration according to the supplier's instructions.

5. According to Frohman et al. (1990), do not use Centricon 30 or Sephadex G-50 columns.

6. Repeat filtration step using 0.2 x TE and collect retained liquid. Concentrate collected fractions in a Speedvac to yield 10μl.

7. Tailing: Add 4μl 5 x tailing buffer (BRL), 4μl of a 1mM dATP solution and 2μl (10 units) terminal deoxynucleotidyl-transferase (BRL).

7. There are several advatages of using a poly(A)-tail. The same primer used for (-) strand synthesis in 3'-RACE, can be used here for (+) strand synthesis. Since A:T binding is weaker than G:C, longer stretches of A residues in the cDNA are required for sufficient binding of the (dT)-adapter primer to an undesired site. The likelihood of the (dT)-adapter primer binding to the cDNA at an undesired location is naturally decreased because 5' untranslated and coding sequences are G/C-rich.

8. Incubate at 37°C for 10min and subsequently inactivate the enzyme at 65°C for 15min.

9. Dilute the "5' cDNA pool" to 500μl with 1 x TE as above.

10. Use 1-10μl of the "cDNA pool" for amplification. Add 5μl 10 x PCR reaction buffer, 2 pmole of the (dT)17-adapter primer for (+) strand synthesis, 25pmol of each primer (5' nested specific primer and adapter primer) for exponential amplification, 200-400μl each dNTP and 2.5 units Taq DNA polymerase.

10. Keep all reaction components and reaction tubes on ice.

11. Overlay with oil and place reaction tubes into a preheated (95°C) thermal cycler and denature for 5min.

12. Anneal at 45-50°C for 2min and extend for 2-4min in the first cycle. Then amplify as follows for 30 to 40 cycles: 94°C for 45sec, 50-58°C for 30-45sec, 72°C for 2-3min and a final extension at 72°C for 5-10min.

13. PCR products can be visualized on an ethidium bromide stained agarose gels or an aliquot subjected to a nested PCR in order to increase specificity or sensitivity.

References

1. Cobianchi F, Wilson SH. Enzymes for modifying and labeling DNA and RNA. 1987, Methods in Enzymology, 152, 94-110.

2. Collins FS, Weissmann SM. Directional cloning of DNA fragments at a large distance from an initial probe: A circularization method. 1984, Proc Natl Acad Sci USA, 81, 6812-6816.

3. Garza D, Ajioka JW, Carulli JP, Jones RW, Johnson DH, Hartl DL. Physical mapping of complex genomes. Nature, 1989, 340, 577-578.

4. Fritz JD, Greaser ML, Wolff JA. A novel 3' extension technique using random primers in RNA-PCR, 1991, Nucl Acids Res, 19, 3747.

5. Frohman MA, Dush MK, Martin GR. Rapid production of full-length cDNAs from rare transcripts: Amplification using a single gene-specific oligonucleotide primer. 1988, Proc Natl Acad Sci USA, 85, 8998-9002.

6. Frohman MA, Martin GR. Rapid amplification of cDNA ends using nested primers. 1989, Techniques, 1, 165-170.

7. Frohman MA. Rapid amplification of cDNA ends (RACE): User-friendly cDNA cloning. 1990, Amplifications: A Forum for PCR Users, 5, 11-15.

8. Jones DH, Winistorfer C. Sequence specific generation of a DNA panhandle permits PCR amplification of inknown flanking DNA. Nucleic Acids Research, 1992, 20, 595-600.

9. Korenberg JR, Rykowski MC. Human genome organization: Alu, Lines and the molecular structure of metaphase chromosome bands. Cell, 1988, 53, 391-400.

10. Nelson DL, Ledbetter SA, Corbo L, Victoria MF, Ramirez-Solis R, Webster TD, Ledbetter DH, Caskey CT. Alu polymerase chain reaction: A method for rapid isolation of human-specific sequences from complex DNA sources. Proc Natl Acad Sci USA, 1989, 86, 6686-6690.

11. Ochman H, Ajioka JW, Garza D, Hartl DL. Inverse polymerase chain reaction. in PCR technology: Principles and Applications for DNA Amplification. ed Erlich HA (Stockton Press, New York, NY) 1989, 105-111.

12. Ochman H, Gerber AS, Hartl DL. Genetic applications of an inverse polymerase chain reaction. Genetics, 1988, 120, 621-623.

13. Ochman H, Ajioka JW, Garza D, Hartl DL. Inverse polymerase chain reaction. Biotechnology, 1990, 8, 75-76.

14. Ochman H, Medhora MM, Garza D, Hartl DL. Amplification of flanking sequences by inverse PCR. in PCR protocols: A guide to methods and applications, eds Innis MA, Gelfand DH, Sninsky JJ, White TJ (Academic Press, New York, NY) 1990, 219-227.

15. Parker JD, Burmer, GC. The oligomer extension "hot blot": A rapid alternative to Southern blots for analyzing polymerase chain reaction products. BioTechniques, 1991, 1, 94-101.

16. Parker JD, Rabinovitch S, Burmer, GC. Targeted gene walking polymerase chain reaction. Nucleic Acids Research, 1991, 19, 3055-3060.

17. Sambrook J, Fritsch EF, Maniatis T. Molecular cloning: A laboratory manual. Cold Spring Harbor Lab, Cold Spring Harbor, New York, 1989.

18. Silver J, Keerikatte V. Novel use of polymerase chain reaction to amplify cellular DNA adjecent to an integrated provirus. J Virol, 1989, 63, 1924-1928.

19. Silver J. Inverse polymerase chain reaction. in PCR: A practical approach, eds McPherson MJ, Quirke P, Taylor GR (Oxford University Press, Oxford, UK) 1991, 137-146.

20. Singer MF. SINEs and LINEs: Highly repeated short and long interspersed sequences in mammalian genomes. Cell, 1982, 28, 433-434.

21. Triglia T, Peterson MG, Kemp DJ. A procedure for in vitro amplification of DNA segments that lie outside the boundaries of known sequences. Nucleic Acid Research, 1988, 16, 8186.

16. Quantification of PCR Products

Polymerase chain reaction has, over a short space of time, proved to be one of the more essential techniques in the fields of molecular biology, microbiology and oncology.

As outlined in earlier chapters, the crucial advantage of this method over conventional biochemical laboratory methods is its high sensitivity. This sensitivity also makes it possible to use PCR as a method for the detection of rare DNA or mRNA species. However, since most PCR assays only allow qualitative statements, their area of use is mostly limited to applications where only the presence or absence of a specific DNA or RNA molecule has to be determined. The major uses of quantitative PCR to date have been to monitor gene dosage, viral infection, and gene expression.

The herpes virus group shows us, for example, with regard to the high incidence of latent infections, that a simple examination of the pathogen DNA/RNA by means of PCR technology is not sufficient for the application of any pathogen activity parameters on the genomic level. Identification of the pathogen's genome on the RNA or DNA level allows no conclusion regarding the transcription activity and therefore no answer to the amount of the specific genome inside the patient's sample.1

It has been shown that, with PCR assays of high sensitivity, positive detection of CMV DNA is possible even in CMV-antibody-positive subjects displaying no accompanying signs of active CMV infection (Schumacher 1991). In all HIV-I-positive groups, nearly 50 % of all asymptomatic, CMV-culture-negative subjects were positive on the DNA level in the CMV-PCR assay. Even the investigation of the RNA level of specific targets yields no clear distinction between latent and active infection: 60 % of all CMV-culture-positive subjects were PCR-RNA-positive, as opposed to only 7 % which were asymptomatic and CMV-culture-negative.

There is substantial evidence that the change from the latent state of herpes infection to an active phase is not merely an on/off phenomenon, but rather, that the viral gene is in permanent, slow, dynamic replication and therefore steadily producing specific RNA below a specific cut off (RNA leakage).

A contribution to solving the problem of how to get exact data about the acitivity of an infection or the expression level of an oncogene etc. is made by the quantification of PCR products (QPCR). This method allows conclusions as to the amount of specific PCR amplificates in relation to the available in-vivo RNA quantity.

Such quantification assays are very important for many clinical applications. They are the only method to compare the initial amounts of the template DNA or RNA in two different samples. For ease of use, they should be simple, non-isotopic, and accurately reproducible.

In order to quantify PCR products, the following considerations should be taken into account: for cycles 1 to 20-22, in vitro DNA amplification results in an exponential reaction with a replication factor in the region of 2 per cycle. The detection of PCR fragments

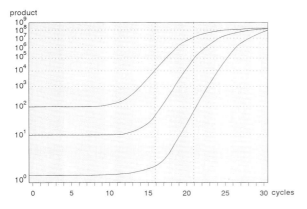

Figure 16.1: Schematic depiction of the rise of amplification products (three different intiail amounts of target: 10^0, 10^1, 10^2) depending on the cycle numbers. Note the plateau at about 10^8 amplification molecules and the linear range about between the 15th and 20th cycle (see also chapter 1.2.5).

using non-radioactive test systems produces problems because of the linear signal enhancement system of these tests in comparison to the exponential PCR system. Through the combination of both techniques, it might be possible, with good test sensitivity and amplification dynamics, to examine a single copy gene with roughly 22 to 26 PCR cycles. However, after about 20-22 cycles we find in some cases that PCR hits a plateau and doesn't allow linear models to be applied. To quantify after 18 to 22 cycles instead of 28 cycles requires a detection system with a sensitivity about 500 times higher. This clearly leads to a desire for a steady and continuous, extremely sensitive detection system to be linked with any QPCR undertaking.

The methods best-described for quantifying specific DNA or RNA in PCR reactions, in addition to amplifying the target DNA proper, use a sample-internal standard (control fragment) of known amount that is coamplified using the same primers. The coamplification of the standards serves as a sample-internal control in order to arrive at statements on the amplification efficiency, by comparing the known original amount of the standard to its final concentration measured after PCR has finished. Since target DNA and standard compete for the same primer, their molar quotient should remain constant over the whole amplification reaction.

A remaining problem for the subsequent detection reaction is the distinction between the signals of the standard amplificate and the target DNA proper.
Previously published papers have already dealt with the problems inherent in QPCR (Wang 1989, Lundeberg 1991, Katz 1990, Gilliland 1990, Chelly 1990); these partly concern variations in the size of internal standards and target DNA and they deal partly with the detection of amplificates using immunoassays. But what are the requirements one should meet when at a later date QPCR becomes part of the routine clinical techniques?

All QPCR methods must:
a) exclude radioactivity and be easily carried out,
b) manage without time-consuming gel systems (PAGE, agarose),
c) conform to standardized measurement systems that are already available in many laboratories,
d) be internally and externally standardized
e) be able to accommodate large numbers of test samples
f) include the ability to produce internal results from a standard sample as reference.

Again, a decisive factor in understanding a quantitative PCR assay is the inclusion of internal sample standards because of the reaction-to-reaction variation in amplification efficiency. To derive the original from the amount of the amplified PCR product to the initial target concentration in the patient's sample is only possible if the amplification grade, or efficiency, is known. Amplification efficiency of the same target DNA might differ between several reaction assays by a factor of about 5×10^2 to 10^5.

Use of an internal standard seems uncomplicated in gene dosage and expression studies, since the molar quotient of target and internal standard can be fixed within a relatively narrow dynamic range. The monitoring of infectious diseases with an internal standard is more difficult, since the molar quotient of specific target DNA and nonspecific background DNA (e.g., host DNA) can differ by several powers of ten. There is the danger that in the course of competitive PCR (specific target vs. internal standard), a quantitative overpowering of the target amplification may occur.

Finally, it has to be taken into account that the internal standard must bedesigned so that target and standard will be present in similar structures that will experience similar strand-separation, primer-annealing, and primer-extension kinetics during the critical first 2 to 5 amplification cycles, before short PCR products begin to accumulate.

In an ideal, though theoretical situation, we are able to calculate the factor of multiplication of the original segment with the formula

$$y = a \times 2^n \qquad [1]$$

where a is the concentration of the original product and n the number of cycles. However, the efficiency of amplification in any given test is never perfect, a complete doubling with each cycle step is not achieved, and the amplification efficiency of each experiment is furthermore dependent upon any inhibitor, primer design, primer T_m-value, cation concentrations, DNA purity and concentration, etc. From our own experiments, we know that the factor of 2 in the formula above is - even in optimized cases - in reality a value between 1.48 and 1.76. These limits mean that there is an ever present difference in the efficiency of amplification between identical assays by a factor of 250.

A more realistic formula for the calculation of the efficiency of PCR amplificates should, after adjustment, read:

$$y = a(1 + F)^n \qquad [2]$$

where a is the original concentration of the target fragment, F the efficiency factor (between 0 and 1), and n the number of cycles. From this, we derive the necessity to use an internal sample standard of known concentration as a reference, which runs alongside the amplification. From the amount of the standard, it is possible to determine the amplification efficiency in individual samples and to subsequently determine the original quantity from the amount of amplified target DNA in it. This, however, requires two preconditions:
1. The amplification efficiency of the standard (ST) must be absolutely identical to that of the target DNA inside the patient sample (PS).

2. The amplification products of ST and PS should be very nearly identical, i.e., they should differ only by a few base pairs, but not in any larger numbers. In preliminary experiments, it has been shown that the efficiency factor F is largest with amplification products of less than 150 bp.

Amplificon size	Efficiency factor F
106 bp	0.76
179 bp	0.68
286 bp	0.57
388 bp	0.49
606 bp	0.48

These results verify that the model, to differentiate between ST and PS in quantification assays on the basis of different lengths, is not useful: the difference in length between ST and PS causes itself different amplification efficiencies. This means that any model that tries to calculate the initial amount of ST using the amplification efficiency of PS is not authoritative.

Previously published methods of QPCR have the following disadvantages:
- large difference between ST and PS (Wang 1989, Lundeberg 1991)
- necessity of money and time consuming gel or HPLC systems and therefore no "routinely measured" usage (Wang 1989, Katz 1990, Gilliland 1990, Warren 1991)
- application of radioactivity (Chelly 1990, Choi 1989, Neubauer 1990)
- difficult to standardize (Lundeberg 1991)
- low sensitivity of the detection system (Ribeiro 1989)

The following assay seems to provide a possible solution to the problem: **Differential Liquid Phase Hybridization.**

Following the assay principles of immunochemical quantification techniques using a 96-well microtiter plate, investigations on PCR amplificates can be carried out.

Along the usual procedure of a PCR assay, a standard (ST) is processed of which the amount is known und which differs only slightly (by 1 to a maximum of 2 base pairs) from the gene sequence obtained from the patient under examination (PS):

```
ST-sequence: 5'...TGA ACG CGA ACG TCG |AT|C TGA GTC TGG GAT ..3'
                  ||| ||| ||| ||| |||  |  ||| ||| ||| |||
PS-sequence: 5'...TGA ACG CGA ACG TCG |CG|C TGA GTC TGG GAT ..3'
```

For the target DNA (PS), the following primer sequences results:

(+) primer: 5' TGA ACG CGA ACG 3'
(-) primer: 5' ATC CCA GAC TCA GCG 3'

The corresponding primer sequences for the internal standard DNA (ST) are as follows:

(+) primer: 5' TGA ACG CGA ACG 3'
(-) primer: 5' ATC CCA GAC TCA GAT 3'

Thus, the amplification system contains three primers: the (+) primer is the same for both ST and PS, and the (-) primers (differential primers) for ST and PS differ by two base pairs at their 3' end. When selecting those mismatches that provide for the respective primer to specifically amplify only PT or ST, the studies by Kwok et al. (cited in Gelfand 1990) must be taken into account. They show that, when using Taq polymerase in the context of an allele-specific assay, only the 3' mismatches A-G, A-A, G-A, and C-C dramatically inhibit amplification efficiency. With all other mismatched base pairs, no relevant reduction in amplification efficiency occurs, so that, in these cases, the ST primer could also produce PS amplificates.

Common to the primers used for amplification are, on the one hand, the lower concentration (0.1 to 0.3 µM) in which they are used in comparison to conventional PCR approaches and, on the other hand, the 5'-end labeling with a fluorescent dye. Here, already during oligonucleotide synthesis (see chapter 20) or by using a linker, a FITC (Fluorescein, Peninsula Lab., Inc. N4044) molecule is synthesized at the ST (-) primer, as well as a rhodamide molecule (Peninsula Lab., Inc. N4045) at the PS (-) primer. Thereby, both amplificons (rhodamide-coupled PS product and FITC-coupled ST product), due to their different fluorescent spectra, are detectable in the same tube by a fluorescence-detecting system (e.g., Fluoroskan II™, Flow laboratories) using different wavelengths. The PCR is stopped between the 20th and 22th cycles, since it is then still within a linear amplification range. The fragment length of ST and PS is in both cases 141 bp. Experiments have shown that the amplification efficiency of both sequences (ST and PS) is identical (F = 0.74). After successful PCR reaction, the amplificates are detected in a 96-well microtiter plate. The microtiter plate we have used is a Covalink NH plate manufactured by Nunc. Covalink NH has been developed to bind compounds covalently to a plastic surface. The plate is a polystyrene surface grafted with secondary amino groups (NH) that can serve as bridgeheads for further covalent coupling and allows a carbodiimide-mediated condensation of DNA onto the microwells. The density of the grafted complexes is about $10^{14}/cm^2$. Rasmussen et al. (1991) have shown that a selective binding of DNA occurs via the 5' end. By applying 1-methyl imidazole, pH 7.0, 50 mM ethyldimethylaminopropyl carbodiimide (EDC) and 50°C for 5 hours, the plate binds a maximum of about 60 pmoles of ssDNA.

This plate meets all the requirements of a solid-phase hybridization system, the covalent binding of the target DNA by a phosphoramidate bond selectively between the 5' end of the DNA and the Covalink NH surface. This type of binding was first described by Gilham (1968), who, by using carbodiimide, was able to link DNA molecules covalently to paper via the 5'-end terminal phosphate group. Various other research groups applied the method published by Chu et al. (1983), condensation of amines with the 5'end of polynucleotides using carbodiimide as the coupling agent, and achieved covalent carbodiimide-mediated binding to latex particles (Wolf 1987), magnetic polystyrene beads (Lund 1988), controlled pore glass (Ghosh 1987), and dextran supports (Gingeras 1987), respectively. The covalent binding of DNA to microwell supports, compared to methods involving a passive absorption of the probe, has the advantage of a more uniform coating of the well, resulting in a more uniform binding of the DNA fragments to be detected. The carbodiimide binding in the Covalink NH plate admits a 96% covalent attachment of DNA, of which about 85% are exclusively linked via the 5' end (Rasmussen 1991).

In preparation for hybridization of the double-strand PCR amplificates to the covalently linked capture probe in the 96-well micrititer plate, the plate is incubated for 30min at 45°C with 500µl of hybridization buffer (0.75M NaCl, 5mM sodium phosphate [pH 7.0], 5mM EDTA, 0.1% Tween 20, 50% formamide, 100µg/ml herring sperm DNA). Thereafter, an aliquot of the final PCR reaction (1µl and 10µl, respectively, of a 50µl sample) is incubated for 4 hours at 45°C, in each case together with 100µl of hybridization buffer. After incubation, the plate is washed 4 times for 20min each at 58°C with 6xSSC, 0.1% SDS. Then, detection of the hybridized ST and PS amplificates in the same well follows, at two different excitation wavelengths (517nm [FITC] and 610nm [Rhodamin]) in fluoroscence detector. The detection threshold, without further amplifier systems, is around 20 to 200 fmol of amplificate, which, taking into account amplification efficiency (see formula 2) and number of cycles run, requires in the original sample a minimum of about 100 copies of the target per 0.1µg of total DNA.

The hybridization of both amplificate products (ST and PS) - differential fluid phase hybridization (DFPH) - at a solid phase-bound probe does not only allow an answer with regard to the specificity of the amplification product, but, using the signal intensity of the standard (F1 - ST), makes it possible to calculate the efficiency of the amplification reaction and thereby to calculate the target concentrations in the original patient sample. Completion of the detection assay requires about 6 hours.

The crucial advantage of the system can therefore be summarized as follows:
1. Specific detection of the amplificates
2. Quantitative evaluation of the assay, with calculation of the original amount of the in-vivo sample
3. Rapid, non-radioactive test systems validated by an internal control
4. Practicability by every laboratory experienced with ELISA equipment and fluorometers.

Newton et al. (1989) describe a comparable system, in which the amplificates are made visible through fluorescence-marked primers, then separated in a sequencing gel and, during electrophoresis, quantified using a laser fluorimeter. Using this technique, the authors were able to detect the product in a phase of PCR in which less than 1/10,000 of the employed primer had been incorporated. However, since this method requires quite an expense in equipment and the parallel processing of several samples is limited by the capacity of the gel, use of this system, e.g., in clinical diagnostics, is hardly feasible. The same applies to capillary gel electrophoresis, a technique capable of detection in the attomolar range. By combining PCR with a sensitive secondary detection method without additional detection-amplification techniques, quantification of DNA sequences becomes possible. Besides the effectiveness of the PCR as a result of complete specific primer annealing (see also chapters

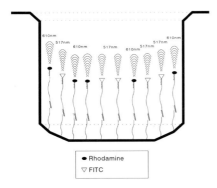

Figure 16.2: Schematic depiction of a single well of a titer-plate. The probe - identical for ST and PS - is bound covalently on the surface of the plate. Each, ST and PS will be detected by different dyes using a fluoroscence detector (rhodamine emission wavelength 610nm, FITC 517nm).

1, 2, 20), enzyme concentration, and purity of the template, among other things, pipetting mistakes during withdrawal of the original DNA sample, with volumes of 1-2µl, also play a significant role. This is a further important reason for using an internal standard pipetted together with the original DNA - and, possibly, also reversely transcribed if one is dealing with an reverse transcriptase-PCR (RT-PCR, for details see chapter 8 and 9).

Becker-André (1989) and Gilliland (1990) describe a system comparable to the one referred to above. With it, the standard sequence differs from the patient sequence by an artificially added restriction site. After amplification of both systems with the same primer pair, the PCR product is cleaved by a restriction endonuclease (see also chapter 11) and the products are separated electrophoretically and quantified densitometrically. In these studies, to date, a problem still inherent in all systems using an internal standard is that since the template integrity has influence on the amplification efficiency in the first cycles (see above), the short standard template may be amplified preferentially, thereby mimicking a lower concentration of the patient template. This error could well be in the order of a power of ten.

Even though a fairly reliable quantification of PCR products is possible by fluorescence measurement, some problems still persist. The critical plateau phase of PCR is caused by limitation of the Taq polymerase and will constitute a fundamental problem of all quantitative assays. Here, it is to be hoped that other polymerases will bring further advantages. Despite current difficulties, it has to be assumed that a detection procedure on the basis of those described above will prevail as a simple and quick standard procedure in clinical diagnostics.

References

1. Becker-André M, Hahlbrock K. Absolute mRNA quantification using the polymerase chain reaction (PCR). A novel approach by a PCR aided transcript titration assay (PATTY). 1989, Nucl Acids Res 17, 9437-9446

2. Bergh St, Hultman Th, Uhlen M. Colorimetric quantification of in vitro-amplified template DNA to be used for solid phase sequencing. 1991, DNA Sequence - J DNA Sequenc Mapp 2, 81-87

3. Chelly J, Montarras D, Pinset Ch, Berwald-Netter Y, Kaplan JC, Kahn A. Quantitative estimation of minor mRNAs by cDNA-polymerase chain reaction. Application to dystrophin mRNA in cultured mygenic and brain cells. 1990, Eur J Biochem 187, 691-8.

4. Choi Y, Kotzin B, Herron L, Callahan J, Marrack P, Kappler J. 1989, Proc Natl Acad Sci USA 86, 8941-8945

5. Gelfand DH, White Th J. Thermostable DNA polymerases. In: PCR protocols. A guide to methods and applications. Eds.: M.A. Innis, D.H.Gelfand, J.J.Sninsky, Th.J.White. 1990, Academic Press, San Diego, pp129-141

6. Gilliland G, Perrin ST, Blanchard K, Bunn HF. Analysis of cytokine mRNA and DNA: Detection and quantitation by competitive polymerase chain reaction. 1990, Proc Natl Acad Sci USA 87, 2725-2729

7. Katz E, Haff LA. Rapid separation, quantitation and purification of products of polymerase chain reaction by liquid chromatography. 1990, J Chromatogr 512, 433-44

8. Kemp DJ, Churchill MJ, Smith DB, Biggs BA, Foote SJ, Peterson MG, Samaras N, Deacon NJ, Doherty R. Simplified colorimetric analysis of polymerase chain reaction: detection of HIV sequences in AIDS patients. 1990, Gene 94, 223-228

9. Lundeberg J, Wahlberg J, Uhlen M. Rapid colorimetric quantification of PCR-amplified DNA. 1991, Biotechniques 10, 68-75

10. Neubauer A, Neubauer B, Liu E. Polymerase chain reaction based assay to detect allelic loss inhuman DNA: loss of beta-interferon gene in chronic myelogenous leukemia. 1990, Nucl Acids Res 18, 993-998

11. Newton C, Kalsheker N, Graham A. Use of polymerase chain reaction and direct sequencing for prenatal diagnosis of α1-antitrypsin deficiency. 1989, Biochem Soc Trans 17, 367-368

12. Ribeiro EA, Larcom LL, Miller DP. Quantitative fluorescence of DNA-intercalated ethidium bromide on agarose gels. 1989, Anal Biochem 181, 197-208

13. Schumacher HC, Rolfs A, Würdemann M. Rapid detection of CMV-specific DNA and mRNA by PCR in immunocompromised patients. In: PCR topics. Usage of polymerase chain reaction in genetic and infectious diseases. Eds.: A Rolfs, HC Schumacher, P Marx. 1991, Springer Verlag, Berlin, pp117-24.

14. Syvänen A-C, Bengtström M, Tenhunen J, Söderlund H. Quantification of polymerase chain reaction products by affinity-based hybrid-collection. 1988, Nucl Acids Res 16, 11327-11338

15. Wahlberg J, Lundeberg J, Hultman Th, Uhlen M. General colorimetric method for DNA diagnostics allowing direct solid-phase genomic sequencing of the positive samples. 1990, Proc Natl Acad Sci USA 87, 6569-6573

16. Wang A, Doyle MV, Mark DF. Quantitation of mRNA by the polymerase chain reaction. 1989, Proc Natl Acad Sci USA 86, 9717-21.

17. Warren W, Wheat Th, Knudsen P. Rapid analysis and quantitation of PCR products by high-performance liquid chromatography. 1991, BioTechniques 11, 250-255

17. Cloning Methods Using PCR

The polymerase chain reaction has contributed to bypassing many applications for which a cloning procedure had hitherto been necessary, as amplification products can be analyzed directly (e.g., by sequencing, see chapter 14). Nevertheless, numerous amplification strategies lead to complex mixtures of products, requiring a cloning step for further molecular analysis of the specific target sequence. For the performance of classical cloning experiments, too, the PCR has contributed to many simplifications. The most often used method for cloning PCR products is to design flanking restriction sites onto the ends of the primers. After completed amplification, the DNA is purified, then restricted by suitable endonucleases and ligated to a compatible vector. But already with this simple step of modifying the 5' end of the primers by adding a specific restriction site sequence, various problems can arise, depending on whether a sticky-end or blunt-end cloning procedure is used. Taq polymerase as well as Thermus flavus and Thermococcus litoralis DNA polymerases (neither of the three enzymes exhibits 3'-to-5' exonuclease activity) add a non-template-dependent base at the 3' end of the strand that is synthesizing (Clark 1988, Mead 1991). The ability to polish is differently marked for Klenow fragment and T7 polymerase, since the latter has no 3'-5'-exonuclease activity, but is able, as is Klenow enzyme, to fill 5' overhangs. When carrying out blunt-end cloning reactions, the Taq polymerase should therefore be inactivated by heating the reaction mixture to 99°C for 10min, the reaction mixture subsequently cooled slowly to room temperature, the $MgCl_2$ concentration increased to a final 5-10mM, 2U Klenow fragment added and the whole mixture incubated for about 30min at 37°C. If 200µM each of dNTP was used for PCR, more is not likely to be needed. The Klenow enzyme can be inactivated at 95°C for 5min, and the amplified DNA can be precipitated if necessary in order to remove primer and dNTPs. When using a DNA polymerase that exhibits 3'-5'-exonuclease activity (e.g., Vent DNA polymerase), the problem of adding a nucleotide to the 3' end of one or both strands can be bypassed (Lohff 1991). A cloning system offered by the Invitrogen Corporation makes use of this effect of Taq polymerase (the single 3'-deoxyadenylate extension) by getting, in a cloning vector (pCR2001, 2.9kB) after restriction digest, a single 3'T nucleotide at the ends. The two projecting 3'-deoxyadenylate extensions on the amplification product can now be inserted directly by adding a T4 DNA ligase (Mead 1991).

Some observations confirm that Taq polymerase may remain bound to the DNA, preventing restriction endonuclease binding (Crowe 1991), because it may be competing with the endonuclease activity at 37°C. This problem can be bypassed if, after completed PCR amplification, the reaction mixture will be digested with proteinase K. The DNA must be purified anyway after completed amplification and prior to cloning, because dNTPs carried over from the PCR are competitive inhibitors for ATP in the ligation reaction.

For all amplification conditions, it must be noted that, in the later cycles, the elongation time must be sufficiently long, because, if the time allowed for elongation is insufficient, some ends may be frayed and, therefore, cannot be used for cloning procedures. This must especially be noted if the ends of the amplicon are cleaved by restriction endonucleases to generate the desired sticky ends on the PCR product. Some restriction endonucleases are unable to cleave sequences located near the extreme ends of DNA fragments (Kaufman 1990). In most cases, the efficiency of the cleavage activity of the restriction enzyme can be improved by allowing for 2-4 random nucleotides at the 5' ends outside the restriction site proper when designing the primers (Scharf 1986). In the following example, a cap of 3 nucleotides (AGT) has been attached to the SacI restriction sequence at the 5' end of the primer used for the amplification of a gene fragment from the nucleocapsid region, which drastically increased the efficiency of cleavage in our experiments (data not shown):

5' AGT <u>GAG CTC</u> ATG CTA CCT GAG TAC CGT AGA 3'

As enzymes that are unable to digest a site located at the extreme end of a fragment, SalI, HindIII and XbaI could be identified (Kaufman 1990), whereas, e.g., KpnI and SacI can be employed without problem.

A method published by Shuldiner and co-workers (1990) describes a ligase-free subcloning procedure. In it, the first step in PCR-induced subcloning comprises an amplification of the DNA of interest, with oligonucleotides being used that carry at their 5' end a 24-nucleotide sequence complementary to the 3' end of the desired linearized plasmid vector. After completed PCR reaction, excess dNTPs and primers are removed and 50 to 100ng of the PCR product are filled in each of two tubes. Here, the target is to achieve, in tube 1, annealing of the 3' end of the PCR product (+)strand to the 5' end of the linearized plasmid (+)strand and, in tube 2, annealing of the 3' end of the PCR product (-)strand to the 5' end of the linearized plasmid (-)strand. Through suitable choice of new primers in this reaction, according to the desired orientation of DNA fragments, an exponential amplification of the recombinant vectors can be achieved. By terminating the 2nd PCR reaction, 10µl each of tubes 1 and 2 are united, double-stranded DNA denatured in 0.2M NaOH and subsequently neutralized with 400ml boiling Tris. Incubation for several hours results in reannealing of complementary heterologous strands, followed by cyclization.

Method: Cloning and purification of a partial gag sequence of HIV-1 using PCR

In the following method, the combination of PCR with a cloning step, followed - after expression - by a fast and reliable protein purification method, is to be presented. The fundamental principle of this protein purification-step with the help of PCR is the use of a calcium-dependent antibody for the identification and purification of the recombinant protein (Prickett 1989). The model is shown using the example of a partial gag sequence of the HIV-1 virus. The antibody published by Prickett and co-workers recognizes, in the presence of Ca^{2+}, a short hydrophilic octapeptide, Asp-Tyr-Lys-Asp-Asp-Asp-Asp-Lys. If the antibody is used in the context of immuno-affinity column chromatography, it can, in the presence of Ca^{2+} ions, recognize and bind the specifically expressed protein from the bacterial lysate. If the calcium is removed or chelated from the washing buffer, the protein can be eluted from the column. If desired, the sequence of the octapeptide, which is still attached to the recombinant protein, can be removed by a protease. Such approaches for the facilitating of the purification of recombinant proteins have increasingly found their way into the literature in the last few years (cf. also Hochuli 1987, 1988).

The system presented here makes special demands upon the design of the primers, since the primers must contain the following information: 1. sequence for the restriction site for the cloning; 2. sequence for the

Partially overlapping primer 1 + 2 at the 5'end of the template

<u>NcoI</u>
5' C CCC ATG GAC TAC AAA GAC GAT GAC GAT AAA ATG CAG AGA GGC AAT TT 3'
                5' GAC GAT GAC GAT AAA <u>ATG</u> CAG AGA GGC AAT TTT AGG AAC CAA AGA AAG A 3'
codon   Asp Tyr Lys Asp Asp Asp Asp Lys

                                          initiation site

Partially overlapping primer 3 + 4 at the 3'end of the template

<u>HindIII</u>
5' GGA AGC TTG <u>TTA</u> CTG ATG TTT CTG CTA CTG CTA TTT TTG TGA CGA GGG GTC GTT 3'
                  5' TTT CTG CTA CTG CTA TTT TTG TGA CGA GGG GTC GTT GCC AAA GAG TGA TCT GAG
codon   Asp Tyr Lys Asp Asp Asp Asp Lys
         stop codon

Table 17.1

octapeptide.
The starting site of the sequence is at nucleotide 1918 (HIV-1 nomenclature) and the stop codon at nucleotide 2323. To modify the ends of the gene sequences subsequently to be expressed, two nested PCR reactions are carried out with partially overlapping primers. The design of the primers is represented in Table 17.1. The final amplicon has a size of 473bp (incl. the sequences for the restriction sites and the octapeptide).

Procedure

1. Performance of a 25µl standard PCR (see chapters 1 and 2), adding 1µl primer 2 (10pmol/µl) and 1µl primer 4 (10pmol/µl), 100ng BH10-HIV-1 DNA, 2U Taq polymerase.

2. Demonstration of the amplicon in 1.6% agarose gel.

Comments

1. Thermoprofile: initially 4min 95°C, followed by 30 cycles: 90sec 92°C, 45sec 50°C, 90sec 72°C. 10min 72°C.

3. 2µl of the original PCR mixture are pipetted into fresh PCR reaction mixture as new template and 1µl each of primers 2 and 3 (10pmol/µl) added. 2U Taq polymerase.

3. Thermoprofile: initially 4min 95°C, followed by 30 cycles: 90sec 92°C, 45sec 50°C, 90sec 72°C. 10min 72°C.

4. Demonstration of the amplicon in a preparative 1.6% agarose gel. Cutting-out of the bands from the gel.

5. Isolation of the DNA from the agarose gel fragment, using a BIOTRAP™ electro-separation system (Schleicher & Schüll).

5. After elution of the DNA has been completed, eluate will be removed using a Pasteur pipette re-aspirating the fluid from the chamber a few times to collect sample material on the surfaces of the device.

6. Phenol-chloroform extract PCR reaction (for details, see chapter 7).

7. The DNA is precipitated using ice-cold ethanol (for details, see chapter 7) and, after drying, resuspended in 20µl aqua bidest.

8. Restriction cleavage of the PCR amplification products: 10µl amplicon, 3µl 10x buffer H (Boehringer Mannheim), 16µl aqua bidest., 1µl NcoI (12U/µl, Boehringer Mannheim). Incubation at 37°C for 2 hours.

9. Ethanol precipitation of the restriction assay (for details, see chapter 7). Resuspend the pellet in 30µl aqua bidest.

10. Second restriction cleavage of the precleaved amplicon: 30µl DNA, 5µl 10x core-buffer (Boehringer Mannheim), 12µl aqua bidest., 3µl HindIII (10U/µl). Incubation at 37°C for 2 hours.

11. As cloning vector, the pKK233-2 expression vector is used, which has an NcoI, PstI, HindIII cloning site.

11. The plasmid contains the highly expressed trc promoter, the lacZ ribosome binding site and the ATG initiation codon. The NcoI recognition sequence, CCATGG, commonly occurs at the initiation codon of eucaryotic genes, allowing direct ligation to the vector.

12. The vector is also cut with NcoI and HindIII in two reactions separated by an ethanol precipitation: 4µl vector (0.5µg/µl), 6µl 10x buffer H, 46µl aqua bidest., 4µl NcoI. Steps analogous to points 8-10 follow.

Procedure(cont.)

13. The two HindIII restriction assays from points 10 and 12 are phenol/chloroform-extracted and ethanol-precipitated. The amplicon is resuspended in 10µl aqua bidest., and pKK233-2, in 1.5µl aqua bidest.

14. Ligation: 10µl amplicon (NcoI, HindIII cleaved), 1.5µl pKK233-2 (NcoI, HindIII cleaved), 1.5µl 10x ligation buffer, 1.0µl ligase (1U/µl).

15. Preparation of competent cells (JM 109): Preparation of an overnight culture (37°C). 1ml o/n culture + 40ml TY until the optical density of the culture reaches about 0.600. 10min at 4°C. Centrifuge for 10min at 6,000 rpm and 4°C. Siphon off supernatant. Add 20ml 50mM $CaCl_2$. Incubate at 42°C for 15-20min. Centrifuge again for 10min at 6,000 rpm and 4°C. Resuspend cells in 2ml 50mM CaCl2, o/n at 4°C.

16. To 200µl of the competent cells, the ligation assay from point 14 is added. 45min at 4°C, then 2min at 42°C. Addition of 1ml TY medium + 50µg/ml ampicillin. 2 hours at 37°C. 100µl of the suspension are distributed evenly on an agar plate. Incubation at 37°C.

17. After 24 hours, mini-prep DNA preparations from the grown cultures are carried out according to Davis (1986). Positive clones will be restricted with NcoI and HindIII after they have been RNase-digested and ethanol-precipitated.

18. According to standard methods (for details, see Davis 1986), 50µl of the mini-prep culture from positive clones were suspended in 20ml TY, or 20ml of minimum medium 008 plus 50µg/ml ampicillin, resp.

19. When cells reach an OD of about 0.1, induction will be done using 1mM IPTG (isopropyl-ß-D-thiogalactopyranoside). To check the effectivity and specificity of the induction, it makes sense to carry out time kinetics with measurement of OD.

20. After successful growth of the cells, the cells are

Comments(cont.)

14. T4 DNA ligase (Promega M1801). 10x reaction buffer: 300mM Tris-HCl, pH 7.8, 100mM $MgCl_2$, 100mM DTT, 10mM ATP. Fresh ATP is crucial for the ligase reaction.

15. TY medium: bacto-tryptone 10g, bacto-yeast 10g, NaCl 5g ad 1,000ml aqua bidest.

18. Minimum medium 008: 2g NH_4Cl, 6g Na_2HPO_4 x $2H_2O$, 3g KH_2PO_4, 3g NaCl, 0.175g $MgSO_4$ x $7H_2O$. Dissolve in 900ml H_2O, adjust pH to 7.4 with 10N NaOH. Sterilize. Add 7.5ml 20% glucose, 7.5ml 2% yeast extract. Adjust to 1,000ml.

Procedure(cont.)	Comments(cont.)

frozen in a dry ice-methanol bath, then allowed to thaw.

21. The cells are resuspended in 50ml PBS (pH 8.4)/lysozyme.

21. Bring 50ml of PBS to pH 8.4 with 5M NaOH; add 12.5mg of lysozyme (Sigma L-6876) to this solution to get a 0.25mg/ml lysozyme solution.

22. Freeze and thaw (37°C) three more times.

23. Bring the mixture to 1.0mM Ca^{2+} with 1M $CaCl_2$ and then pour into a Dounce homogenizer and dounce to achieve a uniform suspension. Incubate at 37°C for 30min with douncing every 5min.

24. Centrifuge at 25,000g for 60min at 4°C and remove the lysate supernatant.

25. Apply the lysate supernatant to the column which is already packed with antibody-containing gel. Packing is done as follows: after the antibody-containing gel has been mixed thoroughly and loaded into the column, wash the gel by loading three sequential 5ml aliquots of glycine HCl, followed by 3 sequential 5ml aliquots of PBS.

25. Glycine HCl: 0.1M glycine, titrate to pH 3.0 with HCl. Antibody is purchased as Flag™ Technology from Immunex Corporation. It is important to make sure that the lysate is present at about the following concentrations: 0.15M NaCl, 0.01M sodium phosphate, 1mM $CaCl_2$, pH 7.4.

26. Load the supernatant into the antibody column under gravity flow. Wash column with at least three aliquots of 3ml of PBS/Ca.

26. PBS/Ca: Phosphate-buffered saline with 1mM $CaCl_2$ included.

27. Elution of the protein is carried out by rinsing with PBS/EDTA. For this, aliquots of 1ml each are run through the column in intervals of 10min. As a rule, six elution steps will be necessary.

27. PBS/EDTA: Phosphate-buffered saline with 0.02% sodium azide included.

28. If the eluted protein is to be used further specifically (e.g., antibody production, etc.), the octapeptide can be split off by enterokinase, a specific protease. When doing so, of course, care must be taken that no further cleavage site for this protease occurs in the rest of the specific protein.

28. Enterokinase is a highly specific protease that removes the Asp-Asp-Asp-Asp-Lys sequence found at the N-terminal of the zymogen.

Procedure(cont.)

Comments(cont.)

Using this procedure, it has been accomplished within a few days to successfully express and purify the partial gag-protein of HIV-1. The specificity of the product after purification is demonstrated using the western blot (Figure 17.1).

References

1. Clark JM. Novel non-templated nucleotide addition reactions catalyzed by procaryotic and eucaryotic DNA polymerases. 1988, Nucl Acids Res 16, 9677-9686

2. Crowe JS, Cooper HJ, Smith MA, Sims MJ, Parker D, Gewert D. Improved cloning efficiency of polymerase chain reaction (PCR) products after proteinase K digestion. 1991, Nucl Acids Res 19, 184

3. Davis LG, Dibner MD, Battey JF. Basic methods in molecular biology. Elsevier, Amsterdam 1986, pp102-104

4. Hochuli E, Bannwarth W, Döbeli H, Gentz R, Stüber D. Genetic approaches to facilitate purification of recombinant proteins with a novel metal chelate adsorbent. 1988, BioTechnology 6, 1321-1325

5. Hochuli E, Döbeli H, Schacher A. New chelate adsorbent selective for proteins and peptides containing neighbouring histidin residues. 1987, J Chromatogr 411, 177-184

6. Kaufman DL, Evans GA. Restriction endonuclease cleavage at the termini of PCR fragments. 1990, BioTechniques 9, 304-305

7. Lohff CJ, Cease KB. PCR using a thermostable polymerase with 3' to 5' exonuclease activitiy generates blunt products suitable for direct cloning. 1991, Nucl Acids Res 20, 144

8. Mead DA, Pey NK, Herrnstadt C, Marcil R, Smith L. A universal method for the direct cloning of PCR amplified nucleic acid. 1991, BioTechnology 9, 657-663

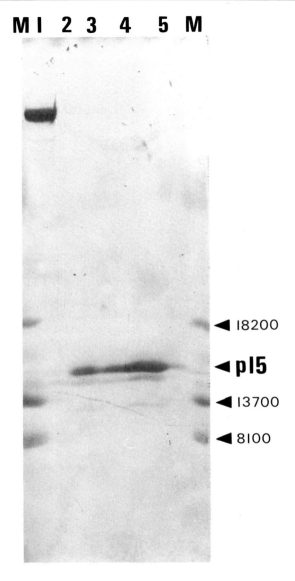

Figure 17.1. Demonstration of the partial gag-HIV-1 protein (15kD molecular weight) in the western blot using 50µl sheep anti-HIV-1 p15 antibody (Biochrom, FRG) as monoclonal antibody. Incubation for 2 hours, followed by a second antibody (rabbit anti-sheep) and a third antibody for detection (anti rabbit-alkaline phosphatase conjugated antibody). M = marker; lane 1, gag-lysate for positive control; lane 2, JM109 + insert after 2 hours IPTG induction; lane 3, JM109 after 3 hours IPTG induction; lane 4, JM109 + insert, no induction; lane 5, JM109 without an insert for negative control.

9. Prickett KS, Amberg DC, Hopp TP. A calcium-dependent antibody for identification and purification of recombinant proteins. 1989, BioTechniques 7, 580-585

10. Scharf SJ, Hron GT, Erlich HA. Direct cloning and sequence analysis of enzymatically amplified genomic sequences. 1986, Science 239, 487-491

11. Shuldiner AR, Scott LA, Roth J. PCR-induced (ligase-free) subcloning: a rapid reliable method to subclone polymerase chain reaction (PCR) products. 1990, Nucl Acids Res 18, 1920

18. Site-Directed Mutagenesis Using the PCR

Changes in genes and/or proteins coded for by them, by substitution of specific nucleotides within a sequence through site-directed mutagenesis, is one of the most important tools of recombinant DNA technology (for a review, see MJ McPherson 1991). The method is important, on the one hand, for investigating the structural basis of genes and proteins and, on the other hand, also for generating functionally and/or structurally new proteins. Hitherto classical methods with which these experiments had been carried out were time-intensive and often little efficient (Wu and Grossman 1987); as a rule, the mutant products, after completed cloning procedure in the bacteriophage or vector system, were only present in low frequency. An important step towards simplification in the creation of a site-directed or (semi-)random mutagenesis within a DNA sequence employs the PCR technique (Hemsley 1989). The simplest way to do this using the PCR is to modify the 5' ends of the primers (see also chapters 14, 17) or - as long as this does not collide with annealing of the immediately 3'-located bases - to perform base exchanges within the primer sequence. Since, however, due to the design of a PCR, the desired base change cannot take place in the region of the primer sequence located at the ends of the targeted template, this kind of site-directed mutagenesis is of limited value. During the last three years, various experimental approaches have been published to bypass this problem (see also page A60, contribution by Landt Hahn). Crucial for the success of site-directed mutagenesis experiments using the PCR is the design of primers and the selection of the restriction enzymes (see chapter 17) - we have found recommendable, e.g., BamH1 and EcoR1. Thus, Ho and co-workers (1989), using the technique of "overlap extension", have produced, cloned, and analyzed 3 variants of a mouse major histocompatibility complex class-I gene. For this, two adjacent fragments having overlapping ends from the interesting DNA sequence are amplified. Annealing of the two fragments ("fusion reaction") leads to the 3' overlap of each strand serving as a primer for the 3' extension of the complementary strand, creating a recombinant molecule. This concept of joining two DNA fragments together by overlap extension allows the introduction of mutations into the center of the PCR fragment. A detailed protocol for this procedure has been described by McArn Horton (1991). If the 5' end of a primer is altered such that it becomes complementary to the sequence in another gene, it is possible to overlap any PCR product with any other gene segment, so that they can be recombined. Site-directed mutagenesis approaches using the PCR reaction are, however, limited by the maximal size of the fragment to be amplified.

Perrin and Gilliland (1990) have simplified the method to create site-directed mutagenesis by using two mutant primers. For this, a large single-stranded mutant primer (100-1,400bp) is produced using an asymmetric PCR by means of a short mutant primer and wildtype 5' primer. After removal of incorporated primers, the large mutant primer of a standard PCR is added with wildtype 3' primer and a sufficient amount of wildtype template. The following PCR reaction generates the mutant DNA fragment of desired length.

Mikaelian and Sergeant (1992) have published a method by means of which site-directed mutations can be performed using three universal primers chosen in the vector and one specific primer for each mutation (M). This method requires two simultaneous PCR reactions. The first reaction is carried out with two primers that are homologous to the vector sequence, of which, however, primer 2 contains a mismatched 3' end. The second PCR is carried out using primer 3 and primer M. The latter contains the mutation (deletion, insertion, substitution). The amplified products of the two PCR reactions are gel-purified, mixed, and subjected to another round of PCR with external primers 1 and 3. Since, in this second PCR reaction, the one hybrid containing the 3' mismatch of primer 2 cannot be amplified because of lacking complementary to the DNA fragment, only the mutated strand is amplified. After completed reaction, the fragment can be digested and ligated into the appropriate vector.

Another interesting development is the so-called "recombinant circle PCR" (RCPCR) (Jones and Howard 1990). This method is carried out using two different PCR reactions to generate products that, when combined, denatured, and reannealed, form a double-stranded DNA with discrete, cohesive single-stranded ends. This requires that the mutant primer amplifies the (+)strand in one mixture and that, in the second reaction, the (-)strand and the corresponding primers are present staggered at exactly the same location. The cohesive ends are designed such that they would anneal to form circles of DNA. It should be stressed that these circles form without the use of restriction enzyme digestion and ligation and that they can be transfected directly into E. coli, leading to a considerable simplification of the cloning procedure for PCR-generated site-directed mutants. With appropriate modification of the employed primers in this reaction, mutagenesis by PCR can serve to generate insertions or deletions (Vallette 1989).

For the generation of random mutagenesis by use of PCR, various methods are available. Leung and co-workers (1989) have chosen experimental conditions that reduce the fidelity of the Taq polymerase. For this, the DNA is amplified in the presence of a PCR buffer with manganese and un-equal molar concentration of dNTPs.

Zhou and co-workers (1991) have somewhat modified this method in that they carry out a four-step procedure. They start with a standard PCR of 30 cycles, 200µl volume, 5U Taq polymerase and overall long reaction periods, which, due to the error rate of Taq DNA polymerase, lead to a random mutagenesis. The amplicon is subsequently cleaved using two restriction endonucleases that cut at each end of the DNA sequence of interest. Then, the DNA fragment of interest is ligated with restriction endonuclease-digested vector DNA and the resulting recombinant DNA molecules are introduced into cells by transformation. This is the simplest procedure for high-frequency, random mutagenesis of gene-sized DNA sequences. According to the authors, the mutant frequency is about 35%, and thus close to the ideal for most applications. All four transition substitutions and one transversion substitution were observed.

References

1. Hemsley A, Arnheim N, Toney MD, Cortopassi G, Galas DJ. A simple method fo site-directed mutagenesis using the polymerase chain reaction. 1989, Nucl Acids Res 6545-6551

2. Ho St N, Hunt HD, Horton RM, Pullen JK, Pease LR. Site-directed mutagenesis by overlap extension using the polymerase chain reaction. 1989, Gene 77, 51-59

3. Horton MR, Pease LR. Recombination and mutagensis of DNA sequences using PCR. In: McPherson MJ (Eds.). Directed mutagenesis - a practical approach. Oxford University Press, New York 1991, pp217-246

4. Jones DH, Howard BH. A rapid method for site-directed mutagenesis and directional subcloning by using the polymerase chain reaction to genrete recombinant circles. 1990, BioTchniques 8, 178-183

5. Leung D, Chen E, Goeddal D. A method for random mutagenesis of a defined DNA segment using a modified polymerase chain reaction. 1989, Technique 1, 11-15

6. McPherson MJ (Eds.). Directed mutagenesis - a practical approach. Oxford University Press, New York 1991

7. Mikaelian I, Sergeant A. A general and fast method to generate multiple site directed mutations. 1992, Nucl Acids Res 20, 376

8. Perrin S, Gilliland G. Site-directed mutagensis using asymmetric polymerase chain reaction and s single mutant primer. 1990, Nucl Acids Res 18, 7433-7438

9. Vallette F, Mege E, Reiss A, Adesnik M. Construction of mutant and chimeric genes using the polymerase chain reaction. 1989, Nucl Acids Res 17, 723-733

10. Wu R, Grossman L. Site-directed mutagenesis and protein engineering. 1987, Methods Enzymol 154, 329-429

11. Zhou Y, Zhang X, Ebright RH. Random mutagenesis of gene-sized DNA molecules by use of PCR with Taq DNA polymerase. 1991, Nucl Acids Res 19, 6052

19. In-Situ Polymerase Chain Reaction

A current limitation of PCR with isolated DNA is the fact that the results of amplification cannot be brought into a direct relationship with the specific cell type that is responsible for the amplification signal. Moreover, all quantitative assays are expensive methods, prone to disturbances if not carried out extremely accurately, and based on theoretical, mathematical premises. Insofar, the performance of the PCR reaction in single cells, followed by a detection in the corressponding cells, would be desirable in order to be able to demonstrate, by a subsequent in-situ hybridization, which and how many cells really carry the sequence to be detected. The problem becomes clear in the context of an HIV-1 infection: in-situ hybridization experiments demonstrate HIV-1 RNA in about 1 in 10,000 to 1 in 100,000 peripheral-blood mononuclear cells (Harper 1986). The use of quantitative PCR in combination with cell sorting (Schnittman 1990) shows that about 1% of all CD4-positive lymphocytes are infected with HIV-1. However, cell sorting followed by a PCR means numerous procedures that involve losses of material and error possibilities. Therefore, it should be strived for to directly in cell smears or paraffin-embedded tissues using PCR.

However, the practical implementation of this "in-situ polymerase chain reaction" poses numerous problems:
1. Amplification of the target DNA, associated with denaturation steps, must not destroy cell morphology in order to be able to assess the cells after detection of the amplicons in the context of in-situ hybridization.
2. For all reagents (Mg^{2+}, Taq polymerase, primer, etc.), the optimal concentrations must be exactly determined by tests.
3. It must be prevented that amplified DNA diffuses out of the cell.
4. Tissue drying and loss of tissue adherence during the amplification procedure must be prevented.

In the last two years, some publications have devoted themselves to this problem of directly detecting target DNA in the cell while preserving cell morphology. Haase and co-workers (1990) were the first to describe the amplification of the LTR-gag transition region (1,200bp) of the Visna virus in a cell suspension of sheep choroid plexus cells. For this, after fixation for 20min in freshly prepared 4% paraformaldehyde (a cross-linking fixative), the cells were washed in Ca^{2+}- and Mg^{2+}-free phosphate-buffered saline (PBS-CMF) and suspended in 100µl of a PCR reaction mixture (10mM Tris-HCl (pH 8.3), 50mM KCl, 1.5mM $MgCl_2$, 0.01% gelatin, 200µM dNTPs, 0.1µM primers). Altogether 9 primers were used simultaneously that generate DNA segments with overlapping cohesive termini, creating a 1,200bp fragment. Choosing such a large amplification product prevents the PCR products from diffusing out of the cell. Prior to adding 2.5U of Taq polymerase, the cells were heated for 10min to 94°C. A thermoprofile of 2min 94°C, 2min 42°C, and 15min 72°C follows. After 25 cycles, a further 2.5U Taq polymerase are added and another 25 cycles carried out. After completed amplification, the cells were centrifuged, deposited on a slide by cytocentrifugation and detected by a ^{125}I-labeled virus-specific probe. The authors report an amplification factor of 300 for 50 cycles. The reason for the limitation of amplification effectiveness must be seen in the diffusion obstacles for PCR reagents in the nucleus. Nuovo and co-workers (1991a) point out that, when carrying out a so-called hot-start in-situ PCR, it is possible, with a single primer pair using a non-isotopic PCR, to detect a single viral copy in the cell, even when amplifying a fragment only 115bp in size. This finding would be of special value, since it is known that probes with sizes of 100-200bp are most efficient for in-situ hybridization. What Nuovo et al. mean by "hot-start" is the procedure of heating the slides to 82°C with the PCR buffer, but without primer and without Taq polymerase, to lift the coverslip at that temperature, and to only then add enzyme and primers. Kuo-Ping (1992) investigated different techniques to maintain the localization of the amplified DNA. Among other things, they investigated the effectiveness of a method that makes use of complementary tails at the 5' ends of the primers, resulting in the synthesis of high-molecular-weight amplification products that contain several times the specific sequence. This procedure permits the detection of a 167bp fragment from the mouse mammary tumor virus genome. Besides, the authors were able to show that a thin film of agarose (2.5% molten SeaKem GTG agarose), solidified over the tissue section, can serve as a matrix to localize the amplified target.

Bagasra and co-workers (1992) also report that they carried out a sensitive in-situ PCR with an unmodified 115bp fragment, thereby detecting a single copy of HIV-1 provirus per cell.

The critical steps in the performance of the in-situ PCR are, above all, the preparations of the cells, the fixation and permeabilization procedures. In various publications, 1-4% paraformaldehyde has proved worth recommending. It is also important to note that the proteinase-K digestion must be carried out extensively, e.g., 100µl per slide with a 60µg proteinase K/1ml phosphate-buffered saline solution for 4 hours at 55°C. Inactivation of proteinase K is subsequently performed at 96°C for 2min, followed by a wash-step with distilled water. However, some cells do not seem to be accessible to the present procedure of in-situ PCR. Thus, central nervous system cells may possibly not be usable for in-situ PCR, since they may possibly not be permeable to PCR reagents, due to the heavy lipid content of their cell membranes.

The importance of in-situ PCR for the understanding of inflammatory or oncological problems will be great, esp. in the area of pathology. A further development of application will come about when, after completed in-situ PCR and hybridization, it should still prove possible to characterize the cells with monoclonal antibodies.

References

1. Bagasra O, Hauptman St, Harold DO, Lischner W, Sachs M, Pomerantz R. Detection of human immunodeficiency virus type 1 provirus in mononuclear cells by in situ polymerase chain reaction. 1992, N Engl J Med 326, 1385-1391

2. Haase AT, Retzel EF, Staskus KA. Amplification and detection of lentiviral DNA in side cells. 1990, Proc Natl Acad Sci USA 87, 4971-4975

3. Harper ME, Marselle LM, Gallo RC, Wong-Staal F. Detection of lymphocytes expressing human T-lymphotropic virus type III in lymph nodes and peripheral blood from infected individuals by in situ hybridization. 1986, Proc Natl Acad Sci USA 83, 772-776

4. Kuo-Ping Ch, Cohen St, Morris D, Jordan G. Intracellular amplification of proviral DNA in tissue sections using the polymerase chain reaction. 1992, J Histochem Cytochem 40, 333-341

5. Nuovo GJ, Gallery F, MacConnell Ph, Becker J, Block W. Am improved technique for the in situ detection of DNA after polymerase chain reaction amplification. 1991a, Am J Pathol 139, 1239-1244

6. Nuovo GJ, MacConnell Ph, Forde A, Delvenne Ph. Detection of human papillomavirus DNA in formalin-fixed tissues by in situ hybridization after amplification by polymerase chain reaction. 1991b, Am J Pathol 139, 847-854

7. Schnittman SM, Greenhouase JJ, Psallidopoulos MC. Increasing viral burden in CD4+ T cells from patients with human immunodeficiency virus (HIV) infection refelcts rapidly progressive immunosuppression and clinical disease. 1990, Ann Intern Med 113, 438-443

20. Oligonucleotides in the Field of PCR

20.1. Guidelines for designing PCR primers

The efficiency of the PCR and thus, the yield and the purity of the amplicon are influenced by numerous parameters. Above all, the choice of the oligonucleotides used and their annealing temperature are decisive. In simple terms, whether a primer will be elongated or not depends on whether the phenomenon of primer dissociation or that of primer elongation dominates quantitatively. When choosing the primers, the following factors are to be taken into account:
- melting temperature of the oligonucleotides
- length of the primers
- concentration of the primers
- sequence of the primers (ratio of the four bases, wobble position, base modifications)
- salt concentrations of the reaction buffer
- degree of purity of the primers

The usual 0.2µmol scale syntheses result in yields of 200-600µg of a 20mer. The concentrations of the purified primers (see chapter 20.3) are determined measuring their optical density at 260nm. As a rule of thumb, approximately 33µg primer correspond to 1 OD_{260}. The OD can, e.g., be determined by adding 10µl of the synthesis product, resuspended in 300µl aqua bidest., to 300µl aqua bidest. and then measuring the OD of this mixture in a quartz cuvette. For greater precision, the molar extinction coefficient (E_m) should be taken into account. E_m is the optical density of a 1M solution of a primer, determined at 260nm in a 1cm-pathlength quartz cuvette. The formula for determining E_m has already been given on page 11 (chapter 1).

The usual primer concentrations used for PCRs are sometimes also influenced by the design and the goal of the assay. In most cases, 100pmol primer/100µl reaction mixture are used for the preparation of 5-15pmol of a 250-500bp fragment. Generally, primer concentrations should be kept as low as possible, since high concentrations facilitate the formation of primer dimers and non-specific products, and reduce the fidelity of DNA polymerases (for further details, see also pp. 11-12). The optimal annealing temperature (T_{opt}) of oligonucleotides can be approximated mathematically by taking into account the melting temperature (T_m) (for examples of this, see p. 11). The "melting temperature" of an oligonucleotide is the temperature at which 50% of the oligonucleotide duplex dissociates under particular concentrations of duplex and cation. For the determination of the T_{opt} value in the design of various primers in the PCR assay, computer programs have become available, e.g., the OLIGO™ program (Rychlik 1989, 1990).

In addition to the factors that determine the hybridization temperature for Southern and Northern blots, the following factors must be considered for PCR:
1. Due to the decrease in the initial primer concentration and the increase in concentration of the product during the amplification cycles, the T_{opt} value

changes.

2. Not only the sequence of the oligonucleotide itself, but also the sequence of neighboring bases determined the stability of the hybrid at different temperatures.

3. The salt concentrations of the buffer are crucial for the stability of the hybrids. One should remember that most of the formulas are based on 1M Na⁺ concentrations so that corrections with respect to real PCR conditions might be necessary. Rychlik et al. (1990) have tried to do justice to the special PCR conditions by using an optimized equation for calculating T_{opt}:

$$T_{opt} = 0.3\, T_m^{primer} + 0.7\, T_m^{product} - 14.9 \quad [1]$$

where T_m^{primer} is the T_m value of the primer-template couple and Tmproduct is the Tm value of the PCR product. For calculating the value for T_m^{primer}, the authors have used the nearest-neighbor model of Borer et al. (1974) and the thermodynamic values of Breslauer et al. (1986). However, since the latter relate to a 1M Na⁺ buffer, a correction factor must be introduced for the PCR (50mM K⁺):

$$Tm_{primer} = \frac{\delta H}{\delta S + R \times \ln(c/4)} - 273.15 + 16.6 \log [K^+] \quad [2]$$

δH and δS are the enthalpy and entropy of helix formation, resp., R is the molar gas constant (1.987 cal/°C x mmol), and c (the total molar concentration of the annealing oligonucleotide) was empirically determined by the authors to be 250pM.

For the calculation of $T_m^{product}$, the authors took into account the equation of Baldino et al. (1989):

$$T_m^{product} = 0.41\, (\%G + \%C) + 16.6 \log [K^+] - 675/L \quad [3]$$

L corresponds to the length of the PCR product being formed.

Using these equations, the authors calculated T_{opt} values corresponding to the optimized test values with a mean deviation of 0.7°C.

The "detection window" of various oligonucleotides - i.e., the annealing temperature range at which amount and specificity of the amplicon occur at the most favorable ratio - depends on various factors, but essentially on the T_m value of the oligonucleotide. However, in most cases, the annealing temperature of standardizable PCR assays can be varied by 4°C-10°C without the specific band disappearing completely.

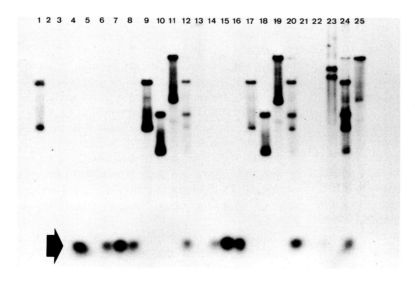

Figure 20.1: Autoradiography (2hrs) of a 6% PAGE, labeling of the products by incorporation of ³²P-dCTP during the amplification reaction. Several amplification products from different gene regions of mycobacteria (lanes **9-12, 17-20**) are demonstrated. Lane **1**, reference with M. tb H37Rv; lanes **7, 8, 14-16, 22**, negative control; lanes **2-6**, Nocardia; lanes **9-13**, M. tuberculosis; lanes **17-20**, M. bovis. In all cases where no or only few specific products are detectable (e.g., lanes **2-6**), distinct primer dimers (arrow) with sizes of about 50bp are formed.

Presently, almost all commercially available programs for the design of primers take into account the problem of 3' homology between the two primers. If the 3' ends of both primers possess complementary base sequences (e.g., -GG 3' vs. -CC 3'), hybridization of the two primers with each other is an almost regular phenomenon leading to the formation of so-called primer dimers. Primer dimers result from the amplification of hybrids between the two primers. This product, upon denaturation, is a perfect template for further primer binding and elongation. If the phenomenon of 3' end complementarity is disregarded in the design of primers the PCR assays may produce primer dimers only. This will, of course, result in complete or near-complete insensitivity to the target sequence. Even without complementarity of the 3' ends, primer dimers may be formed anytime. Interestingly, purine-purine pairings (G-G) yield the least primer dimer artefacts. Even though the primers are increasingly used up in the course of the reaction, primer dimers frequently occur at more than 30 cycle numbers. Although the occurrence of primer dimers is often an indication that the primers were not, or could not be, matched ideally or that experimental conditions were not chosen ideally, the demonstration of primer dimers in the detection gel is always an indication that the amplification reaction has worked, even if no specific amplicon was formed.

Rychlik et al. (1990) have shown that, with fragments smaller than 1kb, increasing the annealing temperature for every second cycle by 1°C each leads to an efficiency of amplification approximately 33% higher than with constant annealing temperature. However, this can only be demonstrated with plasmid DNA, not with genomic DNA. It would therefore offer itself to perform this annealing-temperature modification with nested PCR assays. In contrast, Don et al. (1991) propose, in the "touchdown" PCR named by them, to start with an annealing temperature of 65°C, in order to increase the specificity during the initial cycles, and then to decrease this temperature consecutively over several cycles to the "touchdown" temperature of 55°C, followed by a further 11 cycles at this temperature of 55°C.

The alteration of the annealing temperature in the design of a one-tube nested PCR and the use of the "GC clamp" is described in chapter 3. In situations in which, due to the design of the PCR, the choice of primer is very restricted and the primers in question have strongly different T_m values, it may be advisable to approximate the T_m value for the two primers with additional sequences at the 5' ends.

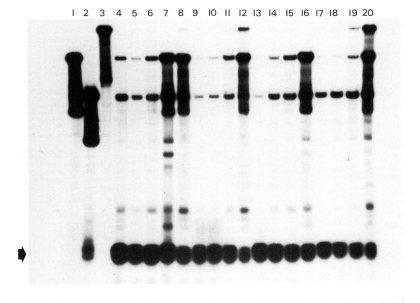

Figure 20.2: Example of an optimization experiment of a multiplex PCR (for details, see chapter 12) in which the ratio of the three primers (formation of a 383bp, 240bp, and 183bp amplification product) was varied with respect to each other. The concentration of primer 1 (383bp fragment) in this mixture remained constant. For details of this experiment, see figure 12.1, chapter 12. The high percentage of primer dimers (arrow) with the use of 3 different primer pairs in a PCR tube is here clearly visible.

In view of the current konwledge it is recommendable to keep the following in mind when designing oligonucleotides:

1. Rule of thumb: The reduction of the annealing temperature reduces the specificity of an assay but in some situations increases the chance to get an amplicon at all. Increasing the annealing temperature increases the stringency of an amplification so that in most cases, up to a temperature limit, a more specific product can be obtained.
2. The ratio of G/C to A/T should be approximately 1:1.
3. The oligonucleotides should not contain secondary structures. If secondary structures are present in the amplicon, the use of 7-deaza-2'-deoxyguanosine triphosphate (c7dGTP) (McConlogue 1988) can be helpful in certain cases.
4. The length should be between 18 and 26bp for standard PCRs. In some cases, lengthening of oligonucleotides contributes in some cases to a higher specificity. With allele-specific PCR assays, shorter (14mer-16mer) primers are to be recommended.
5. The T_m values of the oligonucleotides should be between 65°C and 72°C (for exceptions, see one-tube nested PCR, chapter 3). Conditions for a two-step PCR (annealing and elongation at the same temperature) improve with temperature approaching 72°C.
6. It makes sense to position the 3' end on triplets coding for conserved amino acids with nondegenerate codons.
7. When dealing with unclear template sequences, wobbling of the primer at critical points increases the probability of obtaining a product. Addition of an inosine base at the 3´end might further improve conditions (see chapters 3.9 and 3.10).
8. 3' complementarity must be avoided for all primers under all circumstances. This is all the more true for multiplex PCR assays (cf. chapter 12).

20.2. Synthesis of oligonucleotides

The availability of synthetic oligonucleotides as primers for PCR has become an important factor in performing amplification reactions. Automation of chemical synthesis has considerably simplified the production of these primers. Stepwise automated coupling of base is performed in repeated reaction cycles on a DNA synthesizer. The chemically produced DNA is single-stranded and of authentic base composition and cannot be distinguished from natural nucleic acid. The key to automation is the application of the principle of solid-phase synthesis, which was originally developed for the synthesis of peptides. First attempts at applying this efficient and simple technique to the production of oligonucleotides were made as early as 10 years ago. The oligonucleotide, which is covalently bound to a chemically inert carrier, "grows" by stepwise coupling of individual DNA base monomers. The first nucleoside (A, C, G, or T, 3' end of the sequence to be synthesized) is already bound to the carrier when the synthesis starts. The 5' end of the nucleoside is free for the coupling of the next base (A, C, G, T, or modified bases). The dissolved base monomers for coupling are kept in supply reservoirs connected to the transport system of the synthesizer. These monomers are the "mobile" phase and are transported to the carrier material in a well-defined manner. At the surface of the carrier material, the activated base monomer reacts with the firmly bound first nucleotide to form a dinucleotide. Before the next synthesis round, excessive reagents are rapidly and efficiently removed by washing. This is a decisive advantage of solid-phase synthesis over earlier techniques, which synthesized DNA in solution. Here, the intermediate products had to be separated from the initial reagents after each step, which was time-consuming and reduced the yield. New techniques for the use of oligonucleotides include the incorporation of inosine as a "wobble" base at ambiguous codon positions. The most widely used carrier material for solid-phase synthesis is silicate-based controlled pore class (CPG), an inert material of defined pore size (several hundreds of angstroms in diameter). The pores provide sufficient space for coupling new bases to the

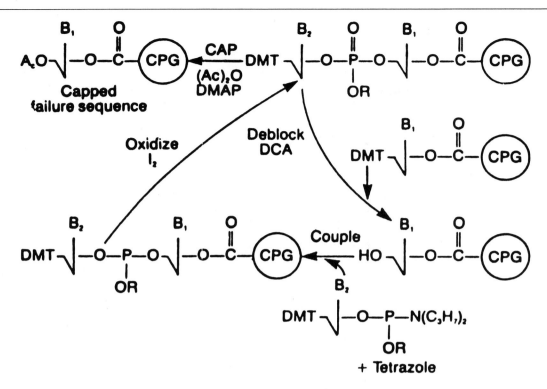

Figure 20.3 shows a diagram of a synthesis cycle. Activation by tetrazol and coupling must be followed by oxidation with an iodine solution in order to produce authentic and stable phosphodiester bonds like in natural DNA. "Capping" is performed to remove those molecules which reacted only incompletely with the activated amidite monomer (<1%): Free DNA ends are modified in a chemically irreversible manner (acetylation) to block further extension of the chain. Without the capping step, shorter DNA molecules with bases lacking in various positions would be formed.

growing DNA chain. Derived CPG material is commercially available, both in bulk and in small plastic columns ready for use on the synthesizer without further preparation.

Various DNA synthesizers are available on the market, ranging from simple devices for the production of DNA primers to large systems for sophisticated applications, i.e., from single- to four-column systems, on which up to four DNA syntheses can be run simultaneously (ABI, Beckman, Millipore). The selection of the most suitable system depends on quantitative requirements and the expected chemical modification capacity of the oligonucleotides to be produced.

DNA synthesizers can synthesize oligonucleotides with a length of up to about 200 base pairs. Nearly 100% coupling is required for efficient synthesis and high yields of raw DNA. The work on the use of deoxyribonucleoside ß-cyanoethyl phosphoramidites for solid-phase synthesis of oligonucleotides in the 80s was a major prerequisite for the advancement of DNA chemistry. The nucleoside - adenosyl, cytidyl, guanosyl, or thymidyl - is bound to the amidite group which, upon activation with tetrazol, reacts with the free end of the growing DNA chain (immobilized at the CPG carrier) with an efficiency of 99%. All amidite monomers are provided with an acid-labile blocking group, dimethoxytrityl (DMT), in the 5' position. After each coupling cycle the blocking group has to be removed for the next step. Diluted acid (deblocking solution, 3% dichloroacetic acid) is added, which removes the DMT groups in less than 30sec. In an acid environment, the free cation DMT shows bright orange staining. The amount of free DMT groups can be determined photometrically to calculate the stepwise coupling efficiency which may vary between 98 and over 99%, depending on the system and the quality of the reagents used. Chemical synthesis runs contrary to enzymatic synthesis: the sequence is built up from the 3' end to the 5' end. Before using the synthesized DNA in biological experiments the DMT group has to be removed automatically by the synthesizer or by incubating in 80% acetic acid for 20min.

When using reverse-phase chromatography, the DMT group must remain in place during purification. In all other cases of chromatographic or electrophoretic separation, the DMT group can be removed by the synthesizer. At the end of synthesis, the completed DNA is removed from its carrier by treating with concentrated aqueous ammonia at room temperature for 30min.

Modern DNA synthesizers are equipped with various synthesis scales, ranging from 0.05 µMol to 15 µMol. Most PCR applications require only low amounts of synthetic primers; several OD_{260} (1 OD = 33µg) is more than enough for multiple reactions. The required amount can easily be generated with a 0.05 µMol synthesis of a 20mer, which yields 5 to 8 OD_{260} of the product. According to the synthesis scale selected, the synthesis columns are filled with corresponding amounts of derived CPG material. The 0.2µMol synthesis scale with about 20 OD_{260} of raw product (approx. 600µg) is often used as a standard. This amount is not only sufficient for many experiments, but also for DNA purification after synthesis. Labeling of oligonucleotides with fluorescent dyes is an alternative to radioactive labeling. The 5' end of the oligonucleotide must be "functionalized" for the coupling of biotin, fluorescein, rhodamine etc. Phosphoramidites with a DNA base replaced by a molecular spacer (hexyl, C6) and the functional group - an amino or thiol group - are used as linkers. Synthesizers can automatically attach the linkers to the 5' end of the oligonucleotides as the last base-coupling step. Premature reactions are prevented by providing the functional groups (amino or thiol) with a blocking group, which is removed manually after synthesis and prior to the coupling of the fluorescent dye.

20.3. Purification of oligonucleotides

After chemical synthesis of an oligodeoxyribonucleoside, it is necessary to analyze the synthesis mixture for assessing whether the desired oligomer has been synthesized at all and, if so, in sufficient amount. In addition, even with quality synthesizers, it is necessary for some PCR applications to separate by-products from the synthesis product properly to allow for a preparative purification. Several purification methods are available: acrylamide gels (Maniatis 1975), reversed- (Zon 1986) or ion-exchange (Scanion 1984), high-performance liquid chromatography (HPLC), and trityl cartridge methods. The last method takes advantage of the hydrophobicity of the 5' dimethoxytrityl group, that was added during synthesis (McBride 1988). After synthesis, the tritylated full-length oligonucleotide is bound to a hydrophobic resin, by interaction with the trityl group. Low-molecular-weight contaminants and untritylated by-products or wrong synthesis products are eluted from the purification support as they remain unbound. The full-length oligonucleotide is detritylated on the solid support and subsequently eluted (for details of the procedure, see Method 3 in this chapter). The trityl cartridge minicolumns, compared to HPLC and PAGE, have the advantage of being not quite as labor-intensive and time-consuming. Before the oligonucleotides are purified using solid supports or gels, it is necessary, in a final deprotection step, to split off the benzoyl and isobutyryl groups protecting the primary amino groups of the bases. The usual protocols achieve this by incubation of the synthesized oligonucleotides in concentrated ammonium hydroxide at 55°C for about 8 hours, or at room temperature for about 16-24 hours (Sinha 1984). A simplification of this lengthy incubation period has been described by Reynolds and Buck (1992), showing that incubation of the synthesized oligonucleotides in concentrated (30%) NH_4OH at 85°C for less than 30 mins has the same deprotection efficiency as the splitting-off at usual temperatures (55°C or room temperature, resp.) over 8-24 hours. This rapid high-temperature deprotection protocol is highly efficient for oligonucleotides with a length of 15-30 bases. Longer nucleotides require a somewhat longer deprotection incubation.

Reverse-phase chromatography

This procedure separates the crude oligonucleotide mixture on the basis of different hydrophobicities of the molecules. Since the technique exploits the nonpolar properties of the above-mentioned 5' terminal DMT blocking groups, these are not automatically removed at the end of synthesis. Complete DNA molecules have the hydrophobic group at the 5' end while all (shorter) molecules are capped and lack this group Therefore they are more hydrophilic than the main DNA product with the complete base sequence. The phase material used in reverse-phase systems (C18) shows stronger interaction with the more hydrophobic main product than with the more hydrophilic shorter sequences. A binary buffer system (aqueous/acetonitrile) elutes shorter molecules first and DNA molecules of complete base length (DMT+) at increasing acetonitrile concentrations. The formation of double-stranded DNA segments from complementary sequence segments, which yields diffuse chromatography profiles, can be prevented by increasing the working temperature of the column (60° to 72°C) using a column oven.

Anion-exchange chromatography

While reverse-phase chromatography separates DMT+ from DMT- molecules, anion-exchange chromatography uses the principle of molecule size. The phase material in the separation column interacts more strongly with molecules carrying a higher negative charge. Thus, since DNA primers with longer base chains contain more phosphodiester anions (i.e., linkages between two DNA bases), longer oligonucleotides are more strongly bound to the column matrix than shorter molecules. Thus this technique first elutes the defective sequences. The longer DNA molecules are eluted at continuously increasing salt concentrations (gradient 0 to 600mM, consisting of a binary system, buffer B: 0.9M NaCl, buffer A: 25mM TE, pH 8.3).

Procedure	Comments

Method 1: Purification of oligonucleotides by gel electrophoresis

1. After the deprotection procedure, dry the deprotected oligonucleotides by evaporation in the vacuum centrifuge. After complete drying of the pellet (yellowish-white, slightly crumbly pellet), solve the oligonucleotide in 60-100µl sterile water.	1. Again and again, it has been discussed whether oligonucleotides can also be used unpurified for the PCR. Even though today's synthesizers yield high qualities for oligonucleotides, failure sequences of about 10% occur as a rule. These undesirable products

Procedure(cont.)

2. Mix an aliquot (e.g., 10µl) with deionized formamide (20µl; for deionization procedure, see chapter 10.4.1) in an Eppendorf tube and denature the mixture at 95°C for 3min. Subsequently, cool rapidly on ice before the sample is loaded on the gel.

3. Pour a 0.4mm-thick denaturing polyacrylamide gel (for details, see chapter 10.4) between siliconized plates with 10mm-wide slots, adding 7M urea.

4. Load about 10µl oligonucleotide solution in each of the slots. It is sufficient to load 5µl formamide dye mixture in one slot as reference.

5. Let the gel run at constant voltage (e.g., 1,000-1,500 V) until the bromphenol marker has reached about 2/3 of the gel length.

6. Carefully transfer the gel to a saran wrap and make the bands visible under 254nm UV light.

Comments(cont.)

are the result of incomplete coupling steps and chemical by-reactions occurring during synthesis (e.g., depurination during strong acid treatment, phosphitylation of O6 in guanosine leading to the formation of branched chains).

2. The remaining oligonucleotide solution can be vacuum-dried for longer storage and subsequently be stored at -20°C.

3. The concentration of the acrylamide (20%, 16%, or 12%) depends on the length of the oligonucleotide. For siliconization, the glass plates should be wiped clean - under a vent! - using a 5% dichlordimethylsilane, 95% chloroform solution. Then rinse the glass plates with water intensively and repeatedly and bake for 2 hours at 180°C.

4. If only an analytical gel was to be performed to check the purity of synthesis, amounts of 0.0015-0.002 OD_{260} suffice in case a radioactive measurement is taken. For this, 0.015-0.03 OD_{260} is resuspended in 1µl 10xkinase buffer, 1µl unlabeled ATP [660µM], 1µl spermidine [10mM], 1µl ^{32}P gamma ATP (3,000Ci/mmol), 5µl aqua bidest., 1µl T4 polynucleotide kinase (2 U). Incubate for 30min to an hour at 37°C. Mix a few microliters of this mixture with 7µl formamide solution.

5. The running length of 2/3 of the gel for bromphenol blue applies to 20% denaturing PAGE. In gels containing less acrylamide, the marker should run further. As an indication for the co-migration of the dye, see also chapter 10.4.1, description of the PAGE method.

6. The desired product should be the least mobile band in the respective slot row. It should show as the most prominent band, indicating it is present in highest quantitiy. For UV shadowing, 1-3 OD_{260} units of crude sample are required. Alternatively, for methylene staining, only 0.05-0.1 OD_{260} units are required.

Procedure(cont.) *Comments(cont.)*

7. Cut out the desired oligonucleotide from the gel using a scalpel.

8. Carefully transfer the gel fragment into a 1.5ml tube, adding 1.5ml elution buffer. Incubate overnight at 37°C with constant shaking.

8. Elution buffer: 0.5M ammonium acetate, 10mM magnesium acetate in aqua bidest.

9. Vortex the sample, then centrifuge at maximum speed (about 13,000rpm) for 10min.

10. Transfer the supernatant (about 1.3ml) into a new tube.

11. Wash the remaining gel with 0.5ml elution buffer, vortex, and centrifuge as under 9. Transfer this supernatant and unite with the supernatant from 10.

11. In order to safely remove all gel fragments, sometimes filtering of the supernatants with a Millipore filter disc (0.45µm) is recommended.

12. Distribute oligonucleotides over three tubes (approx. 600µl per tube) and precipitate each tube with 1ml ice cold ethanol. Store at -70°C for about 30min. Centrifuge at 4°C for 15min with 15,000rpm.

13. Carefully lift off the supernatant, wash the pellet twice with cold 95% ethanol (400µl at 0°C), centrifuge at maximum speed (about 13,000rpm) and 4°C, completely remove the ethanol, and dry the pellet.

14. Dissolve the pellet in 1ml aqua bidest., measure the absorbance at 260nm in order to determine the concentration of the oligonucleotide.

Method 2: Purification of oligonucleotides by reverse-phase HPLC

1. Dry the deprotected and DMT-on synthesized oligonucleotide in the centrifuge at vacuum speed and subsequently dissolve the (yellowish-white) pellet well in 300µl aqua bidest.

Procedure(cont.)

2. Prepare the buffer systems for the HPLC apparatus (Beckman). Solvent: 100mM TEAA, pH 7.0 (A), acetonitril (HPLC grade) (B). Pregasing of the solvents or ultrasound treatment. Prerun with an acetonitril gradient from 0% to 100% in 20min to clean the columns. Then equilibrate the system with 15% B and 85% A.

3. Separation columns: Columns stuffed with a kieselguhr-polydimethylacrylamide support using Hypersil ODS (Knauer Co.), 5µm grain size. Main column 4mm x 250mm, precolumn 4mm x 60mm.

4. HPLC run conditions (pump volume 1ml/min)

The stationary phase is run with 0.1M TEAA, the mobile phase with acetonitril.
- 5min 15% B
- 25min increase in B from 15% to 30%
- 5min plateau at 30% B
- 3min increase in B from 30% to 100%
- 10min plateau at 100% B
- 5min decrease in B from 100% to 15%
- 15min equilibration of columns with 15% B and 85% A

Wavelength for the detection of oligonucleotides 260nm

5. Collect the peak (mostly about 1ml) in an Eppendorf tube.

6. Vacuum-dry the collected peak in the centrifuge. Dissolve in 300µl 80% acetic acid for 20min at room temperature to split off the DMT group. Add 300µl 100% ethanol (p.a.) and vacuum-dry again in the centrifuge. Dissolve in about 100µl aqua bidest., add 1/10 vol. sodium acetate and three times the volume 100% ethanol. Precipitate at -70°C for about 1 hour, vacuum-dry again, dissolve in 300µl aqua bidest., and measure OD_{260} to determine the concentration.

7. With a 0.2µM oligonucleotide synthesis, the yield should be about 20 OD_{260}.

Comments(cont.)

2. Preparation of a 1M triethyl ammonium acetate solution, pH 7.0 (TEAA): drop-by-drop addition of 1M Triethylamin (Merck) into an aqueous 1M (500ml) acetic acid solution in an ice bath (the reaction is exothermic!). Adjust pH value to 7.0 with concentrated TEA or acetic acid, then fill up to 1,000ml.

representing the by-products.

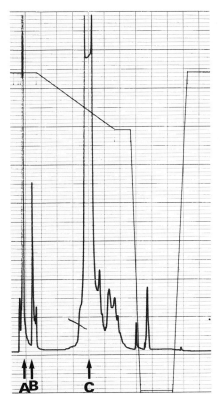

Figure 20.4: Analysis of a crude mixture of a oligonucleotide (using HPLC method): 30mer 5'GAA CTG TTG CAT GGA TCC TGT GTT TGC AAC 3'. Hypersil ODS (Knauer Co.) 4.0 x 250mm column (5µm). **Buffer A:** 0.1M TEAA (pH 7.0). **Buffer B:** 100% acetonitril. Gradient: 5min 15% B; 25min increase in B to 30%; 5min plateau at 30% B; 3min increase in B to 100%; 5min decrease in B to 15%; 15min equilibrating with 15%. The first peak (A) represents untritrylated oligonucleotides, the second peak (B) benzamide residue, and the third (main) peak (C) the oligonucleotide to be purified. Some smaller peaks follow,

The OligoPak™ column from Millipore achieves base-specific separation of oligonucleotide mixtures of 2 to 100 bases at amounts of up to approx. 100µg in about 1 hour. Between 10 and 20 OD_{260} units of crude oligonucleotide can be loaded on one column. The end product is suitable for being used as a primer or probe or for similar applications. The separation principle is the relative hydrophobicity of the different species present in the solution. The least hydrophobic molecules are eluted first. The more hydrophobic molecules are retained on the column longer. For this method, the oligonucleotide must be synthesized in such a way that the 5'DMT group stays on the molecule and is not split off after the synthesis has ended. The DMT group renders the product oligomer more hydrophobic, which makes it possible to separate the desired end product from failure sequences, the latter have free 5' hydroxyl groups and are therefore eluted earlier.

Procedure	Comments

Method 3: Quick purification of oligonucleotides using anion-exchange columns (OligoPak™)

1. Perform a standard oligonucleotide synthesis with the 5' protection group (DMT-on synthesis).

2. Split off the 3' protection group from the oligonucleotide by adding 1.0ml 30% ammonia and incubating for 40min (oligo 15-30mer) at 85°C or, alternatively, for 6-8 hours at 55°C.

2. When handling ammonia, it is imperative to keep in mind that, with repeated opening of the bottle, the highly volatile, highly concentrated ammonia (32%) loses its potency. If lower-concentrated ammonia is used for the deprotection procedure, the removal of the base blocking groups is incomplete, resulting in oligonucleotides with altered hybridization specificity and reduced amplification efficiency. We recommend to always store the ammonia well isolated (sealed with additional parafilm) at 4°C and aliquoted.

3. Preequilibrate the OligoPak™ column with 5ml 100% acetonitril in a 5ml syringe, let the solution run through twice.

4. Rinse the column with 3 x 5ml 1M TEAA, pH 7.0 (see Method 2).

5. Dilute 10-20 OD_{260} (generally corresponding to the amount for a 0.2µM synthesis) of the DMT-on oligonucleotide, now deprotected and dissolved in ammonia, with the same volume (1:1) of aqua bidest.

6. Withdraw this mixture (about 2.0ml) with a syringe and slowly inject it in the OligoPak™ column. Collect the eluate and reinject it in the column twice more.

6. Always store the eluate until final purification and OD measurement of the oligonucleotide, in case problems arise with the coupling of the oligonucleotide to the column.

7. Wash three times with 5ml 3% ammonia each, to remove the short synthesis fragments.

7. 1 part 30% ammonia stock solution, 9 parts aqua bidest.

Procedure(cont.)   *Comments(cont.)*

8. With oligonucleotides shorter than 75mers, subsequently wash using 3 x 5ml aqua bidest.; with longer ones, 4 x 5ml aqua bidest.

9. Wash with 5ml 2% trifluoroacetic acid (TFA) for a period of about 1min, to detritylate the oligonucleotides.

9. 3ml trifluoroacetic acid (100%) + 97ml aqua bidest.

10. Remove leftover TFA by washing with 2 x 5ml aqua bidest.

11. Elute the purified product with 3 x 1ml 20% acetonitril, collecting each 1ml fraction separately.

12. Vacuum-dry the aliquots in the centrifuge. Resuspend the pellets in 300µl aqua bidest. Determine the OD_{260}, store the resuspended oligonucleotide at -20°C.

20.3. Chemical modification of oligonucleotides

With the increase in possible applications for oligonucleotides, there is also an increase in possible modifications that can be made to these short DNA fragments. The modifications represent, on the one hand, a functionalization of the DNA fragment (e.g., the incorporation of biotin at the 5' end for the production of single-stranded DNA in the framework of sequencing; see chapter 14). On the other hand, with a corresponding increase in sensitivity, the modifications make it possible to detect a target in the framework of hybridization or, in the case of direct incorporation, to demonstrate the end product.

In addition to the marking of oligonucleotides with radioactive substances, numerous non-radioactive markers have become available. Marking is here most easily achieved already during synthesis by directly incorporating a dye molecule at the 5' end, e.g., biotin phosphoramidite (e.g., Glen Research Corp., Sterling/USA). Besides biotin, rhodamine-, acridine-, and FITC-amidites are also commercially available for the direct incorporation at the 5' end of the oligonucleotide (Peninsula Corp.). As an alternative to the direct incorporation of the dye marker during synthesis of the oligonucleotide, a functionalization of the 5' end is possible. This is done by employing phosphoramidites that are complemented by a molecule spacer (e.g., hexyl radical, C6) and a functionalized group (e.g., amino or thiol groups). These steps, too, can be performed automatically by the synthesizer during the last step of synthesis, mostly by placing the linker chemicals at the free position (e.g., position X in the Millipore DNA synthesizer). Premature reactions are prevented by providing the functional groups with a blocking group, which is removed manually after synthesis and prior to the coupling of the fluorescent dye.

Besides the functionalization of the 5' end of an oligonucleotide, there is also one available for the 3' end. Here, the marking process is divided into two steps. First, the oligonucleotide is functionalized at the 3' end with a primary aliphatic amine group (e.g., 3'-Amine-on CPG, Cruachem/UK). 3' amine-on CPG is an ordinary CPG fully compatible with the programs of automatic DNA synthesizers, but incorporating a primary amine group at the 3' end. In the second step, the 3' amino-modifier oligonucleotide reacts with biotin-XX-NHS ester or with FITC. When choosing the biotin, one should be aware that quality and quantity of this reaction, as well as the subsequent usability of this biotin group are determined by the length of the biotin spacer on the one hand. On the other hand, the reaction turns out to be very different with different biotin preparations from different manufacturers.

Procedure	Comments

Method 4: Labelling of oligonucleotides by T4 polynucleotide kinase

Synthetic oligonucleotides are synthesized without a 5' phosphate group and can therefore be marked quickly at the 5' OH end by the transfer of $\alpha^{32}P$. This is supplied by $[\alpha^{32}P]ATP$ and catalyzed by the T4 kinase enzyme. As far as the reaction is performed effectively, the labelling efficiency of the oligonucleotide can be identical to that of $[\tau^{32}P]ATP$ itself.

1.	1µl oligonucleotide (0.5µg, or 10pmol/µl) + 2.0µl 10x T4 kinase buffer + 5.0µl [τ32P]ATP (10pmol) [sp. act. 3,000 Ci/mmol; 10mCi/ml] 10.0µl aqua bidest.	1. It is imperative to use gloves and plastic shields for all procedures, because of the handling of radioactive materials. Properly dispose of buffers, tubes, and columns that have contained radioactive agents. Sterilize water and microfuge tubes by autoclaving. $[\tau^{32}P]ATP$ 3,000Ci/mmol, 10mCi/ml (NEN) T4 polynucleotide kinase, 10U/µl (Gibco-BRL) 5ml 10x T4 polynucleotide kinase buffer: 1.25ml of a 2M stock solution of Tris-HCl (pH 7.6) 0.5ml of a 1M stock solution of $MgCl_2$

Procedure(cont.)   *Comments(cont.)*

	0.25ml of a 1M stock solution of 1M dithiothreitol [DTT] Final concentrations: 0.5M Tris, pH 7.4, 0.1M $MgCl_2$, 50mM DTT Optionally, spermidine (final conc. 1mM) and EDTA (pH 8.0, final conc. 1mM) can be added to the buffer. In some mixtures, this contributes to a slight increase in efficiency. The mixture contains equivalent amounts of [^{32}P]ATP and oligonucleotide. The efficiency of the transfer is in most cases about 50%. An increase in efficiency can be achieved by an increase in the amount of oligonucleotide or of [^{32}P]ATP.
2. Mix everything thoroughly and centrifuge. Then, add 1.5μl (15U) T4 kinase, mix again, centrifuge. Incubate the mixture at 37°C for 45min.	2. If the specific activity of the labeled oligonucleotide is too low, the mixture can again be mixed with 10 or 15U T4 kinase and the reaction can ba performed once more at 37°C for 30-45min.
3. Heat the mixture at 65°C for about 5min in order to inactivate the enzyme.	
4. Equilibrate the Sep-Pak C18 column as recommended by the manufacturer.	4. Depending on what the labeled probe is used for, it is necessary to remove the ^{32}P-molecules not transferred. For numerous hybridization experiments, this is not necessary. If the oligonucleotide is larger than 18-22bp, separation can be carried out quickly and easily by ethanol precipitation. With shorter fragments, the use of cetylpyridinium bromide (Maniatis 1982) is recommended. If more stringent conditions for the separation of nonbonded activity are needed, the possibility of separation by a 20% polyacrylamide gel is available, or the use of G-50 Sephadex columns or Sep-Pak C18 columns. Regarding the method of ethanol precipitation, see method 1, chapter 20.
5. Dilute the reaction mixture with 1.5ml sterile aqua bidest. Let the whole mixture run through the column (about 1.0ml/min).	
6. Wash the column with 10ml 25mM ammonium bicarbonate (pH 8.2), subsequently 10ml 25mM ammonium bicarbonate/5% acetonitril, and finally 20ml aqua bidest./5% acetonitril.	

Procedure(cont.) *Comments(cont.)*

7. Elute the radio-labeled oligonucleotides by washing three times with 1ml aqua bidest./10% acetonitril.

8. Vacuum-dry the eluate in a centrifuge until the pellet has dried.

9. Dissolve the pellet in 10µl TE buffer (pH 7.6).

Method 5: Chemical labelling of oligonucleotides using photoactive biotin

1. Dissolve 1mg photoactivable biotin reagent (PAB) by adding 1.0ml aqua bidest. (final concentration: 1µg/1µl). Shake cautiously; if necessary, vortex briefly.

1. E.g., Clontech's photoactivable reagent (Clontech Cat. # 5009-2). The stock solution produced is stable at -20°C for at least one year. However, the solution is very light-sensitive, so that all steps involving this solution should be performed in a darkened room.
In principle, the hybridization kinetics of biotin-labeled probes are the same as with radioactively marked probes. However, since biotinylation lowers the melting point, a slight modification becomes necessary. The use of 35-50% formamide during hybridization at, e.g., 42°C is sufficient for most systems.

2. Mix 1µg/µl oligonucleotides or DNA fragments with 3µl of the prepared stock solution at a volume ratio of 1:3 in a 1.5ml Eppendorf tube. Open the cap of the tube, incubate the mixture on ice while simultaneously lighting it with a 100W lamp for 15min from a height of 10cm.

2. Best results are achieved with the 1:3 ratio. However, ratios of 1:1 are also feasible.

3. For the extraction of the nucleic acids, the whole mixture is mixed with an identical volume of 0.1M Tris-HCl, pH 9.0, and filled up with aqua bidest. to a final volume of 100µl. Add 100µl 2-butanol. Vortex vigorously. Centrifuge the tube briefly to separate the phases. Carefully remove the upper phase (organic phase) with a pipet, discard the organic phase. Repeat the extraction procedure by adding another 100µl 2-butanol. Again, after centrifugation, remove the organic phases.

3. No phenol extraction must be performed with these biotinylated probes, since biotin is soluble in phenol.

Procedure(cont.)   *Comments(cont.)*

4. Add 3.0M sodium acetate, pH 5.6, until a final concentration of 0.3M is reached. Add three times the volume 100% ice-cold ethanol, precipitate at -70°C for 15min and centrifuge with maximum speed (about 13,000rpm) at 4°C for 10-15min. Decant the supernatant, dry the pellet. Dissolve the pellet in 10mM Tris-HCl, pH 7.5, 0.1mM EDTA. Store at -20°C.

Method 6: 3'-end biotin labelling by terminal deoxynucleotidyl transferase

The terminal deoxynucleotidyl transferase (TdT) enzyme (terminal transferase, calf thymus) catalyzes the addition of deoxynucleotides to the 3'-OH end of single- or double-stranded DNA molecules, according to the following formula:

$$ssDNAOH + ndNTP \xrightarrow{Mg^{++}} DNA\text{-}(pdN)_n + nPPi$$

TdT can be used to incorporate fluorescent dNTPs at the 3' end of synthesized oligonucleotides (Trainor and Jensen 1988). Flickinger at al. (1992) have checked the efficiency of coupling biotinylated dCTP and dATP to a 22bp oligonucleotide and were able to show that biotinylated derivatives of dCTP and dUTP are clearly better incorporated by TdT than is dATP. With regard to incorporation, biotin 11-dUTP and biotin dCTP differed in that, when using dCTP derivatives, the majority of the substrate molecules were tailed with multiple biotinylated radicals, whereas, with 11-dUTP, the subtrate was only tailed with one biotinylated radical in all cases. The labelling is fast and completed within about 15min.

1. Add 100pmol oligonucleotide in aqua bidest.

2. Add 4µl 5x cacodylate buffer.

2. 5x cacodylate buffer: 10mM $CoCl_2$, 0.5M potassium cacodylate, 100mM Tris-HCl, 5mM dithriothreitol, pH 7.2.
Caution: Potassium cacodylate, contained in the reaction buffer, is poisonous.
Preparation of the 5x cacodylate buffer: Equilibrate 5g Chelex 100 (Bio-rad) with 10ml 2-5M potassium acetate at room temperature. After 5min, wash Chelex 100 with 10ml water several times. Prepare a 1M potassium cacodylate solution by adjusting the pH value of cacodylic acid to 7.2 with KOH. Equilibrate the potassium cacodylate solution with Chelex for 2-3min at room temperature. Filter the mixture to remove the Chelex 100. Add water, dithiothreitol and cobalt

Procedure(cont.)　　　　　　　　　　　　　*Comments(cont.)*

chloride (in that order!) to the purified potassium cacodylate until final concentrations 5mM dithiothreitol, 0.5M cacodylate and 10mM cobalt chloride, respectively, are reached..

3. Add 300µM biotin 14-dCTP or biotin 7-dCTP.

4. Fill up with aqua bidest. to a volume of 16µl.

5. Add 4µl (40U) TdT (Gibco BRL, #510-8008SB).

6. Incubate whole mixture at 37°C for 30min.

7. Stop the reaction by heating to 65°C for 5min.

8. Separate the non-incorporated dNTPs, e.g., by Sephadex G-25 spin columns or Sep-Pak C18 columns, as described for method 4.

Method 7: Modifications of the 3' terminus with a primary aliphatic amine

In order to label the 3' end of an oligonucleotide non-enzymatically during synthesis, a functionalization of the 3' end is necessary analogous to 5' labelling. This is done through a primary aliphatic amine at the 3' end.

1. For the 3' modification, a so-called 3'-amine-on column (e.g., Cruachem) is used. The latter carries a bifunctional arm in place of the usual 3' base.

2. Enter the oligonucleotide sequence to be synthesized. Note that the 3'-terminal base of the sequence to be synthesized is entered as the second base, counting from the 3' end, and that, for the last 3'-terminal base, a nonsense base is entered. (The synthesizers are designed in such a way that the 3'-terminal base is already determined by the choice of column. However, the 3'-amine-on column does not carry a base - see above.)

3. Perform a trityl-off synthesis.

Procedure(cont.)   *Comments(cont.)*

4. Separate the 3'-amino-modified oligonucleotide from the carrier column by 1ml ammonium hydroxide for one hour at room temperature.

5. Transfer the ammonia solution to a screw cap and incubate at 55°C for 6 hours. Then vacuum-dry the synthesis product in the vacuum centrifuge.

5. Before opening the screw-cap tube for subsequent centrifuging in the vacuum centrifuge, cool to 4°C to prevent ammonia evaporation.

6. Dissolve the dried amino-modified oligonucleotide in 900µl aqua bidest.

7. Add 100µl 10x labeling buffer.

7. 10x labeling buffer: 1.0M sodium bicarbonate/carbonate (pH 9.0).

8. Add 250µl newly prepared biotin-XX-NHS ester, then shake briefly at once.

8. The biotin-XX-NHS solution always has to be prepared freshly: dissolve 5mg biotin-XX-NHS ester in 250µl N,N-dimethyl formamide (DMF) for a 0.2µM synthesis. Alternatively, the marking can be done in the same way by FITC labeling.

9. Incubate the mixture overnight at room temperature in the dark.

9. If precipitation occurs during incubation, the reaction should be continued for 2 hours at 42°C.

10. After incubation, the whole mixture is poured over a Sephadex G-25 (Pharmacia). Elution is done with aqua bidest. The labeled oligonucleotide will elute in the void volume.

10. Prepare the column by equilibrating with 5ml sheared, denatured DNA (1mg/1ml) and subsequently washing with aqua bidest.
The fractions should be collected in 1ml volumes and their absorption measured at UV_{260nm}.
Biotin can be detected by the p-dimethylamino cinnamaldehyde colorimetric test: 5µl of the 30-40 OD_{260}/ml biotinylated oligonucleotide solution are applied to a silica gel TLC plate. Then, an ethanol solution of 0.2% p-dimethylamino cinnamaldehyde and 2% sulphuric acid is sprayed on. With slight warming, a pink-red spot develops in the presence of biotin.
FITC can easily be detected through its absorption maximum at 495nm. If a more stringent purification of the marked oligo should be required, use of the HPLC method is recommended (see above). There, the lipophilic character of the biotin and FITC groups is responsible for the labeled oligonucleotide being retained longer on the column. Thus, its elution requires higher acetonitril concentrations. It can therefore be eluted as the unmistakably last peak in the purification process.

Procedure(cont.)   *Comments(cont.)*

Method 8: 5'-end labelling by an amino linker during synthesis (e.g., Millipore/Biosearch)

1. Dissolve 150mg of the linker in an appropriate volume of amidite diluent, as described by the manufacturer. Linkers are viscous, oily solutions, so that the dissolution will in most cases take a few minutes.

2. Milligen-Biosearch products for the Cyclone are described as an example: The MMT linker (150mg, MW 589.5 [MMT hexylamine linker 0.15mg, GEN 080020]) is dissolved in 4ml amidite (0.063M solution) and subsequently transferred to position 10 (X) of the DNA synthesizer.

2. It is imperative that, for at least 15sec, position 10 is being primed, in order for the dead-space volumes to be filled with MMT linker.

3. Enter the sequence to be synthesized. The linker always has to be at the 5' position and therefore entered first. Example: 5' XTA CCT AGT ...3'.

3. If the 5' amino linker is entered at some other position, this will lead to immediate chain termination.

4. The synthesis must be performed with DMT-on.

5. Standard purification follows, as for all oligos. See methods 1-3.

a) Biotinylation

6. With the usual synthesis, yields of between 150 and 500µg are obtained from 0.2µM syntheses with 20meres. For biotinylation, amounts of $10D_{260}$ per 6-20µl volume should be used. Fill up the purified oligos with 100µl aqua bidest.

7. Take 1.25 OD_{260} oligonucleotides (corresponding to about 37.5µg) to 75µl aqua bidest.

8. Add 75µl 0.5M Tris-HCl buffer (pH 7.6) and 150µl newly prepared 15mM NHS biotin in dimethyl formamide.

8. N-hydroxy-succimido biotin, MW 341.4, e.g., Sigma H-1759, 100mg dissolved in N,N-dimethyl formamide (DMF), e.g., Sigma D-4254. Prepare the solution. Depending on the number of oligonucleotides that are to be biotinylated, dissolve, e.g., 5mg Sigma-NHS biotin in 1.0ml DMF, approximately corresponding to a 15mM solution.

Procedure(cont.)   *Comments(cont.)*

9. Incubate the whole mixture at room temperature for 24 hours.

10. To separate non-bound biotin from the oligonucleotide, the mixture can be poured over
- NAP5 columns (Pharmacia #17-0853-01) or
- NENSORB 20 columns (Du Pont NEN NLP-022X)
or
- Ultrafree-MC units (Millipore, 30,000 NMWL polysulfone, UFC3 TTK25).

10. In our experiments, NENSORB columns have proved most suitable for purification purposes. Ultrafree columns from Millipore yielded the least reproducible data.

b) FITC marking

11. With the usual synthesis, yields of between 150 and 500µg are obtained from 0.2µM syntheses with 20meres. For biotinylation, amounts of $1OD_{260}$ per 6-20µl volume should be used. Fill up the purified oligos with 100µl aqua bidest.

12. Fill up 1.50 OD_{260} (corresponding to about 45µg) to 150µl aqua bidest.

13. Add 150µl fluorescein-isothiocynanate solution.

13. E.g., fluorescein isothiocyanate, FITC, Sigma F-7250, MW 389.39.
Preparation of the solution: 1mg FITC in 150µl buffer consisting of
- 1M Na-carbonate/bicarbonate buffer (pH 9.0),
- aqua bidest.,
- dimethyl formamide,   <u>at a ratio of 5:8:2</u>.

The solution always has to be freshly prepared.

14. Incubate the whole mixture in the dark at room temperature for about 18 hours.

15. Purify as in step 10 of biotinylation.

Procedure(cont.)   *Comments(cont.)*

Method 9: 5'-end biotin labelling by introduction of a sticky-end restriction site in the PCR with subsequent incorporation by Klenow polymerase

Example: An HIV-1-specific oligonucleotide (#520) used in our laboratory has the following sequence:

    5' ata atc cac cta tcc cag tag gag aaa t 3'

By synthesis of a 5' restriction site - for HIV-1, the BstEII enzyme offers itself, since there is no restriction site for it anywhere on the sequence - the following sequence is created:

5' at ggtaacc ata atc cac cta tcc cag tag gag aaa t 3'
   Bst EII

In the course of amplification, the site is incorporated in the amplification product as an originally non-annealing overhang (cf. also chapters 14 and 17). After successful PCR amplification, the fragment is cut with the BstEII enzyme.

Once more, it has to be pointed out that, of course, this site must not occur again in the sequence.
Using the standard protocol with Klenow polymerase, fill in the asymmetrical site at the 5' end - which is located for BstEII between g/gtaacc (+strand) and ggtaac/c (-strand) - with biotin 11-dUTP (e.g., Sigma B 7645), which is incorporated in place of T, while simultaneously adding corresponding concentrations of dATP, dGTP and dCTP.

1. Dissolve 50-100ng amplificate purified by gel in 20µl aqua bidest.

1. For the purification procedure for amplificates, see chapter 2.

2. Add 3µl 10x polymerase buffer, 3µl 10mM DTT, 3µl dNTP mix. Mix well, centrifuge well.

2. 10x polymerase buffer: 700mM Tris, pH 7.4, 100mM $MgCl_2$, 50mM DTT.
In each case, 0.5mM dNTP solution, biotin 11-dUTP in equal concentration.

3. Add 1µl (2U) Klenow polymerase.

4. Mix briefly, centrifuge again briefly.

5. Incubate at 37°C for 15min.

6. Inactivate the enzyme by heating to 65°C for 5min.

7. Purify the mixture as described with the other methods of this chapter.

References

1. Baldino F, Chesselet MF, Lewis ME. High-resolution in situ hybridization histochemistry. 1989, Methods Enzymol 168, 761-777

2. Borer PN, Dengler B, Tinoco I, Uhlenbeck OC. Stability of ribonucleic acid double-stranded helices. 1974, J Mol Biol 86, 843-853

3. Breslauer KJ, Frank R, Blöcker H, Marky LA. Predicting DNA duplex stability from the base sequence. 1986, Proc Natl Acad Sci USA 83, 3746-3750

4. Chollet A, Kawashima EH. Biotin-labeld oligodeoxynucleotides: chemical synthesis and uses as hybridization probes. 1985, Nucl Acids Res 13, 1529-1541

5. Don RH, Cox PT, Wainwright BJ, Baker K, Mattick JS. "Touchdown" PCR to circumvent spurious priming during gene amplification. 1991, Nucl Acids Res 19, 4008

6. Flickinger JL, Gebeyehu G, Buchman G, Haces A, Rashtchian. Differential incorporation of biotinylated nucleotides by terminal deoxynucleotidyl transferase. 1992, Nucl Acids Res 20, 2382

7. Freier SM, Kierzek R, Jaeger JA, Sugimoto N, Caruthers MH, Neilson T, Turner DH. 1986, Proc Natl Acad Sci USA 83, 9373-9377

8. Maniatis T, Jeffrey A, van deSande H. Chain length determination of small double- and single-stranded DNA moleculaes by polyacrylamides gel elctrophoresis. 1975, Biochemistry 14, 3787-3794

9. McBride LJ, McCollum C, Davidson S, Efcavitch JW, Andrus A, Lombardi SJ. A new, reliable cartridge for the rapid purification of syntheitc DNA. 1988, BioTechniques 6, 362-367

10. McConlogue L, Brow MA, Inis MA. Structure-independent DNA amplification by PCR using 7-deaza-2'-deoxyguanosine. 1988, Nucl Acids Res 16, 9869

11. Reynolds TR, Buck GA. Rapid deprotection of synthetic oligonucleotides. 1992, BioTechniques 12, 518-521

12. Rychlik W, Rhoads RE. A computer program for choosing optimal oligoncucleotides for filter hybridization, sequencing and in vitro amplification of DNA. 1989, Nucl Acids Res 17, 8543-8551

13. Rychlik W, Spencer WJ, Rhoads RE. Optimization of the annealing temperature for DNA amplification in vitro. 1990, Nucl Acids Res 18, 6409-6412

14. Scanion D, Haralambidis J, Southwell C, Turton J, Tregear G. Purification of synthetic oligodeoxyribonucleotides by ion-exchange high-performance liquid chromatography. 1984, J Chromatogr 336, 189-198

15. Sinha ND, Biernat J, McManus J, Koster H. Polymer support oligonucleotide synthesis XVIII: use of ß-cyanoethyl N,N-dialkylamino/N-morpholino phosphoramidite of deoxynucleosides for the synthesis of DNA fragments simplifying deprotection and isolation of the final product. 1984, Nucl Acids Res 12, 4539-4557

16. Smith LM, Fung S, Hunkapiller MW, Hunkapiller TJ, Hood LE. The synthesis of oligonculeotides containing an aliphatic amino group at the 5'-terminus: symthesis of fluorescent DNA primers for use in DNA sequence analysis. 1985, Nucl Acids Res 13, 2399-2412

17. Trainor GL, Jensen MA. A procedure for the preparation of fluorescence-labeled DNA with terminal deoxynucleotidyl transferase. 1988, Nucl Acids Res 16, 11846

18. Wu DY, Ugozzoli L, Pal BK, Qian J, Wallace RB. The effect of temperature and oligonucleotide primer length on the specificity and efficiency of amplification by the polymerase chain reaction. 1991, DNA Cell Biology 10, 233-238

19. Zon G, Thompson JA. A review of high-performance liquid chromatography in nucleic acids research. II. Isolation, purification, and analysis of oligodeoxyribonucleotides. 1986, BioChromatography 1, 22-31

21. Review of Different Heat-Stable DNA Polymerases

DNA replicates semiconservatively i.e. the parental DNA double-strand separates longitudinally and each nucleotide sequence serves as a template for the formation of a new complementary polynucleotide strand. This process results in the formation of two identical DNA daughter molecules composed of a parental and a newly copied DNA strand. DNA polymerases - the enzymes that catalyze the synthesis of long polynucleotide chains from monomer nucleotides play a key role in this process. According to the international enzyme nomenclature, DNA polymerases are ligases (synthetases), a class of enzymes that catalyze the formation of a covalent bond coupled with the breakdown of a nucleotide triphosphate bond. Polymerization always proceeds from the 5' phosphate to the 3' terminal OH group of the growing DNA strand. Unlike RNA polymerases, DNA polymerases are not capable of synthesizing DNA strands without a short starter sequence, the primer, which is bound to the template DNA in its complementary site. Deoxynucleotide triphosphates (dATP, dCTP, dGTP, dTTP) can then attach to the free 3' terminal OH group of the primer as specified by the template sequence. When deoxynucleotide triphosphates are polymerized, the ß- and _-phosphate groups are split off as pyrophosphates (PPi).

The following reaction is catalyzed by DNA polymerases:

$$dNTP + (dNMP)_n \longrightarrow (dNNMP)_{n+1} + PPi$$

The DNA polymerases described in the eubacterium *Escherichia coli* occur with three different molecular structures and functions (PolI to PolIII). DNA polymerase I (Kornberg enzyme) has the lowest molecular weight of 109kD but is the most frequent (400 molecules/cell). It is composed of about 1,000 amino acids and, like PolIII, has two exonuclease activities. Partial proteolytic splitting produces two different fragments: a 68kD fragment (Klenow fragment) with 5'-3' polymerase activity and 3'-5' exonuclease activity and a 35kD fragment with 5'-3' exonuclease activity. DNA polymerase II (120kD, 50 copies/cell) can catalyze DNA synthesis even in the absence of PolI and PolIII, though its precise biological function remains to be elucidated. DNA polymerase III consists of at least seven subunits, the largest subunit is polymerase active and has a molecular weight of 130kD. PolIII catalyzes the polymerization of about 1,000 nucleotides per second.

DNA polymerases are also capable of in vitro synthesis of polynucleotide chains on a DNA template in the presence of dNTPs and magnesium chloride. Therefore they can be used in a variety of assays (DNA sequencing, nick-translation). Experiments are carried out at the temperatures at which the DNA polymerases display their highest activity. Those typically range between 28 and 37°C.

The "historical" experiments on the polymerase chain reaction still used the thermolabile Klenow fragment of PolI or the T4 DNA polymerase. These experiments had the disadvantage that new enzymes had to be added to the reaction mixture after each denaturation cycle (Keohavong 1988, Mullis 1987). The identification of thermostable DNA polymerases made it possible to perform in vitro DNA amplification without having to add fresh enzyme after each cycle. Thermostable polymerases show only moderate activity losses when heated to the denaturation temperature (>93°C) (Saiki 1988).

The thermostable DNA polymerase from the eubacterium *Thermus aquaticus* (Taq polymerase) has been most widely studied. The Thermus aquaticus strain YT1 grows at a temperature of 70 - 75°C and was first isolated from a hot spring in the Yellowstone National Park in 1969. The enzyme (molecular weight: 63-68kD) was characterized by Chien et al. (1976) and by Kaledin et al. (1980). Taq polymerase shows maximal activity at about 80°C, a pH of 8.0 and in the presence of all four deoxynucleotide triphosphates. Its activity is decisively influenced by the concentration of Mg^{2+}.

The DNA polymerases of other species of the genus Thermus have also been characterized: *Thermus flavus* (Kaledin 1981), *Thermus ruber* (Kaledin 1981), and *Thermus thermophilus* (Rüttimann 1985, Carballeira 1990). A DNA polymerase (Bst) of 76kD and an optimal temperature of about 60°C was isolated from the mesothermophilic eubacterium Bacillus stearothermophilus (Kaboev 1981).

Archaebacterial thermostable DNA polymerases have been characterized from *Methanobacterium thermoautotrophicum* (Klimczak 1986), *Thermoplasma acidophilum* (Hamal 1990), *Thermococcus litoralis* (Neuner 1990), *Pyrococcus furiosus* (Fiala 1986) and from the two *Sulfolobus species*, *Sulfolobus acidocaldarius* (Salhi 1989) and *Sulfolobus solfataricus* (Rossi 1986). The DNA polymerases of *Methanobacterium thermoautotrophicum* and *Thermoplasma acidophilum* both have 3'-5' exonuclease activity and display optimal activity at 65°C. Their molecuar weight is 72 and 88kD, respectively. The DNA polymerase of *Sulfolobus acidocaldarius* shows optimal activity at 70°C. It remains stable at a temperature of up to 80°C and still retains a polymerization activity of up to 200 nucleotides/sec at 100°C. The purified enzyme has a molecular weight of about 100kD and lacks both exonuclease and primase activity. This polymerase has been used successfully in PCR experiments with single-stranded M13 templates as well as with genomic and plasmid DNA templates (Salhi 1990). The yields at 70°C were comparable to those obtained with Taq polymerase, but required lower magnesium concentrations.

21.1 Taq DNA polymerase

The molecular weight of Taq is 94kD and its specific activity is 200,000 units/mg (Lawyer 1989). The Taq gene is 2,499 base pairs long, which corresponds to 832 amino acids. The sequence shows close homologies to the N-terminal domain of E. coli PolI, where 5'-3'

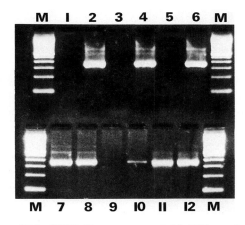

Figure 21.1: 3% NuSieve agarose gel. M: 100bp molecular weight standard. Lanes **2, 4 and 6** demonstrate a 365bp HIV-I amplification product (for details see method 1, chapter 21) from patient samples using 2U/50µl Taq polymerase from different manufactures (Lane 1: Perkin-Elmer Cetus [AmpliTaq], lane 3: Amersham, lane 5: Boehringer). Lanes 1, 3 and 5 are negative controls without DNA template in the amplification assay. Lanes **7 and 8** represent the same 365bp HIV-1-amplification product using 2U/50µl Pfu polymerase (lane **7**: buffer 1, lane **8**: buffer 2, see method 1, chapter 21). In lanes **9-12** different formamide concentrations were added to the Pfu amplification reaction: lane **9**: 20% final concentration, lane **10**: 10%, lane **11**: 1%, lane **12**: 0%. It is clearly seen that the amplification is inhibited by formamide concentrations of 10% and 20%.

exonuclease activity is encoded and to the PolI region coding for polymerase activity. These homologies were confirmed functionally by the demonstration of polymerase and 5'-3' exonuclease activity and the lack of 3'-5' exonuclease activity in purified Taq.

Taq polymerase is available from many suppliers including Amersham, Anglian Biotechnology, Beckman, Boehringer-Mannheim, Cambio, Clontech, IBI, Perkin-Elmer Cetus, Pharmacia, Promega, Stratagene, USB (Table 21.1). One unit is typically defined as the amount of specific enzyme which will catalyze the incorporation of 10nmol of total nucleotide into acid-insoluble material in 30 minutes at 74°C (reaction conditions: 50mM Tris-HCl [pH 9.0 at 25°C], 50mM NaCl, 10mM $MgCl_2$, 200µM dATP, dCTP, dGTP, and 50µM 3H-TTP and 12.5µg activated calf thymus DNA in a 50-µl reaction). Taq polymerase has an optimal extension rate (rate of polymerization) of 35-100 nucleotides/second at 70° - 80°C. Specific Taq preparations are available from different manufacturers. For example USB offers a a Taq polymerase with a molecular weight of a 94kD, Promega an 85kD (*Thermus aquaticus strain YT2*), and Boehringer a 95kD (*Thermus aquaticus BM*, a strain lacking Taq I restriction endonuclease activity). There are no longer any major differences between individual native Taq preparations. Nearly all Taq polymerases synthesize the same amount of DNA in standard PCR assays (amplification product < 500bp, see also figure 21.1). However, wide differences exist in the fidelity of different Taq polymerase preparations, which may differ by a factor of 50-500 (range 1/300-1/18,000), and in the processivity (unpublished data). Processivity is expressed as the average of nucleotides synthesized before the enzyme dissociates from the template. The fact that many Taq polymerase preparations including recombinant Taq polymerase are contaminated by bacterial DNA continues to be a problem, especially in view of false-positive results. When these preparations are used in reaction mixtures to which no DNA is added and exogenous contamination is thus excluded, DNA fragments may nevertheless be visualized on the gel (Böttger 1991, Schmidt 1991). Under modified reaction conditions, Taq polymerase also displays some reverse transcriptase activity besides its DNA polymerase

Thermus aquaticus	Amersham Buchler
	Beckman
	Boehringer Mannheim
	Clontech
	Genofit
	Gibco BRL
	ICN
	Perkin-Elmer Cetus
	Pharmacia
	Promega/Serva
	USB
Thermus flavis	DuPont
Bacillus stearothermophilus	Bio-Rad
Thermococcus litoralis (Vent)	New England Biolabs
Pyrococcus furiosus	Stratagene

Table 21.1: List of different DNA polymerases from several distributors

activity (Jones 1989, Tse 1990).

Taq polymerase has its temperature optimum (T_{opt}) between 75° and 80°C, depending on the template used. At this temperature, the enzyme incorporates about 150-300 nucleotides(nt)/sec/enzyme molecule. Decreasing temperatures will reduce the synthesis rate as follows: 70°C >60 nt/sec/enzyme molecule, 55°C 24 nt/sec, 37°C 1.5 nt/sec and at 22°C 0.25 nt/sec (Gelfand 1989, Innis 1988). The Taq polymerase initially described by Saiki et al. (1988) showed a 50% activity reduction after 130min at 92.5°C, 40min at 95°C and 5-6min at 97.5°C. When the upper temperature of the denaturation step is limited to 95°C for 20 sec, the enzyme has a residual activity of approx. 65% after 50 cycles (Gelfand 1989).

The concentration of magnesium ions has a decisive influence on enzyme activity (for details see also chapters 1 and 2). Since dNTP binds Mg^{2+} optimal magnesium concentration is primarily a function of the dNTP concentration. A 2.0mM magnesium chloride concentration induces maximal Taq polymerase activation at a total dNTP concentration of 0.7-0.8.

Taq activity is reduced by 50% when the Mg^{2+} concentration is increased to 10mM $MgCl_2$ and by 30% when dNTP is increased to 4-6mM.

More recent studies (Chou 1992), using the hot-start PCR method (for details see chapters 1 and 2), suggest that Taq polymerase has a much higher polymerization rate at room temperature than assumed so far. Hot-start PCR largely prevents primer oligomerization. This might indicate that this side reaction is primarily due to incubation at room temperature. There is also some indication that repeated ethanol precipitation of DNA increases the mis-priming rate of Taq polymerase and thus the proportion of PCR by-products.

Modified Taq polymerase preparations

Native Taq DNA polymerase is a thermostable 85-94kD enzyme, isolated and purified from the Thermus acquaticus strains YT1, YT2 or BM. The genetically engineered enzyme AmpliTaq™ offered by Perkin Elmer Cetus is a modified Taq polymerase which has a molecular weight of 94kD and is expressed in E. coli (Lawyer 1989). Its thermal stability is as follows: half-life of 10min at 97.5°C and about 40min at 95°C. The thermostability of the recombinant enzyme (rTaq) is, among other factors, dependent on the KCl concentration: After 10min at 97.5°C and final KCl concentrations of 50mM, 25mM and 10mM, the enzyme has a residual activity of 50%, 30%, and 20%, respectively. The enzyme displays 5'-3' exonuclease activity (0.3pmol/sec/pmol enzyme), has a processivity of 50-60 nucleotides (Abramson 1990) and an elongation rate of 75nt/sec. Deletion of the 289 N-terminal amino acids of the native Taq polymerase preparation (832 amino acids) results in a 61kD active fragment (*Stoffel fragment*, Perkin Elmer Cetus) that lacks any intrinsic 5'-3' exonuclease activity (< 0.00001 pmol/sec/pmol enzyme), but has an approx. two times higher thermostability (half-life of 20min at 97.5°C). Another important advantage of the Stoffel fragment over native Taq polymerase is the fact that it exhibits optimal activity over a broader range of magnesium ion concentrations (2-10mM). The lack of 5'-3' exonuclease activity improves the amplification of circular templates (e.g., plasmid DNA). The higher thermostability allows for PCR cycles with higher denaturation temperatures, which is particularly important for fragments with high proportions of GC and complex secondary structures. The higher range of magnesium concentrations over which the Stoffel fragment is active might contribute toward improving PCR methods and it might also prove useful in the simultaneous amplification of different fragments in a single tube (Multiplex PCR, see chapters 3.4 and 12). Assays using the *Stoffel fragment* in the Taq polymerase buffer (10x Taq buffer: 500mM KCl, 100mM Tris-HCl [pH 8.3] 15mM $MgCl_2$, 0.01% gelatin; 10x Stoffel buffer: 100mM KCl, 100mM Tris-HCl [pH 8.3] plus additional $MgCl_2$) are most suitable for the synthesis of small fragments less than 250bp long (see also figure 21.2.).

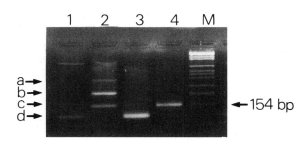

Figure 21.2: Amplification of three different *Mycobacterium tuberculosis* gene regions using 1U Taq polymerase (lanes **1** and **2**) and 1U Stoffel fragment (lanes **3** and **4**). Lane **1**: 111bp fragment [d] (used as a probe for the further detection of the 158bp amplification product), lane **2**: multiplex PCR with a 158bp [c], 240bp [b] and 385bp [a] *Mycobacterium tuberculosis* product (for details see chapter 12). Lanes **3** and **4** represent an amplification assay using the same primers as in lanes **1** and **2** but a 1U/50μl *Stoffel fragment* in Taq buffer instead of Taq polymerase. Stoffel fragment polymerase preferentially amplifies fragments smaller than 250bp and shows good results under ionic conditions like those of the Taq polymerase buffer. This effect is clearly demonstrated in lane **4** where instead of a multiprimer assay (158bp, 240bp, 383bp) and in contrast to lane 2 only the 158bp fragment can be amplified..

21.2. Vent polymerase (Thermococcus litoralis)

Vent DNA polymerase was first isolated from a strain of the thermophilic bacterium *Thermococcus litoralis* which lives at the bottom of the ocean at temperatures of up to 98°C. New England Biolabs has recently cloned and expressed in E. coli the gene coding for Vent DNA polymerase. An exonuclease-deficient genetic derivative of Vent DNA polymerase has also been described (Vent-(exo-)DNA polymerase). Both polymerases are characterized by high thermostability and yield amplification products of 10 - 13 kB. Compared to Taq DNA polymerase, which has a fidelity of 1/290 - 1/2,400, that of Vent-DNA polymerase appears to be 5 - 15 times higher (1/31,000) and that of Vent-(exo-)DNA polymerase two- to-three times higher (Eckert 1991). According to the manufacturer, the absence of exonuclease activity in Vent-(exo-)DNA polymerase affords advantages in the dideoxy sequencing reaction.

With its 3'-5' exonuclease activity, Vent polymerase is capable of removing possible mismatches at the 3' end of the primer. This strand-displacement does not result in degradation of the DNA, thus differing from the 5'-3' exonuclease activity of Taq DNA polymerase. The strand-displacement activity of the Vent polymerase is temperature sensitive: at 72°C, the polymerase will displace more than 100bp of encountered DNA; at 55°C, however, the polymerase will not displace DNA, and polymerization is stopped when the 5'end is encountered.

Since more than 95% of the DNA fragments produced by Vent polymerase are blunt-ended, they can be directly cloned into other structures. Vent-(exo-)DNA polymerase, on the other hand, yields about 70% blunt-ended fragments, and the bulk of the remaining products consists of single base 3'extensions. The enzyme retains about 80% of its initial activity after 10min at 100°C and about 30% after 180min at this temperature. Enzyme activities in relation to reaction temperature are as follows: at 40°C 15% of that seen at 75°C, at 50°C 30%, at 60°C 50% and at 80°C 125%. Vent polymerases display optimal activity in a low ionic strength, sulfate-containing buffer (recommended buffer composition: 10mM KCl, 10mM $(NH_4)_2SO_4$, 20mM Tris-HCl (pH 8.8 at 24°C), 2mM $MgSO_4$, 0.1% Triton X-100); the Taq polymerase buffer inhibits about 80% of the Vent activity. When using Vent polymerases, it is also important to pipette all reaction products at 4°C, since nonspecific annealing of the primers at room temperature may result in their digestion by the proofreading activity of the enzyme. Furthermore, due to the 3'-5' exonuclease activity, prolonged incubation of the reaction mixture will lead to the degradation of nonannealed primers at their 3'ends. It is recommended to optimize the $MgSO_4$ concentration in preliminary assays - comparable to those performed with $MgCl_2$ when using Taq polymerase. Starting from an initial buffer concentration of 2mM $MgSO_4$, a final concentration range of 2 to 8mM $MgSO_4$ should be tested by stepwise addition of defined amounts of 50mM $MgSO_4$ to the buffer. The synthesis of amplification products more than 2,000bp long usually requires a concentration range of 4 to 8mM $MgSO_4$. At a dNTP concentration of approx. 200μM, the proofreading activity of the enzyme will not degrade the DNA products. Such degradation may occur when the dNTPs are completely used up. It is therefore important to use sufficiently high amounts of dNTP to maintain adequate concentrations during all reaction cycles. Such problems can be recognized by gel-analysis of one reaction after completion of 75% of the intended cycles and comparison of the result with the product obtained after the last cycle. According to the manufacturer, addition of bovine serum albumin up to a final concentration of 100 μg/ml can increase enzyme activity by up to 10%. The precise mechanism of this increase is not known; it may be due to the neutralization of enzyme inhibitors in some DNA samples or the prevention of nonspecific adsorption of reagents to the reaction vessels (for more details see also chapter 4).

The following amplification protocol is recommended: 1. initial denaturation at 93 - 95°C for 5min; 2. annealing temperature according to the T_m-value of the primers for 1min (if no product is seen in the analysis of the reaction, the annealing temperature should be decreased in 2-degree steps); 3. elongation of the primers for about 1min per kilobase of extension product at 72-75°C; 4. denaturation at 93-95°C for about 20-40 sec.

Thermococcus litoralis DNA polymerase has a higher thermostability and processivity (amplification of 7-10kb fragments) than Taq DNA polymerase. It is important to note that, because of its proofreading activity, Vent polymerase cannot be used for allele-specific PCR assays (see chapter 13.1). Both Vent DNA polymerase and Vent-(exo⁻)DNA polymerase are particularly suitable for dideoxy sequencing because of the diminished secondary structure effects resulting from the higher reaction temperature.

In a sequencing study, Bergh et al. (1991) showed that Taq polymerase yielded only low amounts of specific product when used for the amplification of a clone containing a high proportion of G-C. These assays were performed at different Mg^{2+} concentrations ranging between 0.8 and 3.2mM with denaturation at 95°C for 1.5min. When the experiments were repeated using Vent polymerase (at a denaturation temperature of either 95°C or 98°C and 5.0mM Mg^{2+}), the yield of specific product was high enough for subsequent sequencing studies. Bergh et al. (1991) mention that later they were also able to obtain a good amplification product of this clone with Taq polymerase when they added formamide in an unknown concentration. additionally added formamide at an unknown concentration (Thomas Hultman/Stockholm, unpublished).

No detailed data can be given for the Deep Vent™ DNA polymerase that was recently put on the market by New England Biolabs. According to the manufacturer, the enzyme displays a 3'-5' proofreading activity and is characterized by an even higher thermostability (approx. 70-80% residual activity after 10 hours at 95°C, half-life of 23 hours at 95°C).

	AmpliTaq	Stoffel	Vent	Pfu
Molecular weight	94kD	61kD	?	92kD
Processivity	50-60 nt	5-10 nt	30-40 nt	?
Extension rate	75nt/sec	>50nt/sec	>80nt/sec	60nt/sec
Thermostability half-life time at - 97.5°C	10min	20min	130min	>3h
- 95.0°C	40min	90min	360min	>2h
- 92.5°C	130min	?	?	?
5'-3'-exonuclease activity (pmol/sec/pmol enzyme)	0.3pmol	<0.00001pmol	?	?
3'-5'-exonuclease activity	no	no	yes	yes
Mg^{2+} optimum	1.5mM	3.0mM	2.0mM	1.5-2.0mM
KCl optimum	50mM	10mM	10mM	10mM
Reverse transcriptase activity	(yes)	?	?	?

Table 21.2: Some characteristics of different polymerases

21.3. Thermus thermophilus DNA polymerase

Tth DNA polymerase is a thermostable DNA polymerase isolated from the thermophilic strain *Thermus thermophilus HB* 8, which is the source of the restriction endonuclease TthI, a thermostable isoschizomer of TaqI (Venegas 1989).

Ruttiman et al. (1985) isolated three DNA polymerases from T. thermophilus (A, B, and C), and Carballeira et al. (1990) described another DNA polymerase from this eubacterium. The latter has a molecular weight of about 67kD, lacks 5'-3' exonuclease activity and has an extension rate of about 25nt/sec. The enzyme seems to be as efficient and specific as Taq polymerase in the PCR assay, amplifying a 1.3kb fragment (Carballeira 1990) and a 405bp fragment (Glukhov 1990). A further Tth DNA polymerase with a molecular weight of 92kD is marketed by USB/USA. This enzyme is devoid of 5'-3' and 3'-5' exonuclease activity. Optimal buffer conditions are: 10mM Tris HCl (pH 8.9 at 25°C), 80mM KCl, 1.5mM $MgCl_2$, 500µg/ml BSA, 1% sodium cholate, 1% Triton X-100. 100min incubation at 85°C reduces the initial enzyme activity to 60%.

Myers and Gelfand (1991) describe a recombinant DNA polymerase from the same species (Tth pol, rTth reverse transcriptase, Perkin Elmer Cetus) which, in addition to its DNA polymerase activity, displays a very high reverse transcriptase (RT) activity in the presence of $MnCl_2$. The use of this thermostable reverse transcriptase may help to solve problems associated with the presence of extensive RNA secondary structures when synthesising cDNA. In coupled RT/PCR assays, Tth pol is about 100 times more efficient than the analogous Taq DNA polymerase. Meyers and Gelfand (1991) show that the sensitivity of the system is sufficient to demonstrate about 100 copies of a synthetic cRNA in the subsequent PCR assay after reverse transcription. The RT activity of rTth reverse transcriptase is dependent on Mn^{++}. The enzyme has a half-life of 20min at 95°C and displays pronounced 5'-3' exonuclease activity, while lacking 3'-5' exonuclease activity. The manufacturers recommend the use of phenol/chloroform-extracted RNA, 35-50 cycles with a total of less than 250 ng RNA and stepwise temperature priming with oligo(dT). The ability of the rTth enzyme to perform both reverse transcription and DNA amplification will certainly help to facilitate the detection and quantification of low abundant viral transcripts.

21.4. Pfu DNA polymerase (Pyrococcus furiosus)

Pfu DNA polymerase is isolated from the hyperthermophilic marine archaebacterium *Pyrococcus furiosus* (Mathur 1991, Lundberg 1991). The multifunctional enzyme shows a 5'-3'-DNA polymerase activity and a 3'-5'-exonuclease activity which results in a 12-fold higher fidelity of DNA synthesis compared to Taq DNA polymerase. The temperature optimum of the enzyme ranges between 72°C and 78°C. After one hour of incubation at 95°C, the enzyme retains more than 95% of its initial activity. It is important to note that, because of its 3'-5'-exonuclease activity, the Pfu DNA polymerase will begin to degrade template DNA in the absence of dNTPs. Therefore, it is essential to always add the enzyme to the reaction mixture last. The recommended 1x buffer composition is: 20mM Tris-HCl [pH 8.2], 10mM KCl, 6mM $(NH_4)_2SO_4$, 1.5-2.0mM $MgCl_2$, 0.1% Triton X-100, 10ng/µl nuclease-free BSA is optional. Because of the much lower KCl concentration in the Pfu buffer (10mM vs. 60mM in the Taq buffer), minor adjustments of the annealing temperature may be required in order to maximize primer extension. The lower salt concentration requires a reduction in the annealing temperature to the range of about 37°C to 45°C. If no amplification product is seen, a further decrease of the annealing temperature is recommended. In contrast, elevation of the annealing temperature may reduce the amount of non-specific products. The addition of 1-5% glycerol or 1-5% DMSO (final concentration) might produce slightly higher yields.

Procedure	Comments

Method: Amplification of a 365bp HIV-1-fragment using Pfu polymerase and influence of DMSO on amplification efficiency

1. All pipetting steps have to be done on ice. Preperation of 6 autoclaved 0.7µl tubes for performing a 50µl PCR assay. Labeling of the tubes with 1-6. Pipette the following volumens of aqua bidest. into the different tubes: tube 1-3 26µl, tube 4 25µl, tube 5 21µl, tube 6 6µl.

2. Addition of 5µl 10xPfu-buffer 1 each to tubes 1, 3-6 and 5µl 10xPfu-buffer 2 to tube 2

2. 10x Pfu buffer 1: 200mM Tris-HCl [pH 8.8], 100mM KCl, 60mM $(NH_4)_2SO_4$, 20mM $MgCl_2$, 1% Triton X-100, 100ng/µl nuclease-free BSA.
10x Pfu buffer 2: 200mM Tris-HCl [pH 8.8], 100mM KCl, 60mM $(NH_4)_2SO_4$, 20mM $MgCl_2$, 1% Triton X-100.
Since the enzyme ist salt-sensitive, the final concentration of KCl should not exceed 10mM. Remember that templates and primers sometimes bind extraneous salt. The Mg2+ concentration is as critical for Pfu as it is for other thermostable DNA polymerases. If a low yield is seen in the PCR results, test a final concentration range between 2.0mM and 6.0mM.

3. Addition of 8µl dNTP mix.

3. dNTPs, equimolar dATP, dCTP, dGTP, dTTP, (Fa. Boehringer, 100mMol, #1051466), 1.25 mM solution.

4. Add 2µl of the HIV-1-primer mixture.

4. Primer 1268 + 1269 (I Weber, unpublished): + primer 7698, - primer 8025, BH10-nomenclature, including the universal M13/rM13 sequence, results in a 365-bp fragment: (+) primer: 5'cag gaa aca gct atg acc (rM13) aga gtt agg cag gga tat tca c 3', (-) primer: 5'taa aac gac ggc cag tgc ca (m13) tga gca agc taa cag cac tat t 3'. Primers are stored in a 15µM stock solution; both primers are mixed together to yield a final concentration in the PCR assay of 0.6µM (= 2µl).
Note that an increased amount of primers may be

Procedure(cont.)

5. Add 1µl formamide to tube 4, 5µl to tube 5 and 20µl to tube 6. Final concentration will be 1%, 5%, and 20%, respectively. Overlay the samples with 50µl Sigma mineral oil.

6. Add 5µl of the DNA template (about 100ng).

7. All tubes are heated to 95°C for 5min followed by a cooling step of 5min at room temperature to anneal the primer.

8. Pipette 4µl diluted Pfu-enzyme (= 2U) through the oil overlay in each tube. Mix all reagents very carefully. Centrifuge for just a few seconds.

9. In contrast to Taq amplification procedures, no initial 5min denaturation step is done. 40 cycling steps. 10 sec 95°C, 20 sec 40°C, 60 sec 72°C, 5min final extension delay at 72°C.

10. Analysis of the amplification products in a 3% NuSieve/agarose gel (for details see chapter 10).

Comments(cont.)

required when using Pfu DNA polymerase for primer extension. A final primer concentration of 0.3 to 1.0 µM (100-250ng for an 18-25-mer primer) is recommended. 0.5µM seems to be optimal for most applications; concentrations below 0.3µM may not produce an amplification.

5. 50% formamide stock solution (Gibco-BRL, 540-5515UA)

8. Pfu DNA polymerase (Stratagene, # 600 136). Avoid excessive amounts of enzyme. Optimal amounts will be 1 - 2.5U. Note: This step is highly susceptible contamination. It migth be essential to use positive-displacement pipettes.

9. If no amplification product is seen in the gel analysis, increase the annealing time and reduce the temperature by about 5°C. An elongation time of 1-2 min at 72°C to 75°C per kilobase of desired product is necessary.

21.5 Bst polymerase

Bst polymerase, a thermostable DNA polymerase I isolated from the mesophilic bacterium Bacillus stearothermophilus T-3468, was first described for DNA sequencing by Ye and Hong (1987). The experience with this enzyme is still limited. Teams from Wisconsin (Mead 1991) and Shangai (McClary 1991) have reported initial results obtained with Bst polymerase in DNA sequencing experiments. The enzyme has a polymerization rate of about 120 nucleotides per second and replicates a template of 7,250bp in 5min at 65°C. In a sequencing experiment, the authors demonstrated that the radioactive incorporation rate was highest at 70°C, though the fidelity of the enzyme remained consistent between 25° and 70°C. The enzyme is capable of incorporating 7-deaza-dGTP and ITP, a property that might prove useful in the analysis of templates with extensive secondary structures. Furthermore, Bst polymerase might turn out to be superior to Taq and T7 polymerase in that lower amounts of enzyme (1/2 U vs. 2.5 U T7 and 8.0 U Taq) and of inital DNA template are required. Mead et al. (1991) report that 50-100 ng template and 2.5 ng/sequencing lane produce sufficiently high signals after 16 h of exposure in a radioactive sequencing procedure. Corresponding amounts are 500 ng and 34 ng/lane for Taq polymerase and 1000 ng and 25 ng/lane for T7 polymerase. Interestingly, Bst polymerase does not require an annealing step in the sequencing reaction: The sample can be incubated at the appropriate temperature directly after mixing of the reagents.

21.6. Fidelity of different heat-stable DNA polymerases

Specific DNA polymerases described in the literature differ in efficiency as well as in fidelity, that is the frequency of enzyme-induced errors. The kind and rate of error depend on the specific DNA polymerase used and the reaction conditions. A high infidelity of the enzyme used in PCR assays might be problematic for different reasons: 1. Each error, once initiated, will be amplified along with the the original DNA sequence and quantitatively increased in an exponential manner with each amplification cycle. 2. The frequency of deletion mutations depends on the template sequence and is increased in repetitive DNA sequences (Kunkel 1990, Ripley 1990). There are some PCR methods which are designed especially to amplify regions of tandem repeat-motifs (e.g. VNTR-PCR, see chapter 3). 3. Allele-specific PCR assays, assays using restriction endonucleases for the subsequent detection or for cloning procedures and assays designed to detect heterozygosity, might give false positive or -negative results because of possible mutations in the sequence of the final amplification product. Depending upon the template copy number and how early in the amplification process the error occurs, individual error-containing amplification products may increase to a significant portion in the reaction sample.

DNA synthesis is a highly ordered and complex molecular process at the center of which is the coupling of deoxynucleotide triphosphate to the free 3' hydroxyl end of the DNA primer/template. The overall fidelity of a DNA polymerase is determined by different properties. A decisive factor is the enzyme's ability to discriminate different dNTPs and to select the proper one for attachment to the primer/template (insertion step). Twelve different types of mismatches can occur during DNA synthesis. Together with the effect of adjacent template sequences this results in a large number of potential molecular structures among which the enzyme must discriminate. Base selectivity during the insertion step is affected by dNTP pool imbalances. Another important factor is the ratio of elongated primer-templates correctly paired to primer-templates with a terminal mismatch (elongation step). The probability of elongating a terminal mismatch increases with the concentration of the nucleotide to be incorporated next. The fidelity of an enzyme is further influenced by the presence or absence of a proofreading activity (3'-5' exonuclease activity) which selectively removes misincorporated nucleotides at the 3' end of a primer. Proofreading activity can be reduced by high dNTP and dNMP concentrations.

The fidelity of specific DNA polymerases is not constant but is influenced by a variety of modifiable factors which will be discussed in detail below. A number of different in vitro assays are available to determine the rate of nucleotides misincorporated by a given enzyme. Of these, the M13mp2 fidelity assay is the one that is most widely used. This assay uses two mutants of the bacteriophage M13mp2 with single-base changes at position 103 in the lacZ_ region to construct a 363bp gapped heteroduplex molecule. The latter contains a 3' terminal cytosine residue in the primer (minus) strand opposite an adenine residue in the template (plus) strand. The minus strand codes for a medium blue plaque phenotype, while the expression of the plus strand yields faint blue plaques. Polymerization to fill the gap without excision of the cytosine will produce a heteroduplex molecule resulting in 50% medium blue and 50% faint blue plaques. If, however, the mispaired cytosine is excised prior to

	error rate	reference
Taq polymerase	2.0×10^{-4}	Keohavong 1989
	2.0×10^{-4}	Saiki 1988
	7.0×10^{-4}	Tindall 1988
	1.1×10^{-4}	Ennis 1990
	8.9×10^{-5}	Cariello 1991
T7 DNA polymerase	3.4×10^{-4}	Keohavong 1989
	4.4×10^{-5}	Cariello 1991
T4 DNA polymerase	0.3×10^{-5}	Keohavong 1989
		Keohavong 1988
Klenow (1µM dATP)	0.9×10^{-5}	Bebenek 1990
(1µM dNTP)	0.7×10^{-4}	Bebenek 1990
Vent polymerase	6.6×10^{-5}	Ling 1991
	2.4×10^{-5}	Cariello 1991
	1.3×10^{-3}	Matilla 1991
Thermus flavis	6.0×10^{-4}	Mattila 1991

Table 21.3: Error rates of several DNA polymerases. The data shown are results of partly different fidelity assays. However, in the majority fidelity was tested using the M13mp2 fidelity assay and by analysis of PCR products using denaturating gradient gel electrophoresis (DGGE).

gap-filling synthesis, the subsequent, correct incoroporation of thymidine opposite the template adenine will result in a homoduplex molecule uniformly encoding faint blue plaques. Plaques can then be isolated and sequenced to confirm the mutant phenotype. The proportion of medium and faint blue plaques obtained upon transfection is a function of the extent of terminal mismatch excision.

The factors influencing the fidelity of a DNA polymerase have been widely studied by the group of Thomas A. Kunkel (National Institute of Environmental Health, North Carolina). Basically, all DNA polymerases that contain a proofreading activity (T4, T7, Klenow and Vent polymerases) have a higher fidelity, while those that do not, have a higher intrinsic infidelity (Taq and Tth DNA polymerases). Besides proofreading activity, the reaction conditions like relative and absolute dNTP concentrations, dNTP pool imbalances, free Mg^{2+} concentration, reaction pH, temperature, enzyme concentration, structure and amount of DNA template influence the proportion of misincorporated nucleotides to varying degrees. The error rate of Taq is increased by high dNTP concentrations, though equimolar Mg^{2+} concentrations also play a role here. Additionally, dNTP pool imbalances also enhance the misincorporation rate of Taq (elongation step). Vent and T7 polymerases show somewhat different behavior. The fidelity of the former slightly improves with increasing dNTP concentrations, but shows no major changes at dNTP concentrations between 0.2 and 0.8mM (Ling 1991). Changes in Mg^{2+} concentration between 2.0 and 10.0mM have little effect on the fidelity of both Vent and T7 polymerase. Taq polymerase produces more mutants at a reaction pH of more than 8.5 or less than 8.0. Vent and T7

	Increasion of fidelity	Increasion of infidelity
pH (37°C)		
Taq:	8.0	> 8.5, < 8.0
Vent:	8.0 - 9.0	> 8.0
T7:	7.0 - 9.0	< 7.0
dNTP (mM)		
Taq:	< 0.1, > 0.5	< 0.05, 0.1 - 0.5
Vent:	0.2 - 0.8	> 0.8
T7:	2.0 - 5.0	< 2.0
Mg^{2+} (mM)		
Taq:	< 0.05, > 8.0	0.1 - 8.0
Vent:	2.0 - 10.0	< 2.0
T7:	2.0 - 10.0	< 2.0

Table 21.4: Factors influencing the fidelity of different DNA polymerases

polymerase, on the other hand, retain their fidelity over a wide pH range of 8.0 - 9.0 and 7.0 - 9.0, respectively. Changes in reaction temperature produce only a moderate increase in the mutation frequency of Taq. These data support the hypothesis that the rate of DNA synthesis as well as duplex stability has only little effect on the nucleotide discrimination of the Taq polymerase. The most frequent error caused by the Taq polymerase is A-to-C and T-to-C transition. These changes are unique among most polymerases studied in the M13mp2 system and suggest specific mispair and site preferences for this enzyme (Tindall and Kunkel 1988). In accordance with these observations, Saiki et al. (1988) report that AT >> GC transition is the most frequently occurring mutant in cloned HLA-DPß sequences after 30 PCR cycles.

Besides enzyme-associated mutations occurring during multiple cycling steps in a PCR assay, it is also important to note that heat treatment of DNA is mutagenic itself (Drake and Baltz 1976). The most frequent heat-induced change is the deamination of cytosine to produce uracil (Lindahl 1979). Since the latter has the same coding potential as thymine, cytosine deamination will produce a transition mutation (C-G >>> T-A). The danger of cytosine deamination is greatest during the denaturation phase of the PCR. The incidence of cytosine deamination is temperature dependent and is approx. 1×10^{-8} at 80°C and approx. 2×10^{-7} at 95°C (Eckert 1991). Furthermore, DNA exposure to heat induces hydrolysis of N-glycosylic bonds. Depurination of native DNA occurs at a rate of about 4×10^{-9} at 70°C and a pH of 7.4. According to Loeb and Preston (1986), the hydrolysis of DNA results in apurinic/apyrimidinic sites and thus impairs DNA polymerization procedures.

Given the importance of reliably detecting point mutations in some PCR procedures, the following recommendations should be followed when using DNA polymerases in PCR assays:

1. Both the number of cycles and the denaturation temperature should be chosen as low as possible.
2. The four dNTPs have to be added in equimolar concentrations and concentrations must be low (i.e., 30-60µM).
3. The $MgCl_2$ concentration is ideally equimolar to that of the dNTPs and also as low as possible relative to the required efficiency (e.g., 1.0-1.5mM).
4. DNA polymerases with a proofreading activity (i.e., Vent) are clearly superior to other enzymes. They usually have a 5-20 times higher intrinsic fidelity. The enzyme concentration should be kept as low as possible, since too high concentrations contribute toward increasing infidelity. If high concentrations are required for technical reasons, it is important to increase the $MgCl_2$ concentration by 0.5-1.0mM.
5. A reaction pH of around 6.0 is optimal at temperatures of 70° - 75°C, which is somewhat lower than the pH of standard PCR assays.
6. Unless required by the experimental set-up, it is recommended to avoid DNA templates with a high proportion of repetitive sequences.

References

1. Abramson R, Stoffel S, Gelfand D. Extension rate and processicity of Thermus aquaticus DNA polymerase. 1990, FASEB J 4, A2293

2. Barballeira N, Nazabal M, Brito J, Garcia O. Purification of a thermostable DNA polymerase from Thermus thermophilus HB-8 useful in the polymerase chain reaction. 1990, Biotechniques 9, 276-281

3. Bebenek K, Joyce CM, Fitzgerald MP, Kunkel TA. The fidelity of DNA synthesis catalyzed by derivaties of Escherichia coli DNA polymerase I. 1990, J Biol Chem 265, 13878-13887

4. Bergh St, Hultman Th, Uhlen M. Colorimetric quantification of in vitro-amplified template DNA to be used for solid phase sequencinv. 1991, DNA Sequence - J DNA Sequenc Mapping 2, 81-87

5. Böttger E. False positive reaction in PCR. In: PCR topics. Usage of polymerase chain reaction in genetic and infectious diseases. A Rolfs, HC Schumacher, P Marx (Eds.), Springer Verlag, 1991, Berlin, 66-68

6. Cariello NF, Scott JK, Kat AG, Thilly WG, Keohavong Ph. Resolution of a misense mutant in human genomic DNA by denaturing gradient gel electrophoresis and direct sequencing using in vitro DNA amplification: $HPRT_{Munich}$. 1988, Am J Hum Genet 42, 726-734

7. Chien A, Edgar DB, Trela JM. Deoxyribonucleic acid polymerase from the extrem thermophil Thermus aquaticus. 1987, J Bacteriol 127, 1550-1557

8. Drake JW, Baltz RH. 1976, Annu Rev Biochem 45, 11-37

9. Eckert KA, Kunkel TA. DNA polymerase fidelity and the polymerase chain reaction. 1991, PCR Methods and Applications 1, 17-24

10. Eckert KA, Kunkel TA. High fidelity DNA synthesis by the Thermus aquaticus DNA polymerase. 1990, Nucl Acids Res 18, 3739-3744

11. Eckert KA, Kunkel TA. The fidelity of DNA polymerases used in the PCR. In: Polymerase chain reaction: A practical approach. Eds.: MJ McPherson, P Quirke, GR Taylor, 1991, IRL Press, Oxford, pp 227-246

12. Fiala G, Stetter KO. Pyrococcus furiosus sp. nov. represents a novel genus of marine heterotrophic archaebacteria growing optimally at 100°C. 1986, Arch Microbiol 145, 56-61

13. Gelfand DH. Thermus aquaticus DNA polymerase. In: Polymerase chain reaction. HA Erlich, R Gibbs, HH Kazazian (Eds.), Current communications in molecular biology, 1989, Cold Spring Harbor Laboratory Press, New York, 11-17

14. Glukhov AI, Gordee SA, Vinogradov SV, Kiselev VI, Kramarov VM, Kiselev OI, Severin ES. Amplification of DNA sequences of Epstein-Barr and human immundeficiency virus using DNA-polymerase from Thermus thermophilus. 1990, Mol Cell Probes 4, 435-443

15. Goodman MF. DNA replication fidelity: Kinetics and thermodynamics. 1988, Mutat Res 200, 11-20

16. Hamal A, Forterre P, Elie C. Purification and characterization of DNA polymerase from the archaebacterium Thermoplasma acidophilum. 1990, Eur J Biochem 190, 517-521

17. Innis MA, Myambo KB, Gelfand DH, Brow MAD. DNA sequencing with Thermus aquaticus DNA polymerase and direct sequencing of PCR-amplified DNA. 1988, Proc Natl Acad Sci USA 85, 9436-9440

18. Jones MD, Foulkes NS. Reverse transcription of mRNA by Thermus aquaticus DNA polymerase. 1989, Nucl Acids Res 17, 8387-8388

19. Kaboev OK, Lochkina LA, Akhmendov AT, Bekker ML. Purification and properties of deoxyribonucleic acid polymerases from Bacillus stearothermophilus. 1981, J Bacteriol 145, 21-26

20. Kaledin AS, Slivusarenko AG, Gorodetskii SI. Isolation and properties of DNA polymerase from the extremely thermophilic bacterium Thermus aquaticus YT1. 1980, Biokhimiya 45, 644-651

21. Kaledin AS, Slivusarenko AG, Gorodetskii SI. Isolation and properties of DNA polymerase from the extremely thermophilic bacterium Thermus flavus. 1981, Biokhimiya 46, 1576-1584

22. Kaledin AS, Slivusarenko AG, Gorodetskii SI. Isolation and properties of DNA polymerase from the extremly thermophilic bacterium Thermus ruber. 1981, Biokhimiya 47, 1785-1791

23. Keohavong P, Kat AG, Cariello NF, Thilly W. DNA amplification in vitro using T4 DNA polymerase. 1988, DNA 7, 63-70

24. Keohavong Ph, Kat AG, Cariello NF, Thilly WG. Laboratory methods: DNA amplification invitro using T4 DNA plymerase. 1988, DNA 7, 63-70

25. Keohavong Ph, Thilly WG. Fidelity of DNA polymerases in DNA amplification. 1989, Proc Natl Acad Sci USA 86, 9253-9257

26. Klimczak LJ, Grummt F, Burger KJ. Purification and characterization of DNA polymerase from the archaebacterium Methanobacterium thermoautotrophicum. 1986, Biochemistry 25, 4850-4855

27. Kunkel TA. Misalignment-mediated DNA synthesis errors. 1990, Biochemistry 29, 8003-8011

28. Lawyer FC, Stoffel S, Saiki RK, Myambo K, Drummond R, Gelfand DH. Isolation, charaterization and expression in Escherichia coli of the DNA polymerase gene from Thermus aquaticus. 1989, J Biol Chem 264, 6427-6437

29. Lindahl T. DNA glycosylases, endonucleases for apurinic/ apyrimidinic sites, and base-excison repair. 1979, Prog Nucl Acid Res Mol Biol 22, 135-189

30. Ling LL, Keohavong Ph, Dias C, Thilly WG. Optimization of the polymerase chain reaction with regard to fidelity: modified T7, Taq, and Vent DNA polymerases. 1991, PCR Methods Applicat 1, 63-69

31. Loeb LA, Kunkel TA. Fidelity of DNA polymerases. 1982, Annu Rev Biochem 52, 429-457

32. Lundberg KS, Shoemaker DD, Adams MW, Short JM, Sorge JA, Mathuer EJ. High-fidelity amplification using a thermostable DNA polymerase isolated from Pyrococcus furiosus. 1991, Gene 108, 1-6

33. Mathur EJ, AdamsMW, Callen WN, Cline JM. The DNA polymerase gene from the hyperthermophilic marine archaebacterium, Pyrococcus furiosus, shows sequence homology with alpha-like DNA polymerases. 1991, Nucl Acids Res 19, 6952

34. Mead DA, McClary JA, Luckey JA, Kostichka AJ, Witney FR, Smith LM. Bst DNA polymerase permits rapid sequence analysis from nanogramm amounts of template. 1991, BioTechniques 11, 76-87

35. McClary JA, Ye SY, Hong GF, Witney FR. Sequencing with the large fragment of DNA polymerase I from Bacillus stearothermophilus. 1991, DNA Sequenc - J DNA Sequenc Mapping 1, 173-180

36. Mullis KB, Fallona FA. Specific synthesis of DNA in vitro via a polymerase-catalyzed chain reaction. 1987, Method Enzymol 155, 335-350

37. Myers TW, Gelfand DH. Reverse transcription and DNA amplification by a Thermus thermophilus DNA polymerase. 1991, Biochemistry 30, 7661-7666

38. Neuner A, Jannasch HW, Belkin S, Stetter KO. Thermococcus litoralis sp. nov.: a new species of extremly thermophilic marine archaebacteria. 1990, Arch Microbiol 153, 205-207

39. Pääbo S, Irwin DM, Wison AC. DNA damage promotes jumping between templates during enzymatic amplification. 1990, J Biol Chem 265, 4716-4721

40. Ripley LS. Frameshift mutation: Determinants of specificity. 1990, Annu Rev Genet 24, 189-213

41. Rossi M, Rella R, Pensa M, Bartolucci S, de Rosa M, Gambacorta A, Raia CA, dell'Aversano Orabona N. Structure and properties of a thermophilic and thermostable DNA polymeraes isolated from Sulfolobus solfataricus. 1986, System Appl Microbiol 7, 337-341

42. Ruttimann C, Cotaras M. Zaldivar J, Vicuna R. DNA polymerase from the extremely thermophilic bacterium Thermus thermophilus HB-8. 1985, Eur J Biochem 149, 41-46

43. Saiki RK, Gelfand DH, Stoffel S, Scharf St, Higuchi R, Horn GT, Mullis K, Erlich H. Primer-directed enzymatic amplification of DNA with a thermostable DNA polymerase. 1988, Science 239, 487-91

44. Salhi S, Elie C, Forterre P, de Recondo AM, Rossignol JM. DNA polymerase from Sulfolobus acidocaldarius. 1989, Mol Biol 209, 635-644

45. Salhi S, Elie C, Jean-Jean O, Meunier-Rotaval M, Forterre P, Rossignol JM, de Recondo AM. The DNA polymerase from the archaebacterium Sulfolobus acidocaldarius: a thermophilic and thermoresistant enzyme which can perform automated polymerase chain reaction. 1990, Biochem Biophys Res Comm 167, 1341-1347

46. Scharf SJ, Horn GT, Erlich HA. Direct cloning and sequence analysis od enzymatically amplified genomic sequences. 1986, Science 233, 1076-1078

47. Schmidt ThA, Pace B, Pace NR. Detection of DNA contamination in Taq polymerase. 1991, BioTechniques 11, 176-177

48. Tindall KR, Kunkel TA. Fidelity of DNA synthesis by the Thermus aqauticus DNA polymerase. Biochemistry 27, 6008-6013

49. Tse WT, Forget BG. Reverse transcription and direct amplification of cellular RNA transcripts by Taq polymerase. 1990, Gene 88, 293-296

50. Venegas A, Vicuna R, Alonzo A, Valdes F, Yudelevich A. A rapid procedure for purifying a restriction endonuclease from Thermus thermophilus (TthI). 1989, FEBS Lett 109, 156-158

51. Ye SY, Hong GF. Heat-stable DNA polymerase I large fragment resovles hairpin structure in DNA sequencing. 1987, Scientia Sinica 30, 503-506

22. Physical Features of Thermocyclers and Their Influence on the Efficiency of PCR Amplification

Besides the heat-stable DNA polymerase, it was, above all, the introduction of microprocessor-controlled machines that made possible the automation of the process of in-vitro amplification - machines that used either metal blocks, water, air or microwaves for the temperature transition. The task of automated PCR systems consists in performing automatically the cyclic temperature changes required for amplification by a thermostable enzyme; specifically, it means three incubation temperatures of about 55°C, 72°C and 94°C with variable ramping time between them and variable times for all temperature ranges.

What are the essential requirements with regard to the physical characteristics of a thermocycler? (i) Great temperature accuracy, uniformity and reproducibility; (ii) ideal well-to-well uniformity and comparability; (iii) minimal temperature overshoot; (iv) high cycling time reproducibility. Since the temperatures must primarily be present in the reaction vessel, and since the block or the water of the machine are merely transfer media, the machine can essentially only be as good as the reaction tubes. The reaction tubes determine under what kinetics "the optimal temperatures get into the vessel in optimal time": the tubes must be maximally thin-walled and in intimate contact with the walls of a heat-transfer block.

After the first introduction of a thermocycler by Perkin-Elmer Cetus, Emeryville, CA, numerous suppliers have followed suit in the last few years, offering modified devices (Biomed; Coy Temp Cycler; Dunn; Eppendorf; Ericomp; Hybaid; Idaho Technology; MJ Research; Polygen; Savant; Techne; etc.). Several studies (Linz 1990, Hoelzel 1990) have demonstrated that even the more modern devices exhibit great variabilities in the well-to-well uniformity and comparability and in some cases do not even reach the preset temperatures. Therefore, instruments should be individually optimized prior to use and to making comparisons. To check well-comparability, two micro-thermocouple devices mounted in the sample tubes should be used. Glass thermometers do not work well, because they respond too slowly and are not accurate when only the bulb is immersed. Stamm and co-workers (1991) describe a thermocouple using a simple electronic circuit that can be connected to a chart recorder to measure the actual temperature inside a PCR tube. This method permits accurate inspection of the thermocycle program and a comparison between thermoprofiles of different thermocyclers. In their paper, the authors report that, during five different thermoprograms in two different thermocyclers, the temperature profile measured in the PCR mixture of a 500µl microcentrifuge tube differed from the theoretically programmed profile in 11 cases. Conspicuously, neither device reached the 94°C denaturing temperature. Moreover, two seemingly identical devices from the same supplier exhibited different temperature profiles in the test tube and gave different PCR by-products. One of the devices differed by maximally 2°C between its corner and center positions. Such disturbances of temperature homogeneity are intolerable for the implementation of diagnostic PCR assays. For the time being, it must still be regarded as a result of these studies, too, that for the standardization of PCR thermoprofiles it seems to be essential for the user to routinely record temperature profiles from thermocyclers in order to verify their correct function.

General problems occurring with metal block PCR machines are problems of inconstant heat transfer from the heating block to the vessels if the contact between the two materials is not very tight, as well as the slowness and high weight of the devices if the performance of the Peltier elements is not sufficient. Devices that are currently available commercially should meet the requirement of achieving heating and cooling rates of 2°C/sec. In order for the "thermal stress" of the Peltier elements not to get too great during short cycle phases, it is necessary that the Peltier elements reverse poles softly, which means that less than the full energy is applied within the first 2 seconds after reversing poles and that the maximally possible and necessary performance is only used after a transitional period under processor control. With such circuits, the power consumption should nevertheless not reach 1,500W - as is the case with some suppliers - but should instead not exceed 300W, in the interest of low operating expenses.

A fundamental problem of PCR machines using water baths with fluidic switching or mechanical transfer is the increased danger of contamination of the samples through coming into contact with water, as well as different temperatures in the water bath occurring whenever the temperature controller and the location

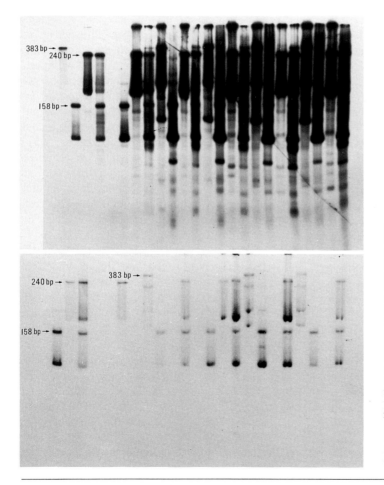

Figure 22.1. Performance of a multiplex PCR in analogy to the data of Figure 12.1, with demonstration of three different amplification products (arrows) having sizes of 383bp, 240bp and 158bp. The amplicon products of both figures (22.1 top and bottom) were produced during a single PCR run. The thermocycler used for this is a water bath machine with fluidic switching, the temperature controller and water inlet to the reaction bath having been installed at diagonally opposed locations, and the transition time between controller signal and water inflow was several seconds. As a reproducible result, there are considerably more reaction products, with a clearly higher percentage of unspecific by-products, in the reaction vessels located near the water inlet (top illustration). In the vessels near the temperature controller (bottom illustration), the signals of the amplification products are considerably weaker and at places even failing.

and extent of water inflow are not ideally matched (cf. Figure 23.1). Also, the water consumption for cooling, or - in the case of a refrigerating unit - the size and weight of the devices, is considerable.

The advantage of PCR machines using a water bath is, however, the fact that the temperature transfer into the tube is limited only by the heat conduction properties of the microfuge tube, whereas the response times of metal blocks are also limited by their heat capacity. Time spent in transition is usually wasted; at the most, a slow transition between annealing and elongation seems to have some significance for the annealing process in the case of difficult primers. On the other hand, long transition times after elongation and denaturation do certainly not have any useful impact on the PCR process: the faster the samples are cooled down after denaturation the shorter the run is, and for the quality of the samples it should only be advantageous (favoring a kinetic process like primer annealing to template/product over the equilibrium process of product dimerization). Since classical kinetic studies of DNA renaturation (Wetmur 1968) show that the fast annealing process is due to high primer concentrations and the denaturation process of DNA is also very fast (Wittwer 1990), both the denaturation and annealing times during the PCR cycle could be significantly shortened if the transition time between tube and block could be reduced and if no advantages for the detection system would result from a long annealing time (cf. chapter 1.2.2). For this, however, changes in the hitherto used vessels would be necessary as well as fast temperature changes in the PCR device. In the meantime, special PCR-designed thin-walled reaction tubes are being offered, e.g., by Perkin-Elmer Cetus (e.g., MicroAmpTM reaction tubes) (Haff 1991). When using the new PCR thermocycler of that company (GeneAmp PCR System 9600), such vessels permit a reduction of almost all standard applications with 30 cycles to times of less than 100min.

Another development direction is the attempt to carry out the PCR reaction in glass or plastic capillaries. A new product from the Corbett Research company (FTS 1S Capillary Thermal Sequencer, distributed in Europe by Labortechnik Fröbel) reduces PCR reaction times (30 cycles) to about 30min (cf. Figure 22.2) through a change in tube techniques: the reaction takes place in a thin-walled plastic capillary which is used as a capillary tip before the start of the amplification and is sealed before amplification and then serves as a capillary. Compared with plastic tubes, capillaries have the advantage of a high surface-area-to-volume ratio, so that heat can be transferred to and from the reaction mixture extremely fast. The walls of the capillary are parallel, so that the reaction mixture is subjected to an exactly uniform temperature transition along the length of the capillary. The capillaries are located in a low-mass circular metal block, which ensures a homogenous temperature distribution. Using this device, RH Symons (Dept. of Plant Science, Waite Campus, University of Adelaide) has amplified a 2.6kB fragment (template bacteriophage SP6 DNA) in 36min.

Even shorter amplification times may possibly result from using air for heat transfer (1605 Air ThermoCycler, Idaho Technology). The fundamental advantage of such an air cycling system for DNA amplification is the simplicity and rapid temperature cycling (Wittwer and Garling 1991). Air is an ideal heat transfer medium that can rapidly change temperatures due to its low density and conductivity. The authors have shown that, using 10µl samples in thin glass-capillary tubes, the following transition times result: denaturation to annealing (92°C-56°C) 9sec, annealing to elongation (56°C-75°C) 4sec, and elongation to denaturation (75°C-92°C) 5sec. The three steps of the PCR reaction

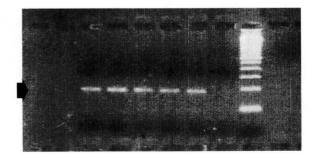

Figure 22.2. Amplification of a 185bp PDH DNA fragment (for details, see Figure 2.1) using an FTS-1S Capillary Thermal Sequencer (Corbett Research) with the following thermoprofile: 3min 95°C initial denaturation; 30 cycles with 5sec 94°C, 5sec 65°C, 20sec 72°C. 5µl per lane.

can be shortened to 1sec (denaturation and annealing) and 10sec (elongation), respectively. Thus, for a 10µl sample, amplification times of 15min are possible for 30 cycles in a 0.52mm-diameter capillary tube. Interestingly, it has become obvious that such rapid cycling procedures require a slightly modified reaction buffer (Wittwer 1991) (increase in the dNTP concentration to 500µM, instead of 200µM dNTPs for conventional slower cycling; addition of bovine serum albumine).

That PCR, in the future, might indeed take place in a teacup (Watson 1990) is borne out by developments that perform the PCR reaction in a microwave oven controlled by a microcomputer (AmpliWaveTM, B. Dunn Labortechnik GmbH).

The purchase of a thermocycler for a laboratory is still a difficult decision today, since numerous devices with different fundamental principles and physical characteristics are on offer on the market. Any purchaser should inquire about the following features of the device: 1. temperature accuracy and uniformity; 2. well-to-well uniformity and comparability; 3. maximum temperature overshoot; 4. cycling time reproducibility; 5. thermal conductivity; 6. controlling of the temperature by a peripheral "in-sample" thermocouple in conjunction with one mounted in the block/water bath; 7. thermal mass; 8. magnitude of internal condensation; 9. possibility of simultaneous performance of different PCR reactions, e.g., in separately controllable thermoblocks within the same device; 10. possibility of using different types of reaction vessel (e.g., 1.2ml or 0.7ml Eppendorf vessel, MicroAmpTM, capillaries, etc.). Items 1-8 are essential, since weaknesses of the device in these respects will contribute to a worsening of the reaction results, whereas the importance of items 9 and 10 must be assessed in relation to the number of samples processed daily, their further use, workload for the device, etc. However, the development trend in diagnostics points clearly away from water-bath machines and towards devices that process small volumes (e.g., 10µl) in capillaries or small vessels under the fastest possible reaction conditions. Nevertheless, it remains to be shown by further studies whether, on the background of well-to-well uniformity, the air-cycling or microwave systems currently offered on the market will keep their promises.

References

1. Haff L, Atwood JG, DiCesare J, Katz E., Picozza E, Williams JF, Woudenberg T. A high-performance system for automation of the polymerase chain reaction. 1991, BioTechniques 10, 102-112

2. Hoelzel R. The trouble with "PCR" machines. 1990, Trends Genet 6, 237-238

3. Linz U. Thermocycler temperature variation invalidates PCR results. 1990, BioTechniques 9, 286-294

4. Stamm St, Gillo B, Brosius J. Temperature recording from thermocyclers used for PCR. 1991, BioTechniques 10, 431-435

5. Watson R. PCR in a teacup. In: PCR protocols - a guide to methods and applications. MA Innis, DH Gelfand, JJ Sninsky, Th J White (Eds.), 1990, Academic Press, San Diego, pp429-434

6. Wetmur JG, Davidson N. Kinetics of renaturation of DNA. 1968, J Mol Biol 31, 349-370

7. Wittwer CT, Fillmore G CH, Garling DJ. Minimizing the time requires for DNA amplification by efficient heat transfer to small samples. 1990, Anal Biochem 186, 328-331

8. Wittwer CT, Garling DJ. Rapid cycle DNA amplification: time and temperature optimization. 1991, BioTechniques 10, 76-83

23. Alternative Methods to PCR

23.1. Ligase chain reaction

The ligase chain reaction (LCR) makes use of the property of thermostable ligases to join two juxtaposed oligonucleotides by the formation of a phosphodiester bond, provided that the oligonucleotides at the junction are correctly hybridized with the template - mainly at 65°C. Provided that altogether four primers are added to the reaction system of which two anneal to the plus strand immediately adjacently and the other two correspondingly to the minus strand of the target (cf. Figure 23.1), an exponential increase in the ligated

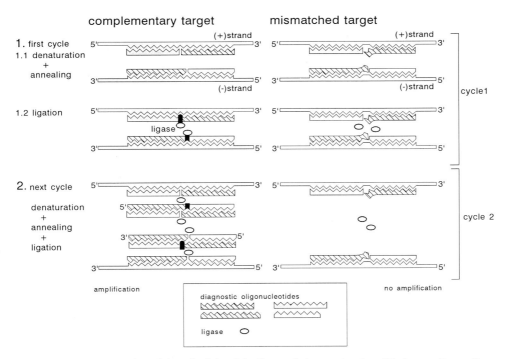

Figure 23.1: Schematic representation of the principle of the ligase chain reaction (modified according to Barany 1991c). The left part of the illustration shows the course with successful ligation. The DNA is heat-denatured and four complementary oligonucleotides anneal to the target at about 65°C. Thormostable ligase will covalently attach only juxtaposed primers that are perfectly complementary to the template at their 3'ends. The products of an amplification cycle in their turn serve as template in the next cycle. The right part of the illustration shows that, with a mismatch at the junction site, no ligation and thus no amplification is possible.

product, consisting of two - originally separated - primers, will result after repeated heating of the reaction mixtures (denaturation) and subsequent hybridization of the primers and covalent joining by the action of the DNA ligase. The ligation event thus identifies DNA sequences that are complementary to the oligonucleotides. It is an essential requirement for the specificity of the reaction to eliminate target-independent ligations completely. To approach this goal, several possibilities are available (Barany 1991b): 1. addition of carrier salmon sperm to the reaction mixture; 2. 5'-phosphorylation of the adjacent (ligating) oligonucleotides only; 3. use of single-base 3' overhangs on discriminating oligonucleotides; 4. selection of temperature cycle conditions near the T_m value of the oligonucleotides used in the assay. At higher temperatures, single-base mismatches form an imperfect double helix at the junction and destabilize the hybridization.

As thermostable ligase, the one from the Thermus thermophilus bacterium is used. For this, Barany and Gelfand (1991a) cloned the DNA ligase-encoding gene (ligT) from Thermus thermophilus in Escherichia coli by genetic complementation of a ligts7 defect in an E. coli host. The sequence analysis of the ligase gene shows a single chain of 676 amino acids with 47% identity and 66% similarity to the E. coli ligase gene. Other working groups (Barker et al. 1988/1989 and Backman et al. 1989) described similar thermophilic genes.

Since the four primers used for the LCR reaction mostly have sizes of about 15-20 base pairs, the ligated products formed have corresponding sizes of 30 to 40 base pairs. The thermocycles performed here essentially correspond to those of a PCR reaction: the prepared reaction sample is heated for 3min at 95°C, subsequently kept at 85°C for 1min and then at 50°C for another 1min; after addition of the enzyme, the tube will be alternated between 85°C and 50°C in the thermal cycler (Hampl 1991). Since the products formed are fairly short, the repetitive denaturing temperature must be chosen correspondingly lower than in the PCR reaction. The denaturation/annealing/ligation steps (see Figure 23.1) are mostly repeated 25-60 times, so that, with the LCR reaction too, exponential growth of the final product results in principle, according to the equation 2^n, where n is the number of cycles. Other working groups report comparable cycle conditions: 94°C 1min, 65°C 4min, 20 or 30 cycles (Barany 1991c); 94°C 1min, 62°C 2min, 30 or 40 cycles (Winn-Deen 1991); 85°C 30sec, 50°C 20sec, 30 or 35 cycles (Bond 1990). In older studies (Landegren 1988) for which thermolabile ligases had still been used the assay was carried out at a constant 37°C. Landegren and co-workers showed in their study that the ligase, in contrast to Taq polymerase (cf. chapters 16, 21), does not amplify 3'-terminal mismatches like T-T, G-T, C-T or C-A, which means that the enzyme is able to discriminate correctly between different alleles (Barany 1991c).

As a rule, the buffer system will contain, in a 10-100µl reaction volume: 100-150mM KCl, 10mM $MgCl_2$, 1-10mM DTT, 1-10mM NAD^+ (for transfer of the adenosyl group from NAD via the e-amino group of a lysine residue to the 5'phosphate of one DNA strand, forming an activated pyrophosphate linkage), 20mM Tris-HCl (pH 7.6) or alternatively 50mM EPPS [N-(2-hydroxyethyl)piperazine-N-(3-propanesulfonic acid)], a carrier (4µg salmon sperm DNA or 10µg/ml BSA), 0.04-1.0 femtomole of each oligonucleotide and about 15 nick-closing units of thermostable enzyme. A nick-closing unit of ligase is defined as the amount of ligase that circularizes 0.5µg of DNase I-nicked pUC4KIXX DNA in 20µl of 20mM Tris-HCl, pH 7.6, at 25°C (cf. Barany 1991b). Any increase in salt concentrations or reduction in enzyme units results in a loss of signal.

The demonstration of ligated products can be done radioactively as well as through an enzyme immunoassay (EIA) using an analyzer with microparticles (Hampl 1991). For this, a capture ligand (e.g., fluorescein) is linked to the two 3'-position primers on the plus and minus strands, and a signal ligand is linked to the corresponding 5'-position primers. When the reaction is completed, only the ligated products will carry both derivative dyes, so that the final product can be bound via the fluorescein molecule and anti-fluorescein antibody-coated latex spheres and detection by anti-biotin alkaline-phosphatase conjugate can follow. The complete measurement can be carried out within 30min. A comparable system has been used by Nickerson and co-workers (1990) in order to detect PCR-amplified DNA: after completed amplification, two neighboring internal primers are added to an aliquot of the PCR reaction mixture and a non-exponential LCR (only one primer set, thermolabile T4 DNA ligase) is carried out, one primer being labeled with biotin and the second one with digoxigenin. The binding to a solid phase (microtiter wells) of the LCR product functioning as a detection system is achieved via streptavidin, while detection is accomplished through an anti-digoxigenin antibody. The essential advantage of this amplification and detection system, which uses both PCR and LCR, must be seen in the fact that the individual steps can be automated to a large degree in order to make possible a high sample-processing rate and to provide a good sensitivity for a non-radioactive system (ca. 3fmol of ligated product).

The system of detection of viral or bacterial DNA or detection of single-base point mutations using allele-specific primers and LCR has hitherto been employed for human papilloma virus (Bond 1990, Hampl 1991), mycobacterium tuberculosis (Barany 1991b, cited as personal communication by DM Iovannisci) and ßA- and sickle ßS-globin genotypes (Barany 1991c). The detection threshold of these systems is around 200-1,000 target molecules.

From the viewpoint of applicability in diagnostics, LCR offers several advantages: at present, it is already fairly well documented, esp. regarding the detection steps; in contrast to Taq polymerase, the ligase does not amplify mismatches at the junction site of the two specific primers; LCR can be performed with 50-70 cycles without considerable growth in unspecific amplification products (H Hampl, personal communication), which means a higher sensitivity. Of course, the application range of LCR is clearly limited compared to PCR (e.g., DNA sequencing, in-vitro mutagenesis, etc.). However, the method offers many advantages in joint application with PCR, such as, e.g., for the performance of genomic sequencing (Pfeifer 1989), in-vivo footprinting (Müller 1989) and cloning of promoter elements.

23.2. Transcription-based amplification system (TAS)

In contrast to PCR and LCR, the transcription-based amplification system (TAS) method proceeds from an RNA matrix as template and thereby makes use of the advantage that RNA molecules transcribed from a gene are present at concentrations 100 to 1,000 times higher, improving from the start - as far as the expression of the gene takes place - the ratio of specific template and possible noise signals. Gingeras and co-workers (1990) published this method for the detection of HIV-1 RNA.

At the start of each cycle of the reaction (cf. Figure 23.2), primer A hybridizes complementarily to the specific sequence. At the 5' end, the primer is modified by addition of a T7-RNA polymerase binding sequence (5' TAA TAC GAC TCA CTA TA 3'). Alternatively, the SP6 (5' CAT ACA CAT ACG ATT GTG ACA CTA TA 3') or the T3-RNA polymerase can be added (cf. also chapter 13.5). Through a reverse transcriptase that uses primer A as the start site, a cDNA is produced as a copy of the existing RNA matrix (step B). After melting open of the cDNA/RNA hybrid and annealing of primer B to the previously produced cDNA, followed by renewed addition of reverse transcriptase, double-stranded cDNA and a new cDNA/RNA heteroduplex are formed (step C, end of cDNA synthesis). From this step onwards, both DNA and RNA are present as matrix for the amplification. The existing double-stranded cDNA is subsequently incubated with T7-RNA polymerase, leading to the synthesis of numerous RNA transcripts from the cDNA which, in turn, again carry the T7-polymerase binding sequence at the 5' end (step D). At the same time, renewed RNA/DNA heteroduplices are synthesized by the reverse transcriptase still present in the reaction, using primer B as start site. Thus, multiplied cDNA and RNA matrices are now available for the second cycle (starting with step E), in turn serving as template in the next cycles.

In the detailed report by Gingeras et al. (1990), the following cycling procedures are used for the implementation of the reaction: 1. Initial heating of the mixture to 65°C for 1min (only from 2nd cycle).

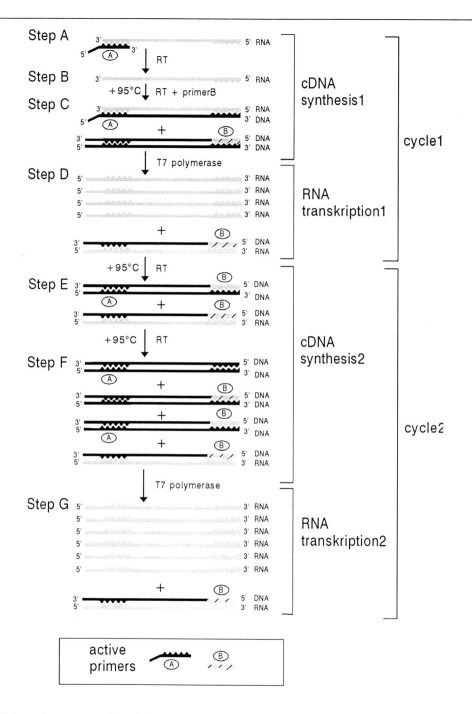

Figure 23.2: Schematic representation of the course of the transcription-based amplification system (TAS) according to Gingeras and co-workers (1990). Details of the course of the reaction are described in chapter 23.2.

2. Cooling for 1min to 42°C, addition of 10U of reverse transcriptase and incubation of the mixture for 12min at 42°C (step A in Fig. 23.2). 3. Melting open of the hybrids by heating of the reaction to 100°C for 1min, then cooling to 37°C for 1min. 4. Renewed addition of 10U reverse transcriptase and simultaneously 100U T7-RNA polymerase, followed by incubation for 30min at 37°C (step D, RNA transcription). All steps are then repeated altogether 10-20 times. As transcription buffer, a buffer with final concentrations of 40mM tris buffer (pH 8.1) with 10mM $MgCl_2$, 31.25mM NaCl, 2.5mM spermidine, 6.25mM dithiothreitol and 0.4mg/ml of bovine serum albumin is used. The amplicons are detected through liquid-phase hybridization with an oligonucleotide bound to a solid phase (sephacryl beads according to Ghosh and Musso 1987). The whole complex (beads plus amplicon) is then detected through hybridization with a second detecting and radioactively labeled oligonucleotide. For this, 0.5-2µl of the amplification reaction are pipetted together with the ^{32}P-labeled oligonucleotide and heated to 65°C for 5min in 10µl TE buffer containing 0.2% SDS. To this, 10µl of a 2x solution hybridization mix (10xSSPE, 10% dextran sulfate) are added. Hybridization takes place at 42°C for 2 hours. After separate pre-incubation of the beads in hybridization solution, the beads are incubated with the detection hybridization mixture at 37°C. After 1 hour, the beads are centrifuged and rinsed (2xSSC) and Cerenkov counts are then measured for 5 to 10min. Using this detection method, the authors were able to detect 1 HIV-1-infected cell in 10^6 cells as a lower detection threshold.

23.3. Self-sustained sequence replication (3SR)

A disadvantage of the transcription-based amplification system (TAS, see chapter 23.2) is the fact that the reaction - similar to the PCR reaction - needs different reaction temperatures, with the denaturation temperature for the melting open of the double-stranded DNA or RNA/DNA hybrid appearing especially critical. With the method of "self-sustained sequence replication" (3SR), this problem is circumvented - similar to NASBA (see chapter 23.4) - by having the hybrids digested by the RNase H of Escherichia coli. We are thus dealing with an isothermal reaction not requiring any instrumentation. During the reaction, three enzymes, viz., avian myoblastosis virus reverse transcriptase (AMV RT), Escherichia coli RNase H and T7 RNA polymerase, produce a tenfold increase in the amplification product every 2.5min within the first 15min, with an amplification factor of 10^7 after 60min (Guatelli 1990) and, after modifications, even 10^8 after 30min (Fahy 1991), resp. Under the optimized reaction conditions of 3SR, double-stranded DNA cannot be used as template, so that this method is well suited for assessing the transcriptional activity of specific genes. The 3SR reaction performs continuous cycles of reverse transcription and RNA transcription to replicate an RNA target, using a double-stranded cDNA intermediate. Transcription-competent cDNAs (including T7 promoter sequence) are used to produce about 50-1,000 copies of antisense RNA transcript of the original template (step G in Figure 23.2).

This method imitates the retroviral strategy of RNA replication by means of cDNA intermediates, resulting in an accumulation of cDNA and RNA copies of the original sequence. Interestingly, HIV-1 copies accumulate - in a 3SR-like mechanism - in chronically infected cells in long-lived, unintegrated and mostly linearized DNA copies, which may be a result of the reverse transcription of newly transcribed, full-length viral RNA. The retroviral RNase H is responsible for the digestion of the RNA/DNA hybrid, so that the second-strand cDNA synthesis can be carried out. Under certain reaction conditions, a partial endogenous RNase H activity is inherent in the AMV RT (Golomb 1979). Fahy and co-workers (1991) have tested in detail the optimized reaction conditions for the implementation of 3SR. For a review, reference can be made to their paper. Surprising is the fact that all three enzymes used here can, at the same time, develop activity in the reaction mixture. It must be mentioned, however, that the concerted multienzyme 3SR reaction requires substrate conditions that are different from those necessary for the individual enzyme reaction.

Table 23.1: 3SR amplification protocol (according to Fahy 1991)

A. Reaction buffer:
1. 20µl 5 x buffer (200mM Tris-HCl (pH 8.1), 150mM MgCl$_2$, 100mM KCl, 50mM DTT, 20mM spermidine)
2. 5µl each primer (0.1µM each, final)
3. 24µl rNTP mix (6mM each, final)
4. 4µl dNTP mix (1mM each, final)
5. 5µl (0.1 amoles) of RNA
6. 36µl aqua bidest. (total volume 100µl)

B. After 1min denaturation at 65°C and transfer to 42°C add enzyme mix:
1. 3µl, 30U AMV RT (Promega, #M5101)
2. 2µl, 4U RNase H (BRL, #510-8021SA))
3. 1µl, 100U T7 RNA-polymerase (USB, #70001)

C. Incubate at 42°C for about 1 hour. Stop the enzyme reaction by freezing the tube at -70°C.

Elongation of the T7 promoter sequence (5' TAA TAC GAC TCA CTA TAG GGA 3') at the 5' end of the primer by 7 bases increases the amplification efficiency.

Through the addition of 10% DMSO and 15% sorbitol to the reaction mixture, the yield in amplicon is increased by a factor of 10 to 1,000. Interestingly, the endogenous RNase H activity of AMV RT (Golomb 1979) is considerably increased in the presence of these additives, so that, in the presence of these subtances, the 3SR reaction can be simplified from a three-enzyme reaction to a two-enzyme reaction by leaving out the RNase H. At the same time, compared to the standard protocol (cf. Table 23.1), less units of the AMV RT (10U) and the T7 RNA polymerase (20U) can be employed without loss of efficiency ($5x10^6$-fold amplification vs. $1x10^7$ for 3-enzyme reaction without additives).

The 3SR reaction has hitherto been used successfully for the detection and characterization of single-base mutations (amino acid positions 67, 70, 215, 219 in the HIV-1 pol gene) of HIV-1 responsible for the zidovudine (AZT) resistance (Gingeras 1991) as well as for the detection of HIV-1 RNA from the plasma of HIV-1-infected infants and children (Bush 1992). In the study by Bush and co-workers, it could be shown that the 3SR method can detect up to about 12 HIV-1 RNA copies, with a 10^{10}-fold amplification level when using purified HIV-1 RNA.

The same principle of primer-directed enzymatic isothermal amplification of specific nucleic acid sequences is also used by the method of "nucleic acid sequence-based amplification" (NASBATM) (van Brunt 1990, Compton 1991, Kievits 1990) developed by the Canadian Cangene concern (Mississauga, Ontario). To our knowledge, there is at present only one publication on the use of NASBA (Kievits 1990) in which the sensitivity and specificity for the detection of HIV-1 and CMV is tested.

23.4. Q-beta replicase

The replication of RNA by bacteriophage Qß replicase (Qß phage RNA-dependent RNA polymerase) follows an interesting pathway in that single-stranded RNA template gives rise directly to a single-stranded RNA product (Axelrod 1991, Palasingham 1992). The fact that special RNA sequences combine in a single molecule the dual function of hybridization probe and amplifiable reporter (Lizardi 1988) seems to be based on several mechanisms: 1. All RNAs that are able to serve in vitro as template for Qß replicase contain an extensive amount of secondary structure. Those RNAs that possess less stable secondary structures exhibit a lower synthesis rate of new RNA strands (Priano 1987), from which can be deduced that the intrinsic structure of a single-stranded RNA template is extremely important for the efficiency of RNA propagation by Qß replicase. 2. Template and product RNAs must form stable <u>intramolecular</u> secondary structures during replication, which are, however, displaced in favor of the formation of local intramolecular pairings after successful replication, due to <u>intermolecular</u> base pair interactions (Axelrod 1991). Double-stranded RNA molecules cannot serve as template in the subsequent cycle of Qß replicase synthesis.

Lizardi and co-workers (1988) were able to show that integration of a sequence specific to Plasmodium falciparum into the sequence of MDV-1 RNA, a natural template of Qß replicase, does not alter the function of the recombinant RNA, viz., to serve as both hybridization probe and template for the exponential amplification. In this connection, the insertion of the probe sequence (Plasmodium falciparum, 58-nucleotide insert) takes place within a hairpin loop that occurs on the exterior of MDV-1 RNA. The MDV-1 cDNA, including the Plasmodium falciparum insert, integrated as a whole in the pT7-MDV-poly plasmid for the purpose of replication, comprises 278 nucleotides. After incubation of different amounts of this 278-nucleotide template (between 1.4×10^{-18} g and 1.4×10^{-10} g of transcript) with 1.2µg Qß replicase at 37°C in 25µl of 400µM ATP, 400µM [α–^{32}P]CTP, 400µM GTP, 400µM UTP, 14mM MgCl$_2$ and 90mM Tris-HCl (pH 7.5), 129ng of recombinant RNA can be detected, after 30min reaction time, in the mixture containing the lowest concentration of the template (about 1,000 molecules). This represents a one-billion-fold amplification.

This ability of the Qß replicase to amplify RNA fragments modified in a certain way can be made use of for diagnostics and the specific detection of RNA or single-stranded DNA. (Knight 1989, Pallen 1991). A prerequisite for this is, comparable to the experiments by Lizardi and co-workers (1988), the insertion into the MDV-1 RNA of a specific probe that can hybridize exclusively with the RNA sequence of the causative agent that one is looking for. In this context, Gene-Trak Systems, exclusive licensee of Qß replicase technology for use in developing diagnostic tests for infectious diseases, is developing a diagnostic system of Qß replicase. For this, RNA is liberated from biological materials (blood, urine, cerebrospinal fluid) by guanidine thiocyanate (cf. chapter 8). Since the Qß replicase does not amplify the specific RNA being looked for, e.g., of HIV-1 in blood, but always only MDV-1 RNA, HIV-1 RNA that is present must be fished out of the biological material highly selectively by a capture probe before the amplification is carried out. This can, e.g., be done by incubating, in a binding

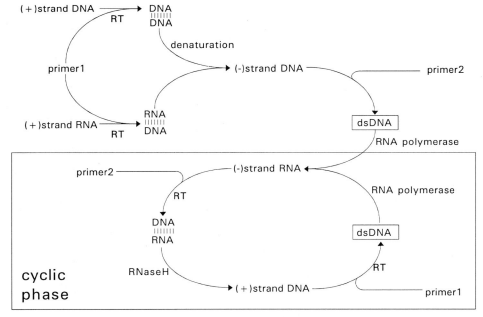

Figure 23.3: Schematic flow-sheet of the self-sustained sequence replication method corresponding to figure 23.2.

buffer with the biological material, paramagnetic particles (cf. chapter 14) that are coated with a specific HIV-1 probe and subsequently removing the non-bound material through a washing buffer. This washing procedure can be carried out repeatedly to increase specificity. Then, this complex of paramagnetic particles, capture probe and fished-out HIV-1 RNA sequences is incubated with MDV-1 RNA carrying a further HIV-1-RNA-specific sequence as a probe. Washing is repeated to remove non-bound MDV-1 RNA. Following that, Qß replicase is added, which recognizes the few MDV-1 RNA molecules specifically bound to the hybrid complex and amplifies the MDV-1 RNA molecule 10^6- to 10^9-fold in about 30min at 37°C. This amplicon can then be detected non-radioactively - e.g., through fluorescent dyes. One essential difference from PCR is, among others, that in this system the specific sequences are first isolated and then amplified, which should contribute to a reduction in unspecific background amplicons. As yet, no tests assessing the validity and reliability of this method have become known. Therefore, it must be shown in the future whether this system has a place beside the other amplification methods. Here, it is a great advantage, however, that on the one hand no instrumentation is necessary and that on the other hand we are dealing with a one-enzyme reaction.

References

1. Axelrod VD, Brown E, Priano Ch, Mills D. Coliphage Qß RNA replication: RNA catalytic for single-strand release. 1991, Virology, 184, 595-608

2. Backman KC, Rudd EA, Lauer G, McKay D. Isolating thermostable enzymes. European patent application (submitted in Deccember 1989)

3. Barany F, Gelfand DH. Cloning, overexpression and nucleotide sequence of a thermostable DNA ligase-encoding gene. 1991a, Gene 109, 1-11

4. Barany F. The ligase-chain-reaction in a PCR world. 1991b, PCR Methods Applicat 1, 5-16

5. Barany F. Genetic disease detection and DNA amplification using cloned thermostable ligase. 1991c, Proc Natl Acad Sci USA 88, 189-193

6. Barker DG, White JHM, Johnston LH. Molecular characterization of the DNA ligase gene, CDC17, fromthe fission yeast Schizosaccharomyces pombe. 1988, Eur J Biochem 162, 659-667

7. Barker DG, White JHM, Johnston LH. The nucleotide sequence of the DNA ligase gene (CDC9) from Saccharomyces cerevisiae: A gene which is cell-cycle regulated and induced in response to DNA damage. 1989, Nucl Acids Res 13, 8323-8337

8. Bond S, Carrino J, Hampl H, Hanley L, Rinehardt L, Laffler T. New methds of detection of HPV. In: J Monsonego (Ed.): Serono Symposia. 1990, Raven Press, Paris

9. Brunt van J. Amplifying genes: PCR and its alternatives. 1990, BioTechnology 8, 291-295

10. Bush CA, Donovan RM, Peterson WR, Jennings MB, Bolton V, Sherman DG, Vanden-Brink KM, Beninsig LA, Godsey JH. Detection of human immunodeficiency virus type 1 RNA in plasma samples from high-risk pediatric patients by using the self-sustained sequence replication reaction. 1992, J Clin Microbiol 30, 281-286

11. Chetverin AB, Chetverina HV, Munishkin AV. On the nature of spontaneous RNA synthesis by Qß replicase. 1991, J Mol Biol 222, 3-9

12. Compton J. Nucleic acid sequence-based amplification - Product review. 1991, Nature 350, 91-92

13. Davis GR, Blumeyer K, DiMichele LJ, Whitfield KM, Chappelle H, Riggs N, Ghosh SS, Kao P, Fahy E, Kwoh DY, Guatelly JC, Spector SA, Richman DD, Gingeras TR. Detection of human immunodeficiency virus type 1 in AIDS patients using amplification-

mediated hybridization analyses: Reproducibility and quantitative limitations. 1990, J Infect Dis 162, 13-20

14. Fahy E, Kwoh DY, Gingeras TR. Self-sustained sequence replication (SR): an isothermal transcription-based amplification system alternative to PCR. 1991, PCR Methods Applic 1, 25-31

15. Gingeras TR, Davis GR, Whitfield KM, Chappelle HL, DiMichele LJ, Kwoh DY. A transcription-based amplification system. In: MA Innis, DH Gelfand JJ Sninsky, TH J White (Eds.): PCR protocols - a guide to methods and applications. 1990, Academic Press, San Diego, pp245-252

16. Gingeras TR, Prodanovich P, Latimer T, Guatelli JC, Richman DD, Barringer KJ. Use of self-sustained sequence replication amplificiation reaction to analyze and detect mutations in zidovudine-resistant human immunodeficiency virus. 1991, J Infect Dis 164, 1066-1074

17. Golomb M, Grandegenett DD. Endonuclease acitivity of purified RNA-directed DNA polymerase fromavian myeloblastosis virus. 1979, J Biol Chem 254, 1606-1613

18. Gosh SS, Musso GF. Covalent attachment of oligonucleotides to solid supports. 1987, Nucl Acids Res 15, 5353-5372

19. Guatelli JC, Whitfield KM, Kwoh DY, Barringer KJ, Richman DD, Gingeras TR. Isothermal, in vitro amplification of nucleic acids by a multienzyme reaction modeled after retroviral replication. 1990, Proc Natl Acad Sci USA 87, 1874-1878

20. Hampl H, Marshall RA, Perko T, Solomon N. Alternative methods for DNA probing in diagnosis: Ligase chain reaction (LCR). In: A Rolfs, HC Schumacher, P Marx (Eds.): PCR topics - Usage of Polymerase chain reaction ingenetic and infectious diseases. 1991, Springer, Berlin-Heidelberg, pp15-22

21. Kievits T, Gemen van B, Sooknamen R, Lens PF. Enzymatic amplification of nucleic acids in vitro at one temperature. VIIIth International Congress of Virology. Berlin, August 1990, Abstract P30-024, p290

22. Knight P. Amplifying probe assays with Q-beta replicase. 1989, BioTechnology 7, 609-610

23. Kwoh DY, Davis GR, Whitfield KM, Chappelle HL, DiMichele LJ, Gingeras TR. Transcription-based amplification system and detection of amplified human immunodeficiency virus type 1 with a bead-based sandwich hybridization format. 1989, Proc Natl Acad Sci USA 86, 1173-1177

24. Landegren U, Kaiser R, Sanders J, Hood L. A ligase-mediated gene detection technique. 1988, Proc Natl Acad Sci USA 241, 1077-1080

25. Lizardi PM, Guerra CE, Lomeli H, Tussie-Luna I, Kramer FR. Exponential amplification of recombinant-RNA hybridization probes. 1988, BioTechnology 6, 1197-1202

26. Müller PR, Wold B. In vivo footprinting of a muscle specific enhancer by ligation mediated PCR. 1989, Science 246, 780-786

27. Munishkin AV, Voronin LA, Chetverin AB. An in vitro recombinant RNA capable of autocatalytic synthesis by Qß replicase. 1988, Nature 333, 473-475

28. Nickerson DA, Kaiser R, Lappin St, Stewart J, Hood L, Landegren U. Automated DNA diagnostics using an ELISA-based oligonucleotide ligation assay. 1990, Proc Natl Acad Sci USA 87, 8923-8927

29. Palasingham K, Shaklee PN. Reversion of Qß phage mutants by homologous RNA recombination. 1992, J Virol 66, 2435-2442

30. Pallen MJ, Butcher PD. New strategies in microbiological diagnosis. 1991, J Hosp Infect 18 Suppl A, 147-158

31. Pfeifer GP, Steigerwald SD, Müller PR, Wold B, Riggs AD. Genomic sequencing and methylation analysis by ligation mediated PCR. 1989, Science 246, 810-813

32. Priano C, Kramer FR, Mills DR. Evolution of the RNA coliphages: The role of secondary structure during RNA replication. 1987, Cold Spring Harbor Symp Quant Biol 52, 321-330

33. Winn-Deen ES, Iovannisci DM. Sensitive fluorescence method for detecting DNA-ligation amplification products. 1991, Clin Chem 37, 1522-1523

Addendum:

Methodological examples for the application of the Polymerase chain reaction

A) Characterization of oncogenes

Detection of Mutations at Codon 61 of the c-Ha-ras Gene in Small Precancerous Liver Lesions of the C3H Mouse

R Bauer-Hofmann, A Buchmann, F Klimek, M Schwarz

Mutational activation of one of the three *ras*-proto-oncogenes, c-Ha-*ras*, c-Ki-*ras*, and N-*ras*, by point mutations at either codons 12, 13, and 61 has been shown to occur with high frequency in both human and animal tumors (Balmain 1988, Bos 1989). Although it is generally assumed that these mutations represent an important step in tumor formation there is some uncertainty as to whether they are an early or a late event during the carcinogenic process. To address this question we have analyzed the frequency and pattern of mutations in the c-Ha-*ras* gene in small precancerous liver lesions of male C3H mice which were induced by a single administration of the hepatocarcinogen diethylnitrosamine (DEN).

1. Histological preparation

For mutation analyses in precancerous liver lesions, 10 mm serial sections were prepared from frozen liver tissue with a cryostat microtome and stained enzyme-histochemically for the activity of glucose-6-phosphatase (Wachstein 1957), which is known to be absent in precancerous liver lesions (Friedrich-Freska 1969a, 1969b). Thereafter, tiny tissue samples were taken from both enzyme-deficient lesions and from normal parts of the liver using small punching cannuli (Fig. 1). Tissue samples from lesions smaller than approximately 0.5 mm in diameter were microdissected out of the liver sections by use of a micro-preparative laser device (Klimek 1988).

2. PCR procedure

In vitro amplification of DNA by PCR was carried out directly on punched or microdissected tissue samples without prior isolation of DNA as recently described (Buchmann 1989). For analyses of ras-mutations in later appearing liver tumors, genomic DNA was isolated and 500 ng of purified nucleic acid were used for PCR. The primers used for amplification (Amp 61/A: 5'-GAG ACA TGT CTA CTG GAC ATC TT-3' and Amp 61/B: 5'-GCT AGC CAT AGG TGG CTC ACC TG-3') yielded a DNA-fragment of 166 bp around codon 61 of c-Ha-ras exon 2.

Following PCR amplification mutations in the c-Ha-ras gene were detected by allele-specific oligonucleotide hybridization using 5' ^{32}P-labeled oligonucleotide probes diagnostic for either the wild-type sequence of c-Ha-ras codon 61 or for 7 different types of mutations within this codon.

Our results show that 12 out of 127 precancerous liver lesions (9%) of male C3H mice occurring 11-29 weeks after a single application of DEN contain either C -> A transition at the first base or A -> G transitions at the second base of codon 61 of the c-Ha-*ras* gene (Table 1). At the first analysis (11 weeks), one focal liver lesion was already mutated in this proto-oncogene.

Since we prepared serial liver sections we were able to reconstruct the actual 3-dimensional sizes of all enzyme-altered lesions by use of a computer-assisted digitizer system (Schwarz 1987). We found that the

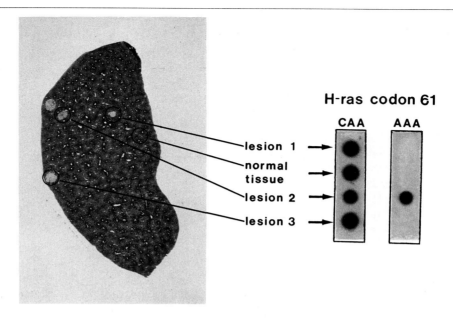

Figure 1. Analysis of mutations at codon 61 of the c-Ha-*ras* gene in small precancerous liver lesions. A 10 mm liver section from a DEN-treated mouse was stained for glucose-6-phosphatase (G-6-Pase) activity. Tiny tissue samples from three G-6-Pase-deficient liver lesions and from normal liver tissue were punched out of the liver section and used for *in vitro* amplification of DNA by PCR. Analysis of mutations at codon 61 of the c-Ha-*ras* gene was performed by allele-specific oligonucleotide-hybridization.

smallest lesions, where we detected c-Ha-*ras* mutations, had sphere diameters of only 0.2-0.4 mm. This relates to values of less than 1,000 cells per lesion. In the mutated liver lesions the signal intensities for the normal and the mutated sequences at c-Ha-*ras* codon 61 were almost identical. Since precancerous liver lesions have been shown to be monoclonal in origin (Rapos 1982, Williams 1983), this finding together

Table 1. Mutations at codon 61 of the c-Ha-*ras* gene in small precancerous liver lesions and later appearing liver tumors of male C3H mice.

Age at-sacrifice, weeks[1]	Number of lesions analyzed	Number of lesions with the mutated sequence at codon 61 of the c-Ha-*ras* gene[2]			
		AAA	CGA	CTA	Total (%)
11-29 127	5	7	0	12	(9)
42-52 50	11	12	2	25	(50)

[1]Precancerous liver lesions and liver tumors were induced by a single i.p. injection of diethylnitrosamine (20 mg/kg body weight) on day 15 after birth.
[2]Analyses for additional types of mutations at codon 61 did not give any positive results.

with the fact that a c-Ha-*ras* mutated lesion could already be detected 11 weeks after a single carcinogen treatment suggests that these mutations have occurred during the first rounds of cell replication and may therefore represent an early, perhaps the first critical event during hepatocarcinogenesis in the C3H mouse.

In contrast to the relatively low mutation frequency in the precancerous enzyme-altered lesions, 50% (25 out of a total of 50) of later appearing liver tumors of mice of the same strain showed mutations at codon 61 of the c-Ha-*ras* gene (see Table 1). This observation indicates that the mutations in this proto-oncogene confer a certain selective advantage to the affected progenitor cells leading to a preferential clonal expansion of the mutated cell population.

References

1. Balmain A, Brown K. Oncogene activation in chemical carcinogenesis. 1988, Adv. Cancer Res 51, 147-182.

2. Bos J L. *Ras* oncogenes in human cancer: a review. 1989, Cancer Res 49, 4682-4689.

3. Buchmann A, Mahr J, Bauer-Hofmann R, Schwarz M. Mutations at codon 61 of the Ha-*ras* proto-oncogene in precancerous liver lesions of the B6C3F1 mouse. 1989, Mol. Carcinogenesis 2, 121-125.

4. Buchmann A, Bauer-Hofmann R, Mahr J, Drinkwater N R, Luz A, Schwarz M. Mutational activation of the c-Ha-*ras* gene in liver tumors of different rodent strains: correlation with susceptibility to hepatocarcinogenesis. 1991, Proc Natl Acad Sci USA 88, 911-915.

5. Friedrich-Freksa H, Gössner W, Börner P. Histochemische Untersuchungen der Cancerogenese in der Rattenleber nach Dauergabe von Diäthylnitrosamin. 1969a, Z Krebsforsch 72, 226-239.

6. Friedrich-Freksa H, Papadopulu G, Gössner W. Histochemische Untersuchungen der Cancerogenese in der Rattenleber nach zeitlich begrenzter Verabfolgung von Diäthylnitrosamin. 1969b, Z Krebsforsch 72, 240-253.

7. Klimek F, Moore M A, Schneider E, Bannasch P. Histochemical and microbiochemical demonstration of reduced pyruvate kinase activity in thioacetamide-induced neoplastic nodules of rat liver. 1988, Histochemistry 90, 37-42.

8. Rabes H M, Bücher T, Hartmann A, Linke I, Dünnwald M. Clonal growth of carcinogen-induced enzyme-deficient preneoplastic cell populations in mouse liver. 1982, Cancer Res 42, 3220-3227.

9. Schwarz M, Schael S, Scholz W, Buchmann A, Pearson D, Kunz W. A computer program for the analysis of marker enzyme patterns in preneoplastic and neoplastic liver lesions. Proceedings of the SEK-Meeting Heidelberg 1987. 1987, J Cancer Res Clin Oncol CANC 42.

10. Wachstein M, Meisel E. Histochemistry of hepatic phosphatases at a physiologic pH. 1957, Am J Clin Pathol 27, 13-23.

11. Williams E D, Wareham K A, Howell S. Direct evidence for single cell origin of mouse liver cell tumours. 1983, Br J Cancer 47, 723-726.

Isolation and Direct Sequencing of PCR-cDNA Fragments from Tissue Biopsies

H Klocker, F Kaspar, J Eberle, G Bartsch

The past two or three years have seen a boom-like increase in the use of the polymerase chain reaction (PCR) due to the manifold technical applications and the extraordinary sensitivity of this method which can also be used to investigate specimens unsuitable for conventional molecular biological tests due to quantity-related problems. This has made PCR a valuable tissue-examination method for clinical diagnosis and research. The availability of specimens is often limited, as biopsies are usually performed on a small scale to avoid unnecessary strain on patients. In a study performed on biopsies from prostatic carcinoma patients, we investigated the transformation of androgenic tumors into malignant tumors which were no longer responding to hormone therapy. Possible pertinent factors are the androgen receptor, growth factors, oncogenes and tumor-suppressing genes. We investigated these in fine-needle and hollow-needle biopsies using a PCR technique specially developed for the isolation of cDNA fragments, which were subsequently examined for mutations by direct sequencing or other methods. In general this method can be used to isolate cDNA fragments from very small specimens (tissue or cultured cells). To obtain the highest possible amount of cDNA fragments from small initial quantities, we tried to find optimal conditions for each step (RNA isolation, cDNA synthesis and PCR).

1. Isolation of total RNA

On of the most economic and safety methods to isolate RNA is acid-phenol extraction using guanidinium thiocyanic acid to inhibit RNAses (for details: chapter 8). Extraction of proteins and DNA is followed by RNA precipitation. The precipitate is then washed with 75% ethanol and immediately used for cDNA synthesis. For small specimens, glycogen is recommended as a carrier for alcohol precipitation, as this increases RNA yields and prevents loss of the specimen to alcohol rinses (a perceptible precipitate is always found). cDNA synthesis and PCR are not impaired by glycogen.

Using commercially available kits with poly-T attached to the carrier material for direct isolation of mRNA (e.g. Serva, Polytract™) on prostate biopsies, we did not succeed in adequately isolating mRNA for our purposes. We found such kits unsuitable for small biopsies. Isolating mRNA after total RNA appears to be unnecessary as this leads to significant losses of the small mRNA quantities.

2. cDNA synthesis

cDNA synthesis was achieved with AMV reverse transcriptase. The specific primers first used for each fragment were later substituted by randomized hexanucleotide primers with which cDNA from a single specimen can be used to amplify several different fragments. With hexanucleotides, longer synthesis times and four different temperature cycles, yields similar to those using specific primers were obtained. For the amplification of larger PCR fragments (1.4 Kb), results using hexanucleotides were also comparable to specific primers.

3. Amplification of cDNA fragments

PCR was performed with the standard buffer (pH value: 9.0-9.1) at 25°C. 1-3 µl cDNA solution and 25 pMol of each primer was used per specimen in 50 µl of PCR starting solution. The cDNA solution used directly for PCR should not exceed this quantity, as this would have a negative influence on amplification. This seems to be due mainly to changes in magnesium ion concentration and pH value. If larger quantities of cDNA are needed, cDNA should first be precipitated with ethanol, followed by direct solution in the PCR buffer. We used 30 temperature cycles for amplification. The results are not usually significantly improved by more cycles. In our experiences, the important factors for efficient amplification of cDNA fragments are: the concentration of magnesium ions, the pH value of the PCR buffer and the denaturation temperature. These parameters are particularly important if fragments are difficult to amplify. In such cases, we obtained better results with a pH value of 9.0-9.1 (at 25°C) instead of 8.5-8.8. Choosing the right denaturation temperature is a difficult compromise between complete DNA denaturation and heat-induced inactivation of the Taq DNA polymerase. Initially we chose 94°C and briefly increased this to 95°C or 96°C before cooling. However, these conditions do not guarantee satisfactory yields of cDNA-fragment amplification which may prove particularly difficult with fragments containing G/C rich regions. The total G/C content is less important than whether or not the fragment contains any regions composed exclusively or almost exclusively of G and C. A good example of this is the median cDNA fragment of the androgen receptor, which contains a polyglycin-coding region with 20 consecutive GGC triplets. DMSO had to be added to the PCR buffer to successfully amplify this fragment. We presume that this succeeded because of the lower melting temperature of DNA as a result of adding DMSO, a small quantity of which suffices. The optimal range of dilution is 2-5%. Using more is inadvisable as this does not improve amplification but enhances the background (for details see chapter 4). We also tested other agents which lower melting temperatures. Glycerin (5-10%) was also suitable, while formamide had no positive effect.

The size of amplifiable fragments which produce satisfactory results is limited. In many cases, amplification of several overlapping fragments is necessary to isolate a complete cDNA or at least a complete coding region. This also applies to our androgen-receptor cDNA. The size of the coding region was almost 3 Kb. We amplified this region and part of the adjacent untranslated region by using three overlapping fragments. The size of the two terminal fragments was 1.4 Kb, while that of the median fragment containing the above-described G/C region was 646 bp. Using cultivated prepuce fibroblasts, we determined the number of cells necessary to isolate all three fragments. The minimum was 1,000-3,000 cells. However, lower numbers will frequently have to suffice due to a weak androgen-receptor expression in these cells, in which amplification of the N-terminal and the median fragment is also rather difficult.

If several cDNA fragments are to be investigated, these can be isolated from a single initial solution of cDNA if random primers are used for cDNA synthesis. Simultaneous amplification of two fragments in a single PCR is also possible. This has to be tested in each individual case, but is usually successful according to our experience. Examples are shown in Figure 1: Total RNA was isolated from prostate biopsy specimens, prostate cell lines and primary fibroblast cultures, followed by transcription to cDNA. Six different cDNA fragments were then amplified from each specimen in three PCR solutions. Two were androgen-receptor cDNA fragments, the third a cDNA fragment of the 'housekeeping' enzyme glyceraldehyde 3-phosphate dehydrogenase (GAPDH), which we used as an internal control, the fourth a cDNA fragment of prostate-specific antigen (PSA), the fifth a cDNA fragment of the epidermal growth factor receptor, and the sixth a cDNA fragment of the transforming growth factor ß2 (TGF ß2). .

Further amplification is necessary for more detailed examination of the PCR fragments. In some cases, aliquots from the first reaction can be used directly for a second PCR. However, it is often advisable to purify the fragments beforehand, either by gel permeate columns, ion exchange columns or preparative electrophoresis in an agarose with a low melting point.

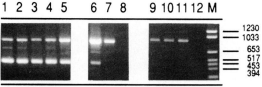

androgenreceptor, hormone binding domaine, 893 bp
prostate specific antigen, 449 bp

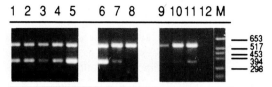

glyceraldehyde phosphate dehydrogenase, 554 bp
androgen receptor, DNA binding domaine, 361 bp

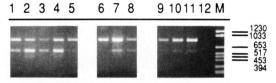

epidermal growth factor receptor, 863 bp
transforming growth factor TGF-ß2, 572 bp

Figure 1: Amplification of cDNA fragments from tissue samples and cultured cells.
Total RNA was isolated from the specimens and transcribed into cDNA by AMV reverse transcriptase using hexanucleotide primers. Six different cDNA fragments were then amplified from each specimen in three PCR solutions and 30 cycles. A 10 µl aliquot of each reaction solution was dissolved in 2% agarose gel and visualized by adding ethidium bromide.
Lanes 1 and 2: prostate tissue obtained during open surgery; lanes 3 and 4: hollow-needle prostate biopsies; lane 5: prostate fine-needle aspiration biopsy; lanes 6-8: prostate cell lines; lane 9: prepuce biopsy, lane 10: prepuce fibroblasts from cell culture, lane 11: cell-culture skin fibroblasts; lane 12: negative controls.

The last method is especially recommendable if additional bands are present.

4. Direct sequencing of PCR-cDNA fragments

The cloning procedure and the problems often involved in cloning PCR fragments can be avoided by direct sequencing. The widely discussed higher failure rate of Taq polymerase is irrelevant here as errors rersist without statistical significance. Only cloning and separation reveals such errors in sequencing. For DNA sequencing, we used an automatic sequencer based on fluorescence detection (see also chapter 14). Taq polymerase was also used for the sequencing reaction with kits supplied by Applied Biosystems. Marking was done either with M13 primers (primer sequencing) or with di-deoxynucleotide triphosphate (terminator sequencing) marked by fluorescence. Both methods can be performed with single-stranded as well as double-stranded fragments. We first sequenced single strands with marked M13 primers. The single-stranded fragments were produced by asymmetric PCR (Fig. 2). The two primers were used in the ratio of 50:3. Asymmetric PCR was applied simultaneously for primer sequencing in order to introduce the (-21)M13 primer sequence into the fragments. The deficient primers were extended by these sequences at the 5' terminal. Amplification was performed under normal PCR conditions, and the single-stranded fragments were then purified with ion exchange columns, concentrated and sequenced. On average, 300 to 500 bases were decoded by the sequencing of single-strands. In case of larger fragments it is necessary to produce overlapping single stranded fragments as described in Figure 2. As you can see, control sequencing of the complimentary strand was always performed.

Sequencing of PCR fragments has been further simplified by the introduction of terminator sequencing kits. Individual sequencing reactions for each base are no longer needed and any primer can be used. Furthermore, these kits yield good results for double-stranded DNA and PCR fragments can be used immediately after purification.

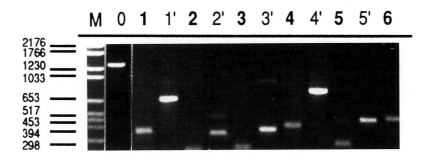
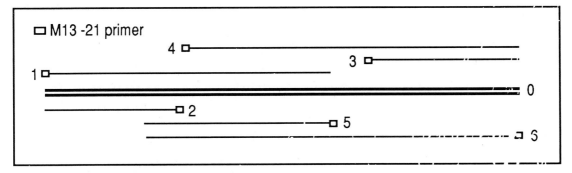

Figure 2: Sequencing strategy for the 1,399 bp androgen-receptor fragment.
Using asymmetric PCRs, three overlapping single-stranded fragments were amplified from strands and complimentary strands of this fragment. The primer ratio was 50:3. The deficient primers had been extended by the (-21)M13 primer sequence (sequence see chapter 13), which was thus introduced into the fragments as a starting point for the sequencing reaction. Following asymmetric amplification, single and double strands were purified with ion exchange columns and then separated and concentrated by alcohol precipitation. The purified fragments are shown above after electrophoresis in 2% agarose gel. 0:1,399 bp androgen-receptor fragment, 1-6 single-stranded fragments, 1'-5' double-stranded fragments.

The methods used here are based on standard procedures as described in the relevant methodology literature, e.g.: Sambrook/Fritsch/Maniatis: Molecular Cloning, ColdSpring Harbor Laboratory Press, 1989, or Davis/Dibner/Battey: Basic Methods in Molecular Biology, Elsevier 1986, and were specially optimized for smaller specimens.

Procedure	Comments
1. Isolation of total RNA from small specimens	This procedure gives best yields when used in fine-needle biopsies, punch biopsies and cell cultures up to approximately 10^6 cells. Isolation should be performed on ice or in a cooling chamber, solutions should be chilled prior to use.
1. Lyse specimen in 0.6 ml GTC buffer in a 1.5-ml airtight tube; if necessary, use an ultrasound disintegrator.	1. GTC buffer: 4 M guanidinium thiocyanate (Merck), 0.5% laurolysarcosine (Boehringer Mannheim), 25 mM trinatrium citrate pH 7.0 (Sigma), 1 drop/100 ml silicon skimmer (Merck). Autoclave solution and add 8 µl/ml ß-mercapto-ethanol (Sigma) and 20 µl/ml glycogen (suitable for molecular biology, Boehringer Mannheim) prior to each use.
2. Add 0.6 ml of water-saturated phenol and 60 µl 2 M sodium acetate (pH 4.0); mix by repeated tilting.	2. Water-saturated phenol: Melt phenol in a water bath. Add 1/4-1/3 volume autoclaved water and a small quantity of 8-hydroxy quinoline (approx. 100 mg/l to prevent oxidation). Mix and cool in refrigerator or on ice. A phenol and a water phase are formed - if not, add a small quantity of water. The solution can be stored in a refrigerator for several months. Sodium acetate solution: Standardize 2 M acetic acid with NaOH to pH value 4.0 and autoclave.
3. Add 130 µl of chloroform, mix vigorously on a Vortex for 10-15 sec, and centrifuge ($\geq$ 12,000 rpm, 10 min). Two phases should be distinguishable after centrifuging (if not, an inadequate quantity of chloroform has been used).	
4. Transfer the water phase into another tube and precipitate RNA with an equal volume of isopropanol. Leave to settle at -20°C overnight or at least for several hours.	
5. Centrifuge (12,000 rpm, 20-30 min) and purify pellet twice with 75% ethanol.	

Procedure(cont.)   *Comments(cont.)*

2. cDNA synthesis with random hexanucleotide primers

1. Dissolve total RNA (entire yield from small tissue sample or 200-500 ng of RNA), boil for 2 min and cool in iced water.

2. Add 35 µl of mixture, mix and perform cDNA synthesis in a thermocycler.

2. Mixture/specimen: 23 µl water, 4 µl 10x AMV buffer (0.5 M Tris-HCl, pH 8.3 (42°C), 0.5 M KCl, 80 mM $MgCl_2$, 1 mg/ml BSA (RNAse- and DNAse-free, Pharmacia), 4 µl dNTP solution (10 mM each), 2 µl random hexanucleotide primer solution (100 pMol/ll, Boehringer Mannheim), 2 µl ß-SH solution (3 µl ß-mercapto-ethanol per 100 µl, freshly prepared), 50 U ribonuclease inhibitor (Boehringer Mannheim), 10 U AMV RT (Promega).
Thermocycler program: 8 min at 20°C, 8 min 25°C, 30 min at 42°C; 4 cycles.

3. PCR amplification

1. Add 1-3 µl cDNA solution to 50 µl PCR mix.

1. Do not use more cDNA solution. If necessary, concentrate cDNA by alcohol precipitation.

2. Amplification (30 cycles): 45 sec at 94°C, 15 sec at 96°C, 1 min at 52-57°C (depending on primer), 1-3 min at 73°C (depending on fragment length); extend initial denaturation cycle by 1 min and final synthesis cycle by 5 min.

3. Inspect 5-10 µl aliquots on 2% agarose gel.

4. Isolate fragments by preparative agarose gel electrophoresis in 2% agarose gel (agarose with low melting point; USB). Following electrophoresis, cut bands from gel, put gel sections in a 1.5 ml tube, centrifuge briefly and freeze in liquid nitrogen. Centrifuge in a cooling chamber for 10-15 min, pour supernatant into another tube. Add the same quantity of TE buffer as agarose pellet, dissolve agarose at 65°C, freeze and centrifuge as before, unite supernatants. If necessary, concentrate the specimen by precipitating with alcohol.

Procedure(cont.) *Comments(cont.)*

5. Second PCR amplification: up to 5 µl fragment solution of the first amplification in a 100 µl PCR preparation. Proceed as above (2.) Again purify PCR fragment by preparative agarose gel electrophoresis or by sepharose G-150 spin column or ion exchange column (e.g., Quiagen Tip-5).

5. PCR mix: 10 µl 10x PCR buffer (100 mM Tris-HCl pH 9.0-9.1 (25°C), 500 mM KCl, 15 mM $MgCl_2$, 1% triton X-100 0.1% gelatin), 50 pMol of primer, 200 µM dNTPs, (2-5 µl DMSO for fragments with GC-rich regions), add water to obtain 100 µl, 2.5 units of Taq polymerase (Promega, Boehringer Mannheim).

4. Asymmetric PCR and sequencing of single strands

1. Approx. 10 ng cDNA fragment + 100 µl PCR mix. Primer ratio 50:3, 30 PCR cycles. For sequencing with M13 primers marked by fluorescence, the deficient primers are elongated at the 5'-end by the M13 universal primer sequence.

2. Isolate and purify single strand with Quiagen-tip 5 ion exchange columns following the Quiagen protocol for ss M-13 DNA.

3. Sequence with Taq polymerase sequencing kits (Applied Biosystems) according to the manufacturer's specifications. The optimal quantity of DNA from single strands should be determined for each individual case (50-100 ng for our fragments).

Using the method described, we started sequencing the androgen-recptor cDNA in prostate cell lines and prostate biopsies. In the LNCaP cell line, we found a mutation within the hormone binding domain of the androgen receptor, probably resulting in the exchange of a threonine for an alanin base and a change in hormone specificity in this receptor. We are currently using the PCR to investigate the possibility of similar mutations in tumor tissue of prostatic carcinoma patients.

Differential PCR: Loss of the ß1-InterferonGene in Chronic Myelogeneous Leukemia (CML) and Acute Lymphoblastic Leukemia (ALL).

A Neubauer, Ch A Schmidt, B Neubauer, W Siegert, D Huhn, E Liu

In the molecular study of the alterations associated with malignant transformation chronic myelogeneous leukemia (CML) serves as a model because a long stable chronic phase is followed by an acute blastic phase. Though the molecular event leading to chronic phase CML is thought to be a rearrangement of the c-abl gene located on chromosome 9 and the bcr gene on chromosome 22 (see Kurzrock, 1988 for a review). The molecular alterations leading to blastic phase are not clear. Loss of tumor suppressor gene function has been implicated in carcinogenesis (see Sager, 1989 for a review). A hint for a presumed tumor suppressor gene is a frequently observed cytogenetic deletion or aberration in certain malignancies. Cells from human ALL and non-Hodgkin's lymphomas and their derivative cell lines frequently exhibit a loss of a band in the short arm of chromosome 9 (9p22) (Diaz 1988, Diaz 1990), a location to which the alpha and ß 1-interferon genes have been mapped (Trent 1982). Besides lymphoblastic cell lines, the CML blastic phase cell line, K562, also carries a homozygous loss of the alpha and ß 1-interferon genes (Diaz 1988). This suggested to us that loss of this locus might be associated with the conversion to blastic phase in CML. To test this hypothesis, we screened a large number of chronic phase and blastic phase CML samples using a newly developed technique, differential PCR (Neubauer 1990, Frye 1989). It is demonstrable that gene amplification can readily be measured using this modification of the PCR techniques (Frye 1989).

The assay is based on quantification of the ratio between a reference gene and the gene of interest and can readily detect subtle changes in the target: reference gene ratios, e.g. ratios of 2:1 and 3:2 (Neubauer 1990). The success of this assay is dependent on the careful adjustment of the PCR conditions. Our current differential PCR conditions are capable of analyzing DNA isolated from minor cell populations by cell sorting or microsurgery. Furthermore, the sensitivity of our assay is not affected by significant fragmentation of DNA as commonly seen in DNA extracted from paraffin embedded tissues. These capabilities make differential PCR superior to conventional Southern hybridization for the analysis of hemizygosity in human tumor samples, especially when only miniscule amounts of cells are available, e.g. from tumor biopsies.

Methods

1. Cells and DNA

The cell line K562 was obtained from the American Type Tissue Collection (ATCC). Patient cells: Diagnosis of CML, and ALL was made using standard blood and bone marrow smears; in ALL, immunological analysis were performed using procedures for the detection of myeloid-antigen expression (Wiersma 1991). The presence of Philadelphia chromosome or bcr/abl rearrangement was required for inclusion in this study. We investigated DNA from 64 CML patients; 49 patients were in chronic phase, and 15 patients were in blast crisis. Uncut placental DNA was purchased from Oncor (Gaithersburg, MD). The DNA concentration was determined by spectrophotometry, and the DNA samples were adjusted to a concentration of 50ng/µl in TE-buffer (10mM Tris Cl, 1mM EDTA, pH 8.0).

2. Polymerase Chain Reaction

PCR was performed with 200ng (4µl) genomic DNA under standard conditions in 50µl (50mM KCl, 10mM Tris Cl pH 8.3, 2.5mM MgCl2, 0.01% (w/v) gelatin (Sigma), 250µM dNTPs (Boehringer), 0.225% Tween 20 (Sigma), 0.225% NP40 (Sigma), 1U AmpliTaq Polymerase (Cetus).

The target gene in all experiments was the ß-interferon gene and the reference (diploid) genes used were gamma-interferon, and the HER-2/neu proto-oncogene. All priming oligonucleotides were 20 bases in length and the sequences for these PCR primers were taken from the published genomic sequences. The sequences of the oligonucleotides used are displayed in Table 1. Optimal concentrations for the priming oligonucleotides in the differential PCR were: 0.5µM for gamma-interferon and neu, and 0.25µM for ß-interferon. The PCR proceeded for 27 cycles in a Perkin Elmer Cetus thermocycler under the following conditions: cycle 1: denaturing at 95°C for 5 minutes, annealing at 55°C for 1 minute, extension at 72°C for 1 minute; cycles 2-27: denaturing at 95°C for 1 minute, annealing and extension under conditions identical to cycle 1. One fifth of the PCR amplification products was electrophoresed on a 12% polyacrylamide gel and stained with ethidium bromide. The relative intensity of the PCR amplified bands was quantitated by densitometry of the photographic negatives of the ethidium stained gels. Results are expressed as the ratio of the area under the

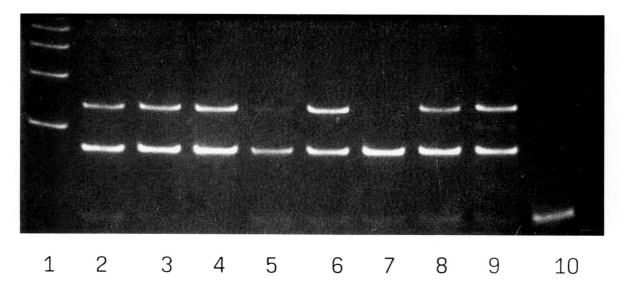

Figure 1: Differential PCR on 5 ALL cases and on a dilution using K562 DNA. Differential PCR was performed as described in the Materials and Methods section. 10ul were electrophoresed on a polyacrylamid gel and stained with ethidium bromide. Lane 1: 123base pair ladder as a molecular size marker; lane 2: bone marrow (BM) patient #605; lane 3: BM #433; lane 4: peripheral blood (PB) #433; lane 5: BM patient # 650; lane 6: PB #650; lane 7: K562; lane 8: 50% K562-50% placental DNA; lane 9: placental DNA; lane 10: no DNA added. The lower ratio in the BM on patient #650 is clearly seen.

Table 1: Sequences of the oligonucleotides used in the study.

Gene	5'primer	3'primer	sequence-region (Ref.)
ß-Interferon	GGCACAACAGGTAGTAGGCG	GCCACAGGAGCTTCTGACAC	-40-130 (1)
g-Interferon 84bp	AGTGATGGCTGAACTGTCGC	CTGGGATGCTCTTCGACCTC	4647-4731 (2)
neu	CCTCTGACGTCCATCATCTC	ATCTTCTGCTGCCGTCGCTT	2122-2219 (3)

(1): Nucl Acids Res 9:1045 (1981); (2): Nature 298:859 (1982); (3) Nature 319:230 (1986).

peak corresponding to the ß-interferon, divided by the area under the peak corresponding to the reference gene.

Results

DNA from 64 cases with CML was subjected to differential PCR: 49 in chronic phase, and 15 in blast crisis. In each PCR run the following controls were performed: K562 DNA alone to test possible contamination, DNA from a normal blood donor, and the 50% mixture thereof with K562 DNA. One of 64 CML cases (CML case # 25) revealed a lower ratio between the reference gene and ß-interferon gene (Neubauer 1990). This finding was corroborated by a differential PCR using primers within the neu oncogene as the reference gene. Here also this patient's DNA revealed a lower ß-interferon/neu ratio. This patient (patient # 25) was in blast crisis and had no apparent cytogenetic abnormality involving chromosome 9. Furthermore, this patient's DNA was not sheared, as demonstrated by a 0.8% agarose gel electrophoresis. Differential PCR on 20 cases with ALL: It has previously been reported that cells from Non-Hodgkin's lymphomas and ALL frequently exhibit loss of the interferon genes (Diaz 1988, Diaz 1990). To test differential PCR in ALL, we screened 20 cases of childhood ALL. We first investigated around 10 cases. However, we did not find allelic loss in any sample. We then figured that differential PCR could yield false negative results if the percentage of blasts was lower than 50%. Thus, we only used cases in which DNA was extracted from samples with a percentage of blasts >50%. Three of 20 cases (15%) displayed an allelic loss within the ß1-interferon gene (Figure 1).

Our data shows, however, that the loss of a ß-interferon allele occurred in only one of 15 patients with blast crisis and none of 49 patients in chronic phase. Though it is possible that deletions at this locus may play a role in the tumor progression of a small number of CML patients, it is not likely that this role is as important as that in acute lymphocytic leukemia, where 28% of patients exhibit some perturbation at the ß-interferon locus.

To test if differential PCR could corroborate these findings obtained by regular Southern blotting, we amplified DNA from childhood ALL cases. Using DNA extracted from specimens with under 50% blasts we did not find any allelic loss; however, when we switched to samples with more than 50% blasts we found 3/20 samples displaying a loss within the ß1-interferon locus (Figure 1). Although our number is somewhat smaller than the number investigated by others (Diaz 1990), we feel that these data show that differential PCR can be used to detect allelic loss. However, the pitfall of this technique is that contamination with normal cells leads to false negative results. This should be circumvented in the future by cell sorting techniques such as flow cytometry or magnetic cell sorting, before the analysis is performed.

REFERENCES

1. Chamberlain JS. Deletion screening of the Duchenne muscular dystrophy locus via multiplex DNA amplification. 1988, Nucl Acids Res 16, 11141

2. Chehab FF. Detection of sickle cell anemia and thalassemias. 1987, Nature 329, 293

3. Diaz MO, Ziemin S, LeBeau MM, Pitha P, Smith SD, Chilcote RR, Rowley JD. Homozygenous deletion of the alpha and beta1 interferon genes in human leukemia and derived cell lines. 1988, Proc Natl Acad Sci USA 85, 5259

4. Diaz MO, Rubin CM, Harden A, Ziemin S, Larson RA, Le Beau MM, Rowley JD. Deletions of interferon genes in acute lymphoblastic leukemia. 1990, New Engl J Med 322, 77

5. Frye RA, Benz CC, Liu E. Detection of amplified oncogenes by differential polymerase chain reaction. 1989, Oncogene 4, 1153

6. Kurzrock R, Gutterman JU, Talpaz M. The molecular genetics of Philadelphia chromosome-positive leukemias. 1988, New Engl J Med 319, 990

7. Maniatis T, Frisch EF Sambrook J. Molecular cloning: A laboratory manual, 2. Cold Spring Harbor Laboratory, Cold Spring Harbor, 1982.

8. Neubauer A, Neubauer B, Liu E. Polymerase chain reaction based assay to detect allelic loss in human DNA: loss of beta-interferon gene in chronic myelogeneous leukemia. 1990, Nucl Acids Res 18, 993

9. Sager R. Tumor suppressor genes: The puzzle and the promise. 1989, Science 246, 1406

10. Trent JM, Olson S, Lawn RM. Chromosomal localization of human leukocyte, fibroblast, and immune interferon genes by means of in situ hybridization. 1982, Proc Natl Acad Sci USA 79, 7809

11. Wiersma SR, Ortega J, Sobel E, Weinberg KI. Clinical importance of myeloid-antigen expression in acute lymphoblastic leukemia of childhood. 1991, New Engl J Med 324, 800

B) Detection of infectious agents

Long-Term Persistence of Borrelia Burgdorferi in Neuroborreliosis Detected by Polymerase Chain Reaction

S Bamborschke, A Kaufhold, A Podbielski, B Melzer, A Porr, B Rehse-Küpper

Infection with the tick-borne spirochete Borrelia burgdorferi (Lyme disease) may be accompanied by nervous system abnormalities in all stages of the disease (Halperin 1988). Diagnosis of neuroborreliosis stage 2 (Bannwarth's syndrome) and 3 (Chronic encephalomyelitis) is usually achieved by detection of specific intrathecal antibody production. However, until now there has been no serological marker for disease progression or therapeutic success.

Therefore, we employed the polymerase reaction (PCR) to look for persistence of B. burgdorferi in CSF and urine samples taken repeatedly during a period of 2 1/2 years in a patient with Bannwarth's syndrome.

Case report

A 58-year-old man suffered from neuroborreliosis with headache, radicular pain, facial paralysis and right oculomotor palsy. CSF pleocytosis and specific intrathecal IgG-production against Borrelia burgdorferi was present. After i.m. treatment with penicillin G, neurological status and CSF values normalized and serum IgG titre against B. burgdorferi fell by 2 dilutions. CSF samples taken 3, 25, and 198 days after onset of illness, and CSF and urine samples from day 906 were examined using the polymerase chain reaction (PCR) for detection of specific bacterial DNA. Specific DNA

FLAG 1 :	5'- GCA GTT CAA TCA GGT AAC GGC - 3'
FLAG 2 :	5'- AGC TTC ATC TTG GGT TGC TCC - 3'
OSP 1 :	5'- GCC TTG ACG AGA AAA ACA GCG - 3'
OSP 2 :	5'- TGA CCC CTC TAA TTT GGT GCC - 3'
FLAG probe:	5'- CCT GAA AGT GAT GCT GGT GTG - 3'
OSP probe:	5'- AAG CGA TGG ATC TGG AAA AGC - 3'
Expected size of the amplified gene segments:	
flagellin gene segment:	273 bp
ospA gene segment:	707 bp

Table 1: Nucleotide sequences of the primers and probes

was detected in CSF on day 3, 25 and 198 and in urine on day 906. After additional i.v. treatment with ceftriaxone, CSF and urine samples were taken on day 946 and found to be negative in PCR. CSF cell counts, specific intrathecal antibody production, and PCR results in CSF and urine during the clinical course are shown in table 2.

Methods

Immunoglobulins in Serum and CSF were determined by lasernephelometry and evaluated according to Reiber and Felgenhauer (1987). Specific IgG against B. burgdorferi was determined in corresponding serum and CSF samples which were diluted to identical IgG concentration (1 mg/ml) using an ELISA as previously described (Rehse-Küpper 1986). Higher titres in CSF than in corresponding serum samples indicate intrathecal specific IgG production.

1. DNA extraction

500 µl samples of CSF or urine or B. burgdorferi ZS7 that served as positive control were boiled for 5 min, centrifuged, and the pellet was resuspended in 400 ul 0.5 % SDS - 10 mM Tris (pH 8.0) - 5 mM EDTA. Proteinase K was added at a final concentration of 200 µg/ml. The mixture was incubated for 3h at 65°C. After purification with phenol/chloroform, yeast tRNA (final concentration 100 µg/ml) was added and the DNA was precipitated with pure ethanol. Finally, the pellet was dissolved in 50 µl distilled water.

2. PCR reaction and blot procedure

For PCR, 10 µl of the resuspended DNA was added as a target. Besides the target DNA, the PCR reaction mixture contained PCR buffer (50 mM KCl, 10 mM Tris-HCl pH 8.3, 1.5 mM $MgCl_2$, 0.001 % gelatine, 200 µM of each dNTP, 1 µM of each primer and 2.5 units Taq polymerase (Boehringer Mannheim, FRG). The mixture was overlaid with 100 µl mineral oil. PCR amplification (45 cycles) was done on an

Table 2: CSF cell counts, intrathecal immunoglobulin production and PCR results during the clinical course

Day	cells/ul	intrathecal production			ELISA (titre) (1 mg/dl IgG)		PCR (flag)		PCR (ospA)	
	CSF	IgG	IgM	IgA	serum	CSF	CSF	urine	CSF	urine
3	128	+	+	+	32	256	+	n.d.	-	n.d.
25	18	-	+	-	32	256	+	n.d.	-	n.d.
198	2	-	-	-	16	64	+	n.d.	+	n.d.
906	3	-	-	-	4	16	-	+	-	-
946	0	-	-	-	4	16	-	-	-	-

n.d. = not done

automated heating block (Techne PHC-1) under the following conditions: 94°C denaturation (1 min), 50°C annealing (1 min), and 72°C extension (2.5 min). A negative control contained all reaction components without the target DNA. Generally recommended precautions were taken to avoid cross contamination between samples (Kwok 1989). PCR products were analysed by electrophoresis on 1 % - 1.5 % agarose gels and staining with ethidium bromide. For Southern blots the DNA was transferred to nylon membranes by vacuum (Vacu-Aid, Hybraid Ltd. Teddington, U.K.). The nucleotide sequences of the PCR primers as well as the oligonucleotide probes that correspond to internal sequences of the amplified fragments are shown in table 1. Primer sequences were selected on the basis of the published gene sequences of the flagellin gene (Wallich 1990) and ospA gene of B. burgdorferi (Bergström 1989), respectively. The oligonucleotides were synthesized on a Beckman 200A DNA synthesizer (Beckman Instruments, Munich, FRG). Further preparation of the oligonucleotides including the labelling of the probes with digoxigenin-dUTP (Boehringer Mannheim) and hybridization assays were performed as previously described (Podbielski 1990). For visualization, the chemoluminescent substrate AMPPD (Boehringer Mannheim) was used.

Results

Using PCR, persistence of B. burgdorferi was detected in CSF (day 198) and urine (day 906) after penicillin treatment and normalization of CSF cell count. Following additional treatment with ceftriaxone (day 946) PCR was negative.

Our results show that B. burgdorferi may persist in patients with neuroborreliosis for years after penicillin treatment even after normalization of neurological status and CSF cell count. Using PCR, in our patient B. burgdorferi was found to persist longer in urine than in CSF and disappeared after additional treatment with ceftriaxone. We conclude, that PCR is a valuable tool for detection of B. burgdorferi in clinical specimens and that it may be used to assess the efficacy of antibiotic treatment.

References

1. Bergström S, Bundoc VG, Barbour AG. Molecular analysis of linear plasmid-encoded major surface proteins, OspA and OspB, of the Lyme disease spirochaete Borrelia burgdorferi. 1989, Mol Microbiol 3, 479-486.

2. Halperin JJ, Pass HL, Anand AK, Luft BJ, Volkman DJ, Dattwyler RJ. Nervous system abnormalities in Lyme disease. 1988, Ann NY Acad Sci 539, 24-34.

3. Kwok S, Higuchi R. Avoiding false positives with PCR. 1989, Nature 339, 237-238.

4. Podbielski A, Kühnemund O, Lütticken R. Identification of group A type 1 streptococcal M protein gene by a non-radioactive oligonucleotide detection method. 1990, Med Microbiol Immunol 179, 255-262.

5. Rehse-Küpper B, Ackermann R. Demonstration of locally synthesized Borrelia antibodies in cerebrospinal fluid. 1986, Zbl Bakt Hyg A 263, 407-411.

6. Reiber H, Felgenhauer K. Protein transfer at the blood cerebrospinal fluid barrier and the quantitation of the humoral immune response within the central nervous system. 1987, Clin Chim Acta 163, 319-328.

7. Wallich R, Moter SE, Simon MM, Ebnet K, Heiberger A, Kramer MD. The Borrelia burgdorferi flagellum-associated 41-kilodalton antigen (flagellin): Molecular cloning, expression and amplification of the gene. 1990, Infect Immun 58, 1711-1719.

Nested Polymerase Chain Reaction for the Identification of B.Burgdorferi in the Tertiary Stage of Neuroborreliosis

H Bocklage, R Lange, H Karch, J Heesemann, H W Kölmel

Lyme borreliosis is a contagious disease transmitted by ticks of the genus Ixodes. Apart from dermatological, cardial and rheumatological manifestations, the multi-systemic disease spectrum also covers affections of the nervous system (neuro-borreliosis), which occur in many different shapes and sizes, frequently resembling the clinical symptoms of other diseases (Pachner 1989). Differentiation is made schematically in three stages, which may be incurred individually, together or even by overlapping them.

The early stage of the disease is as a rule accompanied by unspecific symptoms, e.g. weariness, exhaustion or inappetence. Obvious symptoms of neurological complications cannot be detected. Only headaches and a certain stiffness in the neck may be judged as signs of meningeal irritation and mild encephalopathy.

Characteristic of the second stage of neuroborreliosis is lymphocytic meningopolyneuritis (Bannwarth Syndrome). In addition meningitis, encephalitis, as well as radiculoneuritis may be observed. In the latter stages the clinical findings with neuroborreliosis are predominantly marked by central-nervous system manifestations (Ackermann 1985). The parenchymatous form involves acute, but often chronically progressive meningo-encephalitis or encephalomyelitis. The vascular form is characterized by partially recurrent cerebral circulatory disturbances with varied symptoms and signs within the scope of cerebral vasculitis.

The pathogenesis of neuroborreliosis is still largely unclear. It is known from injection experiments on rats that living spirochaetes induce the synthesis of IL-1 (Garcia-Monco 1990). This leads to increased

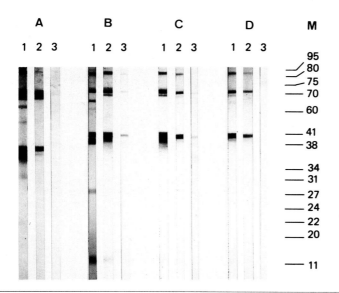

Figure 1: Western blot analysis of CSF and serum 1, 15, 45 and 90 days after the commencement of stationary treatment. Lane 1: serum (1:100), lane 2: CSF (IgG concentration as in lane 3), lane 3: serum (1:500). The molecular weight (Kda) is specified on the right.

permeability in the blood-brain barrier, enabling B. burgdorferi to penetrate the CNS in the early stages of infection.

This observation is also confirmed in man. B. burgdorferi was successfully cultured from the CSF patients with early manifestations of neuroborreliosis and specific B. burgdorferi antigens were cultured (Karlson 1990). This corresponds to the hypothesis that, prior to an immune reaction and the subsequent neurological manifestations setting in, intact spirochaetes have to be present in the brain. The way an infection continues to develop is dependent on whether or not the pathogen manages to withdraw from the immune reaction. Presumably persistent spirochaetes contribute indirectly to subsequent emerging neuroborreliosis. At the present time two hypotheses are being discussed: a) local synthesis of cytokines, b) auto-immune reaction.

To diagnose neuroborreliosis nuclear magnetic resonance (NMR) is increasingly being implemented to detect damage of the brain directly. In individual cases, the results of clinical analysis and NMR may resemble those of multiple sclerosis (MS). For this very reason identification of oligoclonal B.burgdorferi specific antibodies in the CSF of a patient with suspected neuroborreliosis is a fundamental diagnostic parameter. Due to the fact that attempts to culture the pathogen from the CSF of tertiary neuroborreliosis have failed, rapid and direct verification has only become possible with the introduction of PCR. In this paper we are presenting a nested PCR, with which we are able to specifically identify the tiniest quantities of B.burgdorferi. This method puts us in a position to be able to control the effectiveness of antibiotic therapy. To ascertain whether the amplified DNA is specific for B. burgdorferi and not the result of unspecific primer hybridisation, restriction analysis was conducted with sauIIIa. In accordance with the restriction map of the flagellin gene of B. burgdorferi (Gassmann 1991) a 185bp and 105bp sauIIIa fragment occurred (Fig. 2). Due to the unequivocal indications that neuroborreliosis was actually present "Ceftriaxon" was administered intravenously (2g/daily; duration of treatment: 14 days). In the course of this therapy a clear drop in the number of cells and the concentration of protein in the CSF was registered. Subsequent the PCR analysis was negative (Fig. 2). After antibiotic therapy was completed additional treatment was carried out with cortison in order to accelerate a complete recovery. WB-analyses carried out in the course of treatment showed a drop in specific B. burgdorferi antibodies (Fig. 1). In the NMR check-up made 11 months after stationary treatment, no more multiple lesions were detected (Fig. 3b). Additional B-cell mapping showed the absence of antibodies aimed at the flagellin epitope AS 205-225.

Case report and methods

In the spring a rapidly progressive infirmity in both legs in conjunction with dysbasia was observed in a 1-year-old female who displayed no relevant medical case

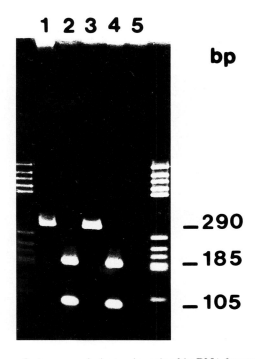

Figure 2: Agarose gel-electrophoresis of the DNA fragments amplified from the CSF. Lanes 1 and 2: positive control from B. burgdorferi B31 (undigested, sauIIIa digested); lanes 3 and 4: CSF sample directly prior to the commencement of antibiotic therapy (undigested, sauIIa digested); lane 5: CSF sample after completion of antibiotic therapy; the outer lanes show the DNA molecular weight marker V of Boehringer.

history. During the summer problems were incurred with incontinence and progressive tetraparesis developed with ataxia. An NMR conducted forthwith revealed a host of lesions in the white matter (Fig. 3a). In addition to an increased concentration of protein the CSF indicated an elevation of the cell number.

The routine laboratory parameters, such as antinuclear antibodies, cytogram, electrolyte content and the sedimentation rate of the blood, were normal. IgM and IgG antibodies to B. burgdorferi could be detected both in the CSF and in the serum with the aid of a flagellin-ELISA (Hansen 1988) and a tricine Western blot (WB) (Lange 1992). It was not possible to culture B. burgdorferi from the CSF. For WB-analysis the sera were diluted to the same IgG concentration of that of the CSF samples (1:400 - 1:500) in order to check whether CSF and serum reactivity with B. burgdorferi proteins varies greatly. The CSF reacted particularly strongly with 80 Kda, 70 Kda, 41 Kda and 38 Kda proteins. On the other hand, antibodies to OspA (31Kda) could not be detected (Fig. 1). Since the CSF in the Western blot had a more conspicuous reaction pattern than the serum it seemed obvious to assume that there was a greater quantity of specific antibodies in the CSF. In order to ascertain the quantity of antibodies, synthesized intrathecally, both the albumin as well as the IgG concentration in the serum and CSF were determined. The IgG/albumin (I/A) index was subsequently determined from these data according to the following formula: ((CSF IgG/serum IgG)/ (CSF albumin/ serum albumin)). The I/A index was raised (Tab. 1). Oligoclonal, specific B. burgdorferi IgG was found by isoelectrical focussing only in the CSF (Tab. 1). B-cell epitope mapping carried out with this patient's serum samples indicated that the antibodies were only directed against the central region of the flagellin (AS 205-225) (Schneider 1991).

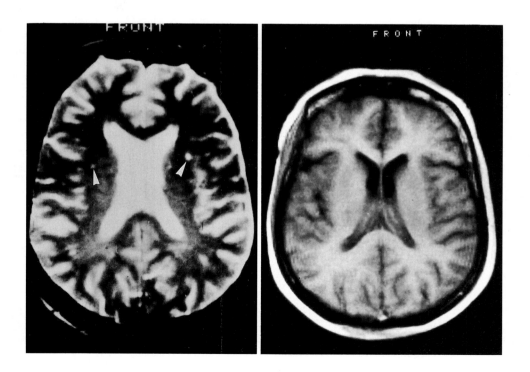

Figures 3a,b. NMR prior (a) and subsequent to "Ceftriaxon" therapy. Prior to treatment lesions can be clearly detected as hyperintensive areas (arrows).

For the PCR procedure 500 µl of CSF was separated by centrifugation and washed. Subsequently the DNA was isolated by proteinase K and phenol/chloroform treatment (Dillela 1985). 20 µl of this DNA was used as a template in a 50 µl PCR preparation with the two external, specific flagellin primers (Wallich 1990), 5'-CTGCTGGCATGGGAGTTTCT-3' and 5'-TCAATTGCATACTCAGTACT-3'. After 40 amplification cycles a second PCR run (25 cycles) was conducted with 5 % of this reaction. Here two oligonucleotides, 5'-AAGGAATTGGCAGTTCAATC-3' and 5'-ACAGCAATAGCTTCATCTTG-3' (Krüger 1991), were implemented, which hybridize within the previously amplified flagellin sequence, so that a subfragment of 290 bp was produced. Specificity of the fragment was shown by restriction fragment analysis using the restriction enzyme sauIIIa.

However, since the reappraisal method we selected resulted in only intact borrelia being recorded, the positive PCR result represents direct evidence of the presence of spirochaetes in the latter stage of neuroborreliosis. Due to the protracted persistence of the humoral immune reaction, the titer course of specific antibodies does not permit any unequivocal conclusions to be drawn regarding the success of this therapy. The PCR is thus a suitable means of checking the effectiveness of antibiotics quickly and reliably.

Apart from the criteria postulated by Pachner (1989), namely (a) damage to the CNS detectable in the NMR, (b) high antibody titer, (c) additional organ manifestations, e.g. ECM, arthritis or meningitis, (d) lymphocytosis in the CSF, (e) response to the antibiotic therapy, the results of a PCR, therefore, represent another significant parameter for identifying tertiary neuroborreliosis.

References

1. Ackermann R, Gollmer E, Rehse-Küpper B. Progressive Borrelien-Enzephalomyelitis. 1985, Dtsch Med Wochenschr 110, 1039-1042

2. Dillela AG, Woo SLC. Cosmid cloning of genomic DNA. 1985, BRL-Focus 7, (2) 1-5

3. Garcia-Monco JC, Fernadez Villar B, Calvo Alen J, Benach J L. Borrelia burgdorferi in the central nervous system: Experimental and clinical evidence for early invasion. 1990, J Infect Dis 161, 1187-1193

4. Gassmann GS, Jacobs E, Deutzmann R, Göbel UB. Analysis of the Borrelia burgdorferi GeHo fla gene and antigen characterisation of its gene product. 1991, J Bact 173, 1452-1459

5. Hansen H, Hinderson P, Pedersen NS. Measurement of antibodies to the Borrelia burgdorferi flagellum improves serodiagnosis in Lyme disease. 1988, J Clin Microbiol 26, 338-346

6. Karlson M, Hovind-Hougen K, Svenungson B, Stiernstedt G. Cultivation and characterization of spirochetes from cerebrospinal fluid of patients with Lyme borreliosis. 1990, J Clin Micobiol 28, 473-479

7. Krüger WH, Pulz M. Detection of Borrelia burgdorferi in cerebrospinal fluid by the polymerase chain reaction. 1991, J Med Microbiol 35, 98-102

8. Lange R, Bocklage H, Schneider T, Kölmel HW, Heesemann J, Karch H. Ovalbumin blocking improves the sensitivity and specificity of IgM-immunoblotting in serodiagnosis of patients with Erythema migrans. 1992, J Clin Microbiol 30, 229-232.

9. Pachner A R. Neurologic manifestations of Lyme disease, the new "great imitator". 1989, Rev Infect Dis, Suppl 6, 1482-1486

10. Schneider T, Lange R, Weigelt W, Kölmel H W. Prognostic B-cell epitopes on the flagellar protein of B. burgdorferi. 1991, Infect Immun 60, 316-319.

11. Wallich R, Moter SG, Simon MM, Ebnet K, Heneberger A, Kramer MD. A Borrelia burgdorferi flagellum - associated 41-kilodalton antigen (flagellin): Molecular cloning, expression, and amplification of the gene. 1990, Infect Immun 58, 1713-1719.

Screnning for CMV Infection Following Bone Marrow Transplantation Using the PCR Technique

H Einsele, M Steidle, M Müller, G Ehninger, J G Saal, C A Müller

Human cytomegalovirus (HCMV) infection is a common complication in immunocompromised patients, particularly after bone marrow transplantation (BMT) (Myers 1984). Fast and sensitive techniques for virus detection are required to allow rapid diagnosis and consequent therapy for the frequent and often symptomatic HCMV infections in these patients. Furthermore, follow-up detection of the virus in bodily excretions, in blood and in the effected organs of the patient could aid in monitoring the efficacy of the different and still largely experimental treatment protocols (Smith 1989). Recent publications have claimed higher sensitivity of hybridization techniques when compared to virus culture for HCMV detection in clinical specimens (Spector 1984, Myerson 1984, Schrier 1985, Saltzman 1988). Furthermore, HCMV can also be readily demonstrated by immunohistological or -cytological techniques (Musiani 1985).

Improvement in virus detection was achieved by the introduction of the polymerase chain reaction allowing highly specific amplification of viral DNA from infected tissues (Salimans 1989). Thus diagnosis of human immunodeficiency virus infection could be established several months before positive reactions in serological assays (Horsburgh 1989).

In this study, the polymerase chain reaction (PCR) was evaluated for its sensitivity and practical value in the diagnosis of HCMV infection after BMT compared to conventional culture tests.

Materials and Methods

1. Patients and clinical specimens

Twenty-eight recipients of an allogeneic bone marrow transplant were followed-up in tests for HCMV infection using various techniques. Only 4 of the patients studied were seronegative when tested for HCMV and received transplants from seronegative donors as well as seronegative blood products. Also 15 patients were followed up after BMT using both culture tests and PCR techniques as well as clinical and biochemical examinations to evaluate these techniques for early diagnosis of CMV disease.

2. Virus strains and control cells

The laboratory HCMV strain AD169, as well as 50 different clinical isolates of HCMV, were amplified by polymerase chain reaction. As a control for non-specific amplification of other viral DNA fragments, other herpes and non-herpes viruses were used. Non-infected human embryonic lung fibroblasts served as negative control cells.

3. Primers and preparation of DNA

For HCMV-DNA amplification, primer I, corresponding to the position between 1767 and 1786 and primer II, complementary to the sense strand between position 1894 and 1913 of the fourth exon of the immediate early gene of AD169 (Jiwa 1989, Einsele 1991), were synthesized. In addition, a 40-mer oligonucleotide homologous to the middle region of the amplified region was also synthesized and employed in slot and Southern blot analysis of PCR products.

DNA was extracted from urine and cells after proteinase K digestion using the phenol/chloroform/isoamylalcohol extraction and precipitation.

4. Polymerase chain reaction

Amplification of a 147 bp DNA fragment between positions 1767 and 1913 of the 4th exon of the immediate early gene of the HCMV strain AD169 using primer I and II has been described before. 100 ng of extracted DNA (after two cycles of phenol/chloroform/isoamylalcohol extraction and precipitation) or the total amount of DNA extracted from 10 ml urine were denatured at 94°C for 5 min and specifically amplified in 50 µl reaction mixture of 10mM Tris-HCl, pH 9.6, 10mM $MgCl_2$, 50mM NaCl, 1mM dATP, 1mM dCTP, 1mM dGTP, 1mM dTTP, 10 µg bovine serum albumin, 0,25 µg of each primer (I and II), as well as of 1 U Taq polymerase (Perkin Elmer-Cetus, Emeryville, California, USA). 32 cycles, each of which included 3 min for annealing and primer extension at 66°C followed by 1 min of denaturation at 94°C.

To minimize the risk of contamination, the PCR technique was physically separated from the DNA extraction, precipitation and DNA recombinant steps. To exclude the presence of polymerase inhibitors and to test the quality of the extracted DNA, a DNA fragment of the human HLA class I gene (4th exon, 129 bp long) was amplified in all samples in parallel.

Detection of the PCR amplification products was achieved after ethidium-bromide stain in a 2% agarose gel or by Southern blot analysis with a gamma ^{32}P-dATP-end-labelled internal oligonucleotide. After prehybridization (20 mM PBS, pH 7.0, 10x Magic Denhardt's, 7% SDS, 5xSSC, 100µg/ml BSA) for 1h at 50°C the filters were hybridized for Southern blot analysis with $5x10^6$ cpm/ml of the gamma ^{32}P-dATP-end-labelled internal oligonucleotide for 16h at 50°C. After two washing steps, each at 50°C for 1h, with 3x SSC, 10x Magic Denhardt's, 5% SDS in PBS first and then with 1xSSC, 1% SDS, the filters were air-dried. Autoradiography of the filters was recorded on an X-Omat AR^R Kodak film at -80°C.

5. Sensitivity and specificity of PCR-analysis of HCMV

After amplification 10 fg of homologous HCMV-DNA were detected by ethidium bromide staining in a 2% agarose gel. With additional hybridization with the labelled detection oligonucleotide, a detection limit of 0.1 fg of amplified homologous HCMV-DNA was achieved. No amplified DNA fragments, usually detectable on agarose gel-electrophoresis could be obtained from clinical isolates of other herpes or non-herpes viruses. Similarly, the control DNA extracted from non-infected fibroblasts gave no results when amplified.

Results

Blood and urine samples from seronegative patients transplanted from seronegative donors, who also received only seronegative blood products, were all negative by PCR and culture techniques.

Twenty out of the 24 seropositive patients analyzed after BMT developed HCMV viremia and viruria one to six weeks post-transplantation as shown by PCR

days after BMT	PCR	Culture	CMV disease
80			o
			o
		o	o
70		o	o
60			oo
		oo	-ooo-
50		oo	o
		-oo-	-oo-
40	o	o	o
	ooo	ooo	
30	ooo		
	—o—	oo	o
20	ooo		
	o	o	
10	o		
	oo		

Figure 1: Fifteen patients were screened for the onset of CMV infection using PCR and culture technique. Also daily clinical examination and screening for biochemical alterations was performed to detect CMV-associated organ dysfunction. In Figure 1 the date of CMV detection by PCR and culture technique are presented as well as the day of onset of CMV disease.

amplification. HCMV was cultured from urine in 16 of these patients and from blood in only nine of the 20 PCR positive cases.

Fifteen patients were followed-up for incidence of CMV infection and CMV disease. As shown in Figure 1 PCR allows virus detection considerably earlier than the culture technique. Only by using PCR CMV infection could be diagnosed prior to the onset of CMV disease and this in all patients analyzed.

The high specificity of the assay was highlighted by the lack of amplification of the DNA of a wide range of other viruses. Because of the sensitive nature of the method, several precautions, which included pretitration of buffer and enzymes for amplification as well as application of several different standardized negative controls and amplification of very small samples of the highly purified DNA of clinical samples, were carried out in each experiment to minimize the risk of false positive results due to minute contaminations.

In the PCR assay 83% of all seropositive patients were found to have HCMV-DNA in the blood and urine after BMT, whereas culture assays revealed 67% of these patients to be viruric and 37% to be viremic. Thus, false positive results of the PCR assay seemed to be unlikely. PCR technique affords detection of the virus considerably earlier and in all patients studied, prior to the onset of CMV disease and might thus help to reduce the still high mortality of CMV infected patients following bone marrow and organ solid transplantation.

References

1. Einsele H, Vallbracht A, Kandolf R, Jahn G, Müller CA. Hybridization techniques provide improved sensitivity for HCMV detection and allow quantitation of the virus in clinical samples. 1989, J Virol Methods 26, 91

2. Einsele H, Steidle M, Vallbracht A, Saal JG, Ehninger G, Müller CA: Early occurrence of HCMV infection after BMT as demonstrated by the PCR technique. 1991, Blood 77, 1104

3. Horsburgh CR, Ou CY, Jason J, Holmberg SD, Longini IM, Schable C, Mayer KH, Lifson AR, Schochetman G, Ward JW, Rutherford GW, Seage GR, Jaffe HW. Duration of human immunodeficiency virus infection before detection of antibody. 1989, Lancet 2, 637

4. Jiwa NM, Van Gemert GW, Raap AK, Van de Rijke FM, Mulder A, Lens PF, Salimans MMM, Zwaan FE, Van Dorp W, Van der Ploeg M. Rapid detection of human cytomegalovirus DNA in peripheral blood leukocytes of

viremic transplant recipients by the polymerase chain reaction. 1989, Transplantation 48, 72

5. Musiani M, Zerbibi M, La Placa M. Alkaline phosphatase staining for the detection of antigens induced by cytomegalovirus. 1985, J Clin Pathol 38, 1155

6. Myers JD, Flournoy N, Thomas ED. Risk factors for cytomegalovirus infection after human bone marrow transplantation. 1984, Transplantation 465, 38

7. Myerson D, Hackman RC, Nelson JA, Ward DC, McDougall JK. Widespread presence of histologically occult cytomegalovirus. 1984, Hum Pathol 15, 430

8. Salimans MMM, Holsappel S, Van de Rijke FM, Jiwa NM, Raap AK, Weiland HT. Rapid detection of human parvovirus B19 DNA by dot-blot hybridization and the polymerase chain reaction. 1989, J Virol Methods 23, 19

9. Saltzman RL, Quirk MR, Jordan MC. Disseminated cytomegalovirus infection. Molecular analysis of virus and leukocyte interactions in viremia. 1988, J Clin Invest 81, 75

10. Schrier RD, Nelson JA, Oldstone MBA. Detection of human cytomegalovirus in peripheral blood lymphocytes in a natural infection. 1985, Science 230, 1048

11. Smith CB. Cytomegalovirus pneumonia. 1989, Chest 95, 1182

12. Spector SA, Rus JA, Spector DH, McMillan R. Detection of human cytomegalovirus in clinical specimens by DNA-DNA hybridization. 1984, J Infect Dis 50, 121

Detection of Spumaviral Sequences by Polymerase Chain Reaction

W Muranyi, R M Flügel

A human spumaretrovirus (HSRV) was isolated from the lymphoblastoid cells of a nasopharyngeal carcinoma patient by Achong et al. (1971). This virus isolate was characterized by nucleotide sequencing, transcription mapping, and molecular biological studies (Flügel 1991). These studies revealed that the HSRV genome encodes the *gag, pol,* and *env* genes typical for all known retroviruses (Cullen 1991) and, in addition, the *bel* genes (Fig. 1). This genomic arrangement indicates that spumaviruses belong to the complex retroviruses (Cullen 1991). The *bel 1* gene was characterized as a transcriptional trans-activator that activates the HSRV long terminal repeat (LTR) region, and to a lesser extent also that of the HIV-1 LTR (Keller 1991). Characterization of the HSRV splicing pattern revealed that part of the *bel 1* gene is combined via splicing with the *bel 2* gene resulting in yet another HSRV gene product, termed Bet, a protein of 56 kD (Muranyi 1991). Besides the *bel 1* and *bel 2* proteins, Bet was indeed identified in HSRV-infected cells by indirect immunofluorescence and protein blotting as an abundantly expressed viral antigen (Löchelt 1991).

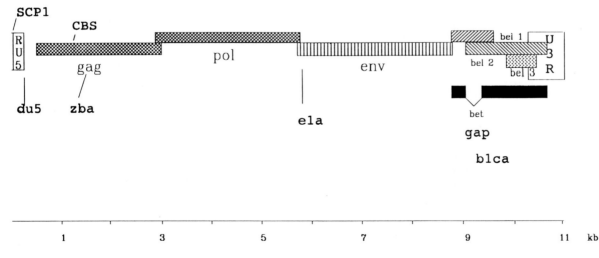

Figure 1. The Structure of the Human Spumavirus Genome. Differently shaded boxes indicate the identified gene products. Sense primers above the boxes are given in capital letters, antisense primers are below the boxes in small letters. For the precise genomic locations of the various primers used, refer to (5).

Spumaviruses were isolated from many different species, most frequently from monkeys and apes. Previous seroepidemiological studies showed the presence of spumavirus antibodies in sera from nasopharyngeal carcinoma patients and in control sera from Kenya (Loh 1980, Mahnke 1991) and in inhabitants of Pacific Islands. To date, spumaviruses also called foamy viruses, have not been unambiguously associated with a defined human disease, and have been described "as viruses in search of a disease" (Weiss 1988).

In an effort to approach this problem, HSRV sequence-specific test sytems are currently being developed in our laboratory by employing defined molecular HSRV clones and expression of recombinant viral proteins. The central part of the HSRV *env* gene was used for the synthesis of a recombinant viral *env* antigen (Mahnke 1990). This *envpx* antigen was used for the development of an HSRV-specific ELISA system. The *env*-specific ELISA detects HSRV antibodies in human sera and has been employed as a first screening test to study the prevalence of HSRV infections in patients. The results of the *env*-specific ELISA clearly show that HSRV infections occurred in individuals with various diseases (Mahnke 1991).

Spumaviruses are complex retroviruses of approximately 12 to 13 kbp in size, since the *bel* genes of spumaviruses contribute substantially to the greater genome size when compared to other retrovirus groups (Flügel 1991). The *bel* genes are characteristic and distinguishing features of the spumaviruses when compared to the other two groups of complex retroviruses. The lentiviruses and the HTLV/BLV group also encode a number of additional and regulatory genes besides the common genes *gag, pol,* and *env* of the simple retroviruses. The *bel* genes, however, are clearly different from the lentiviral accessory genes, although there is a functional equivalence between the transactivators *bel 1* and HIV-1 *tat* (Keller 1991).

Spumaviruses share with other known retroviruses the ability to reverse transcribe a single-stranded RNA genome into a double-stranded DNA. The double-stranded DNA can exist in several forms in retrovirus-infected cells: it is integrated into the host cell genome as provirus and it can occur in an unintegrated form (linear or circular).

HSRV is considered to be the prototype spumavirus since it has been characterized more extensively by nucleotide sequencing and transcriptional mapping (Flügel 1987, Maurer 1988, Muranyi 1991). The results of phylogenetic analyses by several groups unambiguously showed that spumaviruses are clearly distinct from all known retroviruses and distantly related to the complex groups of retroviruses (Maurer 1988, Lewe 1989, Xiong 1988, Doolittle 1989, Myers 1991). The analysis of the splicing pattern revealed that the HSRV genomic RNA is characteristically spliced into a unique arrangement of exons when compared to the transcriptional patterns of the more related lentiviruses, in particular to that of HIV-1 (Schwartz 1990, Muranyi 1991). This finding opens the way for designing and performing diagnostic PCRs that are gene-specific for human spumavirus sequences. Thus, the known HSRV nucleotide sequence can be exploited for the PCR detection of foamy virus RNA and DNA in human tissues.

Procedures

1. Reverse transcription of viral RNA

HSRV cDNA was synthesized with Moloney murine leukemia virus reverse transcriptase for 1 hour at 37°C or with avian myeloblastosis virus reverse transcriptase for 60 min at 42°C from 5 mg total RNA from HSRV-infected cells using the specifications given by the manufacturer (Gibco, Karlsruhe and Boehringer, Mannheim). Reverse transcriptions were started by adding an antisense oligodeoxynucleotide (150 pmol, 20-mer) derived from the 3' region of the HSRV genome and random hexa- oligodeoxynucleotides (0.5 mg/reaction, Pharmacia, Freiburg) according to Kinoshta et al. (1989). Alternatively, reverse transcriptions were started with random hexanucleotide primers only and the sense and antisense primers were added before the

PCR to avoid amplification of false priming events. Concentrations of dNTPs were at 2.5 mM in a reaction volume of 10 µl. The reaction products were denatured at 94°C for five min.

2. Amplification of cDNAs by PCR, gel and blot detection

Viral cDNAs were added to a solution that contained in 90 µl 0.25 mM of the four dNTPs, 150 pmol of a sense primer, and 10x Taq buffer. Primers SCP 1 + DU5 (Table 1) or, alternatively, the gag primers CBS + ZBA, at 50 pmol were used. Primer pairs were chosen by restricting the size of PCR products to about from 150 - 500 bp. In exceptional cases, primer pairs with larger distances of up to 1500 bp between the genetic locations were used. The PCR was started by adding 2.5 units of Taq DNA polymerase (Cetus Perkin-Elmer or Stratagene). Paraffin oil, 50 µl (Merck) was layered on top of the reaction mixture. The reaction mixture was incubated at 94°C, 55°C, and 72°C for one min, two min, and three min. The cycle was repeated 35 times in a DNA thermal cycler (Perkin-Elmer, Cetus). Total RNA from uninfected HEL cells were run as controls under the same conditions, but did not result in any HSRV-specific DNA bands. PCR products were analyzed on agarose gels by visualizing with ethidium bromide or alternatively, by hybridizing with an oligodeoxynucleotide located in both exons. The sequence of the oligonucleotide was derived from a location between the two primers used (inside primers). PCR-amplified DNA bands in the range of 150 to about 1000 bp were isolated by electrophoresing onto DEAE membranes type NA45 (Schleicher & Schüll), purified and cloned into the polylinker site of the Bluescript vector (Davis 1986). Larger and distinct DNA fragments were directly isolated from agarose gels and cloned. Some viral DNAs were pre-checked by restriction enzyme analysis. Nucleotide sequencing was performed with the Maxam and Gilbert method or the dideoxy-mediated chain termination method.

Name of Primer	Sequences of Primer Pairs (5' ---- 3')	Genomic Localisation[a]	Gene Assignment	Size of PCR products in bp
SCP 1	GCTCTTCACTACTCGCTGCGT	3 - 23	LTR (R)	268 (RU5)
DU 5	CACTAGATCTCTCCCTTAGCA[b]	251 - 271	LTR (U5)	
CBS	CTCTATACCTGGGATTCATCC	1066 - 1086	gag	332 (CA)
ZBA	GGAGGCTCTCCAGTTACAGAT	1378 - 1398	gag	
SCP 1	GCTCTTCACTACTCGCTGCGT	3 - 23	LTR (R)	572, 501, 264
E1A	CCAGGCCAATACTCTTGAGCT	5906 - 5929	env	
SCP 1	GCTCTTCACTACTCGCTGCGT	3 - 23	LTR (R)	711, 640, 440
GAP	CAGTCAGGGTCAGTATCTGATTG	9015 - 9038	bel 1	
SCP 1	GCTCTTCACTACTCGCTGCGT	3 - 23	LTR (R)	810, 434
B1CA	ATCGATGGATCGTCTCCTGG	9312 - 9331	bet	
SCP 1	GCTCTTCACTACTCGCTGCGT	3 - 23	LTR (R)	207, 162
B1CA	ATCGATGGATCGTCTCCTGG	9312 - 9331	bel 2	

[a] In nucleotide positions of the HSRV genome (6)
[b] Antisense primer is given as used for PCR

Table 1: Characteristic features of spumaretroviral primer pair sequences

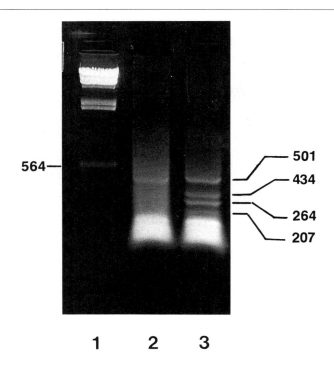

Figure 2. PCR products of HSRV transcripts obtained after reverse transcription and DNA amplification followed by agarose gel electrophoresis. Total RNA (5 mg) from virus-infected cells were reverse transcribed with primers E1A and B2A (which lies about 100 nucleotides upstream of B1CA) in the absence (lane 2) and presence (lane 3) of random hexamers. Viral cDNAs were subjected to 35 cycles of PCR amplification with Taq DNA polymerase in the presence of primer SCP 1 (Table 1). Lane 1 was loaded with lambda HindIII DNA digest as marker. The numbers at the right margin indicate the size of spliced HSRV RNAs that were subseqently amplified into cDNA fragments and sequenced (in base pairs): 501, env mRNA species with a 5' extension; 434, bet mRNA species 1; 264, env mRNA species 3; 207, bel 2 mRNA.

3. Direct detection of spumaviral DNA by PCR

Total DNA (0.1 to 1.0 μg) extracted from patients' biopsies or virus-infected cells was used in a reaction volume of 50 or 100 μl of PCR reaction buffer as given by the manufacturer (Stratagene), dNTPs were added at 250 μM each plus 2.5 units of *Taq* DNA polymerase. Primers (as described above) at 50 pmol were used and overlaid with paraffin oil. The amplification was performed in 40 cycles of 1 min at 92°, 1 min at 50° to 55°, and 2 min at 72°C. PCR products were analyzed as described above.

Results and Discussion

1. General considerations and parameters for HSRV detection by PCR

The specific PCR technique used for the detection of proviral sequences is dependant on the source of the cells or biopsies. The salient point is that if a naturally occurring virus that has never been passaged in in vitro cell cultures is to be detected, it cannot be expected that the sequence of a field virus is identical to that of the known prototype genome. Accordingly, degenerate PCR primer pairs should be designed and used by taking the afore listed parameters into account. In addition to field isolates, this is also valid for variant and defective viruses. Degenerate primers should be invariant at the termini, but can vary in the central part of their sequences (Frohman 1990).

2. Defined primer pairs for the detection of spumaviral sequences by PCR

The genetic structure of the HSRV DNA genome is shown in Figure 1. In general, genomic regions that are required for viral replication and transcription are suitable for PCR amplification. Some examples of sequences of spumaviral primer pairs that were used for PCR amplification of HSRV transcripts from virus-infected human cells are listed in Table 1.

Sense primers that are located at or just downstream of the start site of viral transcription are the more desirable sense primers, since they can be used for the detection of viral DNA, genomic RNA, and subgenomic transcripts. Thus, the SCP 1 sense oligonucleotide is the most frequently used primer (Table 1). The antisense primer should be selected by taking the expected value of the PCR product into account. Product sizes of 150 to 500 bp are optimal and relatively easy to detect on agarose gels. The design of primer pairs that result in PCR products that exceed 900 bp is more difficult, since more sophisticated methods are required for the synthesis and detection of large viral genomic sequences.

The lengths of the primers that were used varied between 18 and 23 bp. The actual lenghts are not of primary importance; however, to adjust the molar (G + C)% contents of a given primer to approximately 55, primers of various lengths can be selected to approach that value (Frohman 1990).

Figure 2 illustrates PCR amplification and the detection of rare and more abundant spumaretroviral transcripts in one set of experiments. The numbers mark four simultaneously detected HSRV cDNA bands. All bands were molecularly cloned and characterized by nucleotide sequencing. It is noteworthy that the sizes are in agreement with the calculated values given in Table 1. The result proved that the DNAs represent *bel 1*-specific mRNAs of different lenghts which is due to the presence of extra small exons derived from the central part of the HSRV genome. This experiment illustrates the advantage of using hexa-random primers that reduces the background level of unspecific PCR DNAs (Fig. 2). The results of the studies revealed novel gene products for both viruses that were subsequently shown to exist (Schwartz 1990, Löchelt 1991). It is also of great phylogenetic interest that several non-coding exons were detected in the central domain of both virus genomes some of which occur in the *pol* gene (Flügel 1991).

In general, PCR primers should be taken from genes that are absolutely required for viral replication, e.g. the *bel 1* gene. Alternatively, genes like HIV-1 *nef* that are necessary for in vivo pathogenesis are also suitable for PCR diagnostics (Kestler 1991).

The methods described above were particularly useful for the detection of HSRV DNA and RNA in virus-infected human cells. Doubtless, improved PCR techniques shaped according to the purpose and to a particular problem will be of great value for identifying spumaviral sequences in patients' biopsies and peripheral blood monocyte lymphocytes.

References

1. Achong G, Mansell PWA, Epstein MA, Clifford P. 1971, J Natl Cancer Inst 42, 299-307

2. Cullen B. Human immunodeficiency virus as a prototype complex retrovirus. 1991, J Virol 65, 1053-1056

3. Davis LG, Dibner MD, Battey JF. Basic methods in molecular biology, 1986, Elsevier, New York, p79-152

4. Doolittle RF, Feng D-F, Johnson MS, McClure MA. Origins and evolutionary relationships of retroviruses. 1989, Quart Rev Biol 64, 1-30

5. Flügel RM, Rethwilm A, Maurer B, Darai G. Nucleotide sequence analysis of the *env* gene and its flanking regions of the human spumaretrovirus reveals two novel genes. 1987, EMBO J 6, 2077-2084

6. Flügel RM. Spumaviruses: a Group of Complex Retroviruses. 1991, J Acquir Immunodef Syndr 4, 739-750

7. Frohman MA. Race: rapid amplification of cDNAs ends. In: Innis MA, Gelfand DH, Sninsky JJ, White TJ (Eds) PCR protocols, a guide to methods aand applications. 1990, Academic Press, San Diego, p 28-53

8. Keller A, Partin KM, Löchelt M, Bannert H, Flügel RM, Cullen BR. Characterization of the transcriptional trans-activator of human foamy retrovirus. 1991, J Virol 65, 2589-2594

9. Kestler HW, Ringler DJ, Mori K, Panicalli DL, Sehgal P, Daniel MD, Desrosiers RC. Importance of the *nef* gene for maintenance of high virus loads and for development of AIDS. 1991, Cell 65, 651-662

10. Kinoshita T, Shimoyana M, Tobinai K, Ito M, Ito S-I, Ikeda S, Tajima K, Shimotono K, Sugimura T. Detection of mRNA for the *tax/rex* gene of human T-cell leukemia virus type 1 in fresh peripheral blood mononuclear cells of adult T-cell leukemia patients and viral carriers by using polymerase chain reactions. 1989, Proc Natl Acad Sci USA 86, 5620-5624

11. Lewe G, Flügel RM. Tracing genetic events in the evolutionary pathway of retroviruses: comparative analysis of the *pol* and *env* protein sequences. 1989, Virus Genes 2, 195-204

12. Löchelt M, Zentgraf H, Flügel RM. Construction of an infectious of the full-length human spumaretrovirus genome and mutagenesis of the bel 1 gene. 1991, Virology 184, 43-54

13. Loh PC, Matsuura F, Mizumoto C. Seroepidemiology of human syncytial virus: antibody prevalence in the Pacific. 1980, Intervirol 13, 87-90

14. Mahnke C, Kashaiya P, Rössler J, Bannert H, Levin A, Blattner WA, Dietrich M, Luande J, Löchelt M, Friedman-Kien, AE, Komaroff AL, Loh PC, Westarp ME, and Flügel RM. Human Spumavirus Antibodies in Sera from African Patients. 1991, Arch Virol, in press.

15. Mahnke C, Löchelt M, Bannert H, Flügel RM. Specific enzyme-linked immunosorbent assay for the detection of antibodies to the human spumaretrovirus. 1990, J Virol Meth 29, 13-22

16. Maurer B, Bannert H, Darai G, Flügel RM. Analysis of the primary structure of the long terminal repeat and the gag and pol genes of the human spumaretroviruses. 1988, J Virol 62, 1590-1597

17. Maurer B, Flügel RM. Genomic organization of the human spumaretrovirus and its relatedness to AIDS- and other retroviruses. 1988, AIDS Res Hum Retrovir 4, 467-473

18. Muranyi W, Flügel RM. Analysis of splicing patterns by polymerase chain reaction of the human spumaretrovirus reveals complex RNA structures. 1991, J Virol 65, 727-735

19. Myers G, Pavlakis GN. Evolutionary potential of complex retroviruses. In: Wagner RR, Frenkel-Conrat H (Eds) Viruses. Levy J (ed) The retroviridae, 1991, Plenum Press, New York, vol 1, p1-37

20. Schwartz S, Felber B, Benko DM, Fenyö E-M, Pavlakis G. Cloning and functional analysis of multiply sspliced mRNA species of human immunodeficiency virus type 1. 1990, J Virol 64, 2519-2529 16.

21. Weiss RA. A virus in search of a disease. 1988, Nature 333, 497-498

22. Xiong Y, Eickbush TH. Origin and evolution of retroelements based upon their reverse transcriptase sequences. 1988, EMBO J 10, 3353-3362

Acknowledgments

We thank Harald zur Hausen for his support. This research project was financed by a grant TS*CT87-0186-D from the Commission of the European Community.

The Use of PCR for Epidemiological Studies of HNANB Viruses in Arthropod Vectors

R Seelig, C F Weisser, H W Zentraf, Cl Bottner, H P Seelig, M Renz

Parenteral transmission of hepatitis C is well documented but in the majority of patients the routes of transmission of hepatitis C virus as well as those of additional infectious agents implicated in hepatitis non-A, non-B (HNANB) remain an enigma. For one of these agents which causes possibly HNANB we proposed the name hepatitis F virus (HFV). This agent first isolated from density gradient fractions (1.3 g CsCl/ml) of stool filtrates (Seelig 1988) represents a virus like particle of 26.7 ± 1 nm in diameter (Fig. 1) which contains a circular double stranded DNA of 5001 base pairs (Fig. 1, insert) with four open reading frames (Fig. 2). The implication of the HFV-DNA presumably representing the genome of a DNA virus in the pathogenesis of HNANB is supported by extended clinical studies (Liehr 1984). HFV-DNA was detected in blood as well as in liver specimens and stool filtrates of patients with hepatitis non-A, non-B in some of which hepatitis C and E could be excluded also. Clinical studies showed further a seasonal accumulation of hepatitis non-A, non-B in

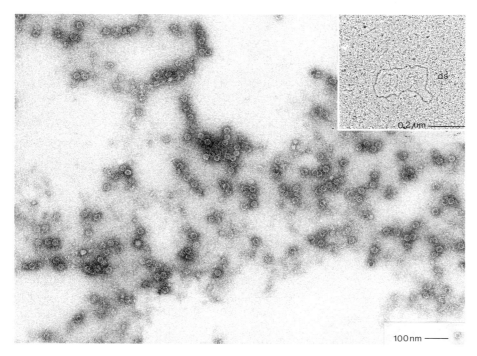

Figure 1: EM picture of HFV particles; the insert shows the DNA of such particles.

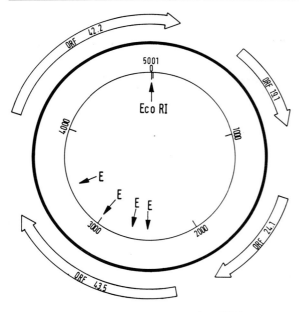

Figure 2: Schematic representation of the HFV genome.

performed some years ago in our laboratory. Epidemics of viral hepatitis occurring at distinct time periods during a year were usually caused by enterically transmitted non-A, non-B hepatitis agents (e.g. HAV) and as recently shown by HEV. Seasonal clustering of nosocomial and posttransfusion non-A, non-B hepatitis, however, was rarely observed or escaped the attention of investigators. A few reports, however, from Japan (Ohori 1983, Dr. Kurahori, Ashiya-City, personal communication), Australia (Cossart 1982) and Western Germany (Liehr 1984) drew the attention to seasonal accumulation of posttransfusion hepatitis non-A, non-B. These observations would indicate a higher infectious contingent of blood units received in these times from donors infected by non-parenteral routes.

By means of PCR performed with primers specific for different coding regions of the genome HFV-DNA was detected in sera, stool and liver specimens, respectively, of patients with hepatitis non-A, non-B, non-C (Seelig 1991).

According to the monthly number of clinically diagnosed HNANB two peaks seem to occur within the year, one beginning in the early summer, the other during autumn (Fig. 3). This fact as well as our impression that patients summer and late autumn, observations which correspond to the seasonal frequency of positive tests for this agent

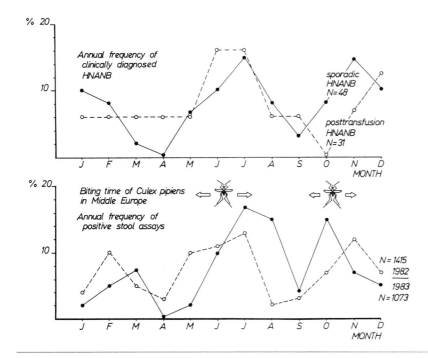

Figure 3: Frequency of clinically diagnosed HNANB (4) in 1984 and frequency of positive assays for the supposed implicated infectious agent in faeces. Concordant peaks of positive stool assays and diagnosed cases corresponding to biting time of Culex p. pipiens.

harbouring sequences of the above mentioned DNA often came from areas generally known as mosquito shelter led us to search in arthropodes as possible vectors for HFV and HCV.

Material and Methods

1. Samples and DNA preparation

Eggs and larvae of mosquitos as well as adult insects (Culex p. pipiens, Aedes vexans, Anopheles maculipennis) were collected from several areas in the upper Rhine valley. Eggs of Aedes ägypti were obtained from a laboratory strain (kind gift of Dr. Ludwig, Heidelberg). Northamerican ticks (Ixodes dammini) were kindly provided by Dr. Calisher (Center of Infectious Diseases, Fort Collins, Colorado, USA). Ixodes ricinus and Rhipicephalus sanguineus were likewise collected in the upper Rhine valley. Each collection of eggs and larvae (in 1 - 2 l water) was subdivided into 50 ml aliquots, centrifuged and washed several times with TE buffer. Nucleic acids were isolated by sonication in the presence of glass beads and RNAsin followed by digestion with proteinase K and organic solvent extraction. Precipitated nucleic acids were redissolved in 500 µl TE buffer, the nucleic acid concentration was about 0.7 µg DNA/µl. Adult Culex p. pipiens were subdivided in four batches of about 25 to 50 insects. DNA and RNA isolation was performed as described above.

2. PCR procedure

The RT-PCR for detection of HCV-RNA was performed with nested primers corresponding to the 5' non-coding region and the NS4 region of the HCV genome (nucleotid positions 34-281 and 5471-5633, respectively (Takamizawa 1991)). The PCR for demonstration of hepatitis F virus DNA was performed with primers derived from different regions of the circular genom encompassing parts of the two open reading frames which code for a 43.5 and 42.2 kD protein, respectively, as well as an intergenic segment. For amplification of the region encoding the 43.5 kD protein primers 5'-TCTCCCTGACGGCTGGGAAGATATGCA-3' (nt 3143-3169) and 5'-GAGGAAAAGCAGCTCAG-GACGATAAAG-3' (nt 3359-3333) were used for the first round (35 cycles with 1 min. at 95°C, 2 min. at 60°C and 2 min. at 72°C) followed by a second round with a nested primer pair:

5'-GGCTGGGAAGATATGCAGTTCGTTACTG-3' (nt 3153-3180) and 5'-CAGCTCAGGACGA-TAAAGCAAAATATCAATG-3' (nt 3350-3320) (30 cycles with 1 min. at 93°C, 2 min. at 62°C and 1.5 min. at 72°C). Similarly, the 42.5 kD protein encoding region was first amplified with primers 5'-CCTGTT-TATTCTGCTTCTGC-3' (nt 4805-4824) and 5'-GCAAATCCTCCGGAGAATCG-3' (nt 4929-4909) for 30 cycles at 95°C for 1 min., 55°C for 1.5 min. and 72°C for 1.5 min. and later with primers 5'-TATTCTGCTTCTGCCTTTGAT-3' (nt 4811-4831) and 5'-CTCCGGAGAATCGGACAGCCA-3' (nt 4921-4901) (33 cycles, 1 min. at 95°C; 1 min. at 52°C; 1 min. at 72°). The region between the genes for the 42.2 kD and 19.1 kD protein was amplified with primers 5'-GATTGGTTGCCATGGTAGAC-3' (nt 271-290) and 5'-TATCACCTCCATCCCAAAGG-3' (nt 444-425) (35 cycles; 1 min. at 95°C; 1 min. at 53°C and 1 min. at 72°C). Amplification products were analyzed by agarose gel electrophoresis and Southern blots probed with ^{32}P-labelled internal oligonucleotides. For DNA sequencing PCR products were excised from agarose gels, blunt-ended and ligated into a plasmid vector for propagation. From each transformation at least two colonies were sequenced. Some sequence data were aquired directly from PCR generated products.

Results

HCV-RNA could not be amplified from the various nucleic acid preparations of mosquitos and ticks. As shown in Tab. 1 and 2 HFV-DNA was detected in larvae as well as in eggs and adult Culex p. pipiens but neither in the larval stages of Aedes vexans and Anopheles maculipennis which were collected at the same time in the same areas nor in the eggs of Aedes ägypti or in the ticks (Ixodes dammini, Ixodes ricinus, Rhipicephalus).

The DNA was found in all developmental stages of a local population of Culex p. pipiens originating from one of the three different collecting areas (Tab. 2), it was not found in the Culex p. pipiens larvae of the two other sampling places. As far as eggs and larvae are concerned in five of the six batches DNA could be amplified. In the case of adult insects one of the four batches containing about 25 to 50 mosquitos was found positive. Of the DNA isolated from larvae three different genomic regions were amplified, of the DNA isolated from eggs two regions, from that of adult Culex p. pipiens one region. Two of the three DNA regions amplified from

Table 1: Arthropodes screened for the presence of HCV-RNA and HFV-DNA by PCR

		HFV-DNA	HCV-RNA
Mosquitos			
Culex p. pipiens	Eggs, larvae, adult animals	positive	negative
Aedes vexans	Larvae	negative	negative
Anopheles maculipennis	Larvae	negative	negative
Ticks			
Ixodes dammini	adult animals	negative	negative
Ixodes ricinus	adult animals	negative	negative
Rhipicephalus sanguineus	adult animals	negative	negative
Aedes ägypti	eggs	negative	negative

Table 2: Culex p. pipiens from different areas of the upper Rhine valley were investigated for HFV-DNA. DNA positive Culex p. pipiens larvae and eggs of two generations were found in one area. Adult insects were collected from farmhouses nearby.

Culex p. pipiens	Area I	Area II	Area III
Larvae I. collection	positive	negative	negative
Larvae II. collection	positive	not done	not done
Eggs	positive	not done	not done
Adult mosquitos	positive	not done	not done

Table 3: Sequence similarities on two open reading frames (ORF) between wild type HFV-DNA and DNA amplified from Culex p. pipiens larvae.

ORF	Position of amplified region (nt)	Similarity (%)
43.5 kD	3153 - 3350	81.0 (larvae) 99.0 (eggs)
42.2 kD	4811 - 4921	97.3

Culex p. pipiens larvae have been sequenced. As shown in Tab. 3 there exists a high degree of homology (81 and 97 %, respectively) with the wild-type DNA (EMBL, data base library X53411). The sequence data of eggs and adult mosquitos showed nearly complete homology with the wild-type.

Although HCV seems to be the major causative agent of hepatitis non-A, non-B more than 30 % of sporadic and parenteral transmitted HNANB infection remain unexplained so that further viruses must be implicated in the pathogenesis of hepatitis non-A, non-B, non-C. The seasonal fluctuation fits well with the biting behaviour of the northern house mosquito Culex p. pipiens which mainly attack their victims in summer and again in late autumn before overwintering in houses.

The genus Culex includes species worldwide known as vectors for several arbo viruses and for avian malaria. Our findings, for the first time described here, would indicate a vertical transmission of a DNA virus in this species. The sequence heterogeneity found in different isolates of Culex p. pipiens might be indicative for the existence of different subtypes of HFV found in an inhomogenous population of Culex p. pipiens.

Because an inhomogenous population have to be considered in countrysite collections, laboratory culture strains should be investigated. These preliminary results call for further extensive epidemiological studies with mosquitos from different regions.

References

1. Cossart Y E, Kirsch S, Ismay S L. Post-transfusion hepatitis in Australia. Report of the Australian Red Cross Study. 1982, Lancet I, 208-213

2. Liehr H, Seelig R, Seelig H P. Hepatitis Non-A, Non-B. Retro- und prospektive Untersuchungen zur Epidemiologie der akuten Erkrankung. 1984, Z Gastroenterol 22, 129-138

3. Ohori H, Nagatsuka Y, Kanno A, Abe Y, Ishida N. Two distinct types of Non-A, Non-B hepatitis in a cardiovascular surgical unit. 1983, J Med Virol 11, 105-113

4. Seelig R, Liehr H, Wildhirt E, Ringelmann R, Hilfenhaus M, Reisert P M, Reitinger J, Burckhardt J, Seelig H P. Hepatitis Non-A, Non-B-assoziierte Substanz im Stuhl bei Patienten mit posttransfusioneller und sporadischer Hepatitis. 1988, Immun.Infekt 16, 85-90

5. Seelig H P, Seelig R, Ehrfeld H, Bottner C, Seelig H P, Renz M. Detection of virus DNA by PCR in Hepatitis Non-A, Non-B. In: Rolfs A, Schumacher HC, Marx P (Eds.). PCR Topics. Usage of Polymerase Chain Reaction in Genetic and Infectious Diseases, 1991, Springer-Verlag, 186-191

6. Takamizawa A, Mori C, Fuke I, Manabe S, Murakami S, Fujita J, Onishi E, Andoh T, Yoshida I, Okayama H. Structure and organization of the hepatitis C virus genome isolated from human carriers. 1991, J Virol 65, 1105-1113

C) Basic methodology and research applications

In vitro Amplification and Digoxigenin Labeling of Single-Stranded and Double-Stranded DNA Probes for Diagnostic in situ Hybridization

U Finckh, P A Lingenfelter, K W Henne, Ch A Schmidt, W Siegert, D Myerson

Non-isotopic DNA-DNA *In situ* Hybridization (ISH) is of increasing value for clinical research and diagnostics (Lichter 1990), eg. virus detection or cytogenetics. With ISH specific hybridization signals can be assigned to single cells in tissue or cell spreads. To avoid the use of bacterial cultures with plasmids, insert preparations, and conventional labeling protocols, we succesfully used the PCR technology, to amplify and to label single-stranded (ss) and double-stranded (ds) DNA probes (Finckh 1991). We performed a two-stage prodedure: In a primary PCR (No 1) a sufficient amount of unlabeled template DNA was produced for a secondary PCR (No 2). PCR No 2 was achieved with the modified nucleotide digoxigenin-11-dUTP (DIG) as label, and with a pair of primers to produce dsDNA probes, and with only one primer to produce ssDNA probes.
It was possible to replace up to 100% TTP with DIG during synthesis. The DIG labeled probes are of unexpectedly sensitivity *in situ* with a colorimetric assay for bright field microscopy.
Synthesis of DIG probes and their application *in situ* will be presented and discussed for the two examples human cytomegalovirus (HCMV) and human Y chromosome (Y body).

As template DNA samples for PCR No 1 we used alternatively
- PCR products (1-50ng)
- 1pg insert DNA form pGEM3 containing the EcoRI/BamHI fragment from EcoRI J of HCMV (IE-1) for HCMV PCR,
- human male genomic DNA or buffy coat leucocytes after alkaline lysis (Jiwa 1989) for Y chromsome PCR.

A complete consumption of nucleotides (dNTP) and primers in PCR No 1 is preferable, to prevent carry over of substrates and non-specific by-products into PCR No 2. With a 0,1 µM concentration of primers (10pmol/100µl), 20 µM dNTP and 55 cycles we received 500 - >1000 ng of specific PCR product that was consistently reamplifiable without prior purification.
In the experiments presented here efficiency of reamplification is increased through the addition of 200ng/100µl salmon sperm DNA (carrier DNA).
For reamplification and labeling (PCR No 2) generally 35% of TTP was replaced with DIG for probe synthesis in PCR No 2. This corresponds to the ratio recommended and distributed by the manufacturer(Biochemica Boehringer Applications Manual). Because of the lower PCR amplification efficiency in the presence of DIG, up to 50 ng product from PCR No 1 was used as a starting template DNA. With the presence of only one primer (instead of a pair of primers) and addition of label to the reaction mixture, synthesis of ssDNA probes is forced. The complementary strand from the initial dsDNA template contains no label. Only in those cases of carry over of primers with original 3'ends from PCR No 1 can some labeled complementary strands be synthesized.
In our examples all parameters, except the partial replacement of TTP with DIG, were identical in PCR Nos 1 and 2. Under nondenaturing conditions in agarose gel electrophoresis, running of ssDNA is influenced by its secondary structure and/or ssDNA tails. Thus the band of interest often does not correspond to the strand

length. Also stainig with ethidium bromide is often insufficient to detect ssDNA in agarose gel. After synthesis of two complementary ssDNA strands in separate tubes and mixing and heating of an aliquot of the two, the known dsDNA is yielded after cooling down the mixture. By analyzing this dsDNA in an agarose gel electrophoresis the amount of the initially produced ssDNA can be estimated indirectly and its specificity assessed. Labeled ssDNA and dsDNA probes are blot transferred from agarose gel directly to a nylon membrane and then cross-linked by UV-radiation. Immunological detection is performed with alkaline phosphatase labeled antidigoxigenin Fab fragment, the chromogen BCIP and NBT according to the manufacturer's instructions.

Specificity Position/Length	Primer	Sequence (5' -> 3')	Ref.
HCMV IE-1 exon 4 2178-2370/198bp	CMV2173 CMV2370c	CTGTCGGGTGCTGTGCTGCTATGTCTTAGA ATGGCCCGTAGGTCATCCACACTAGGAGAG	I) II)
Y chromosome q 3511-100/154bp*	Y 1.1 Y 1.2	TCCACTTTATTCCAGGCCTGTCC TTGAATGGAATGGGAACGAATGG	III) IV) V)

I) Finckh (1991), II) Akrigg (1985), III) Nakahori (1986), IV) Kogan (1987), V) Handyside (1989)
*: The 154bp fragment overspanns the EcoRI site between the Y 3.4 repeat units of Y q.

Table 1: Primers used in PCR No 1 and No 2

Methods

PCR No 1 reaction components
$MgCl_2$	1,5 mM
KCl	50 mM
TrisCl pH 8,3 (RT)	10 mM
Gelatine	0,01 %
carrier DNA	200 ng
Primer No 1	0,1 µM
Primer No 2	0,1 µM
dNTP	20 µM
Taq DNA Polymerase	2 U
mineral oil	80 µl

Template DNA: - 60ng human male genomic DNA for Y chromosome PCR
- 1 pg insert DNA from pGEM3 (EcoRI J of HCMV) for HCMV PCR.
- approx. 1 - 50 ng product from previous PCR.

Reaction volume: 100 µl.

Thermocycle program for PCR No 1 and 2
DNA Thermal Cycler (Perkin-Elmer Cetus):
primary denaturation:	95°C, 5 min
primer annealing:	60°C, 20 sec
primer extension:	72°C, 30 sec
denaturation:	94°C, 20 sec

55 cycles
final annealing and completion: 72°, 15 min.

Agarose gel electrophoresis
For PCR No 1 product analysis 5 µl of the original PCR reaction product is loaded on an agarose gel (see chapters 2 and 10.1 - 10.3 for details).

PCR No 2 synthesis of dsDNA probes
All parameters according to PCR No 1, except:
ATP/CTP/GTP   20 µM   each (100%)
TTP   13 µM   (65%)
DIG   7 µM   (35%)
Template DNA: approx. 50 ng product from PCR No 1.
Equimolar primer ratio.

PCR No 2 synthesis of ssDNA probes
All parameters according to PCR No 1, except:
ATP/CTP/GTP   20 µM   each (100%)
TTP   13 µM   (65%)
DIG   7 µM   (35%)
Template DNA: approx. 50 ng product from PCR No 1.
Alternatively primer No 1 or primer No 2 is used.

Probe purification
0,7 ml Sephadex^R G-50 spin column in H_2O, through Whatman^R glass microfibre filter e.g. in insulin syringe,
1. spin 5 min 400g, discard H_2O
2. add approx. 100 µl PCR product, spin 5 min 400 g
3. add 100 µl H_2O, 5 min 400 g
final volume: 150-200 µl
Expected yield of probe: 100 - 500 ng/100 µl.

Assessment of probe yield and quality
Agarose gel electrophoresis, southern blot and immunological detection: for details see chapter 2 and 10.1 - 10.3).

In situ Hybridization
The ISH's for HCMV and the human Y chromosome were performed with a Histomatic^R histochemistry robot (Fisher Scientific) (Brigati 1988). Automated ISH protocols have been established for hybridization with nick translated and biotinylated plasmid DNA probes (Myerson and Henne 1992). No essential modification was necessary for the PCR synthesized DIG probes. The basic ISH principles are described in Myerson (1988). As standard probe for HCMV we used a plasmid DNA mixture containing approximately 40 kb of the HCMV genome (Enzo Diagnostics), for the human Y chromosome the plasmied pY 3.4 (DYZ1) containing a 3564 bp repeat DNA unit from Yq (Nakahori 1986).

a) Paraffin embedded and formaline fixed tissue
1. Pretreatment of the slides with 0.01% poly-D-lysine, 30 min.
2. Tissue sections are dewaxed repeatedly with Hemo-De^R (Fisher Scientific), 80°C, 40 min followed by rinsing with ethanol 100%, 95% and 2XSSC.
3. 20 min incubation with 1.7mg/ml pronase at 37°C. Rinsing with 2% glycine/25% acetone and 2XSSC.
4. Equilibration with formamide 50%, 2 min, RT and incubation with 100µl probe mixture (10-1000ng probe, 2XSSC, 50% formamide, 400µg/ml SS-DNA, 10% dextran sulfate) 95°C for 15 min.
5. Hybridization for 15 min - 4 h by 37°C.
6. Washing firstly with about 200µl 2XSSC followed by ca. 200µl 0.1XSSC/25% acetone at RT.
7. Blocking of unspecific anitbody binding with goat serum 5%, 10 min, RT.
8. Incubation with antibody-conjugate (sheep antidigoxigenin Fab - alkaline phosphatase) 1:1000, 2 h, RT.
9. Final detection with BCIP/NBT, 1mM levamisole, 2 h, 37°C, pH 9.5 (for details see chapter 10.3, method 1).

b) Interphase and metaphase cell spreads
1. Fixation of the cells with methanol/acetic acid (3:1) for several minutes and completely air drying.
2. Treatment with acetic anhydride/0.1M triethanolamine for 10 min and rinsing with 2XSSC.
3. 15 min denaturation with formamide 70%, 80°C.
4. Dehydration with consecutively increasing concentrations of ice cold ethanol 70%, 95%, 100% and completely air drying at 37°C, 10 min.
5. Addition of the denatured probe mixture (for composition see procedure a) for formaline fixed tissue).
6. Hybridization for 2 h at 37°C.
7. Washing of the slides several times with 50% formamide at 37°C, followed by 2XSSC and 1XSSC at RT. All further steps as described in a) for formaline fixed tissue.

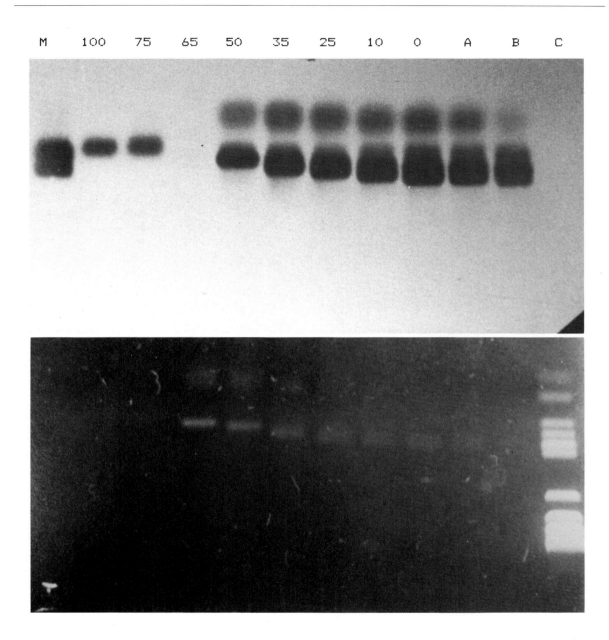

Figure 1. Incorporation of digoxigenin-11-dUTP (DIG). A decreasing percentage of TTP was replaced with DIG. The numbers indicate the % DIG fraction of the DIG/TTP mixture: 100, 75, 65, 50, 35, 25,10, 0%., (9µl/slot). Increasing retardation of the amplified DNA and the primer by-product (running faster) confirms increasing DIG incorporation. Lanes A-C: Single stranded probes, 35% DIG. Lane A: 5µl sense strand probe; lane B: 5µl antisense strand probe; lane C: 5µl sense + 5µl antisense strand probes, low salt, incomplete annealing after 1 min 95°C, slow cooling to RT (30 min), and/ or unequal strand concentrations. Blot transfer of the 1.4% agarose gel to a nylon membrane (Hybond-N^{+R}, Amersham).

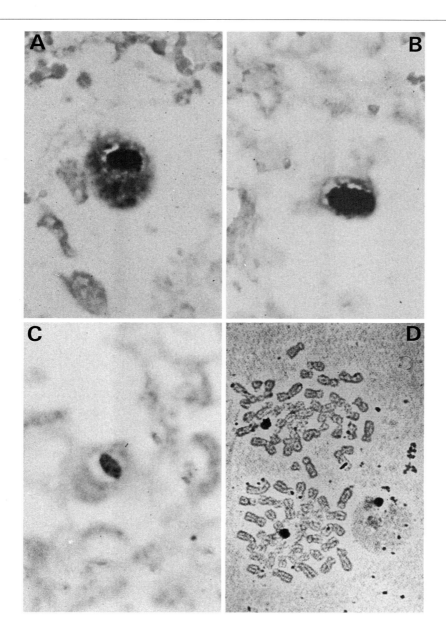

Figure 2. *In situ* hybridization with digoxigenin-11-dUTP (DIG) labeled double-stranded probes, 35% DIG, using the Histomatic[R] histochemistry robot (Fisher Scientific). A,B,C: Detection of human cytomegalovirus (HCMV) in paraffin embedded, formalin fixed lung tissue (40 X, bright field). Probe concentrations and hybridization times were in A: 10ng/ml, 4 h; B: 10ng/ml, 15 min; C: 0,1ng/ml, 4 h. D: Detection of metaphase and interphase Y chromosomal DNA in cells from PHA stimulated, colcemid arrested peripheral blood lymphocytes (100 X, phase contrast, Zeiss Axioskop, digital image). One Y body in an interphase nucleus, and two metaphase Y bodys are shown. Probe concentration: 10ng/ml. Hybridization time: 2 h.

Results and Discussion

Using the protocols described above we are able to produce more than 5 pmol ssDNA or dsDNA probe per 100 µl. Besides the protocol described here there exist different alternative protocols without carrier DNA which are described in chapter 2. In the mean time we have demonstrated that even a hybridization time as short as 15min is sufficient to get a signal without decrease in intensity (fig. 2B). In our ISH experiments 100ng probe was abundant for 10 ml of hybridization solution - sufficient for approximately 200 slides in the histochemistry robot, or up to 1,000 slides in a manually performed ISH.

Compared to the nick translated and biotinylated plasmid probes with the ssDNA and dsDNA PCR synthesized DIG probes, shorter hybridization times (2h vs. 4h) and lower probe concentrations (10 ng/ml vs. 1 µg/ml) are sufficient for optimal results. There are no differences in sensitivity between ssDNA and dsDNA DIG probes. The copy number of the 3564 bp repeat unit on the human Y chromosome (DYZ1 family) varies between 800 and 5000 (Nakahori 1986). This was easily detected with the 154 bp probe (fig. 2D).

With the 198 bp probe for HCMV the same range of sensitivity in detecting HCMV infected cells, with typical morphology in lung tissue, is consistently reached, as with the (approximately 200 times more complex) biotinylated probe described above.

We observed a lower melting temperature and a slowed down reannealing kinetics of DIG labeled DNA compared to unlabeled DNA (data not shown). The melting point of the hybrid is probably between the two. It is possible that the slowed down reannealing kinetics of two DIG labeled complementary strands, and/or their lower melting temperature, make the dsDNA DIG probes behave like ssDNA probes *in situ*. The similar results with ssDNA and dsDNA DIG probes and the very low probe concentrations in the hybridization mixture suggest that networking is not responsible for the high sensitivity *in situ*. For further discussion of the networking hypothesis, see Singer et al (1986).

References

1. Akrigg A, Wilkinson GWG, Oram JD. The structure of the major immediate early gene of human cytomegalovirus strain AD169. 1985, Virus Res 2, 107-121.

2. Biochemica Boehringer Mannheim: DNA labeling and Detection. 1989, Applications manual.

3. Brigati DJ, Budgeon LR, Unger ER, Koebler D, Cuomo C, Kennedy T, Perdomo J Ml. Immunocytochemistry is automated: Development of a robotic workstation based upon the capillary action principle. 1988, J Histotechnology 11, 165-183.

4. Finckh U, Lingenfelter PA, Myerson D. Producing single-stranded DNA probes with the *Taq* DNA polymerase: A high yield protocol. 1991, BioTechniques 10, 35-39.

5. Handyside AH, Penketh RJA, Winston RM, Pattinson J K, Delhanty JD, Tuddenham EG. Biopsy of human preimplantation embryos and sexing by DNA amplification. 1989, Lancet I 1989, 347-349.

6. Jiwa NM, Van Gemert GW, Raap AK, Van de Rijke FM, Mulder A, Lens PF, Salimans MM, Zwaan FE, Van Dorp W, Van der Ploeg M. Rapid detection of human cytomegalovirus DNA in peripheral blood leukocytes of viremic transplant recipients by the polymerase chain reaction. 1989, Transplantation 48:72-76.

7. Kogan S C, Doherty M, Gitchier J. An improved method for prenatal diagnosis of genetic diseases by analysis of amplified DNA sequences. Application to hemophilia A. 1987, New Engl J Med 317, 985-990.

8. Lichter P, Ward D C. Is non-isotopic *in situ* hybridisation finally coming of age? 1990, Nature 345, 93-95.9

9. Myerson D. *In situ* Hybridisation. *In*: Colvin RB, Bhan AK and McCluskey RT (Eds.), Diagnostic Immunopathology, 1988, 475-498. Raven Press, New York.

10. Myerson D, Henne KW. Automation of in-situ hybridization. 1992, Amer J Clin Pathol, in press.

11. Nakahori Y, Kounosuke M, Masao Y, Yasuo N. A human Y-chromosome specific repeated DNA family (DYZ1) consists of a tandem array of pentanucleotides. 1986, Nucl Acids Res 14, 7569-7580.

12. Singer RH, Lawrence JB, Villnave C. Optimization of in situ hybridisation using isotopic and non-isotopic detection methods. 1986, BioTechniques 4, 230-250.

Acknowledgement: We thank E. Bryant, dep. Cytogenetics, FHCRC, for chromosome preparation and digital image processing.

This work was supported by the Deutsche Krebsgesellschaft Berlin and Boehringer Ingelheim Fonds and PHS grants NCI CA18029 and NHLBI HL36444.

Differentiation of Arylsulfatase A Deficiencies Associated with Metachromatic Leukodystrophy and Arylsulfatase A Pseudodeficiency

V Gieselmann

Diagnostic problems due to ASA pseudodeficiency

Metachromatic leukodystrophy (MLD) is an autosomal recessively inherited disease with an incidence of about 1 in 40 000 (for review see Kolodny 1989). Arylsulfatase A (ASA) desulfates the polar glycolipid cerebroside sulfate, which is a characteristic component of the myelin sheaths of the nervous system. This explains why accumulation of cerebroside sulfate in MLD mainly affects the nervous system, where it causes a progressive demyelination. The patients suffer from a variety of neurologic symptoms, like a delay in neurologic development, weakness, ataxia, spastic tetraparesis and dementia. Finally they die in a decerebrated state. Based on the age of onset three different clinical forms are distinguished: a late infantile form starting around the age of two years (60% of all cases), a juvenile form with an age of onset in between 4 and 16 years (30% of the cases) and an adult form starting above the age of 16 years (10% of the cases). Late infantile patients usually die within about 5 years after the onset of the disease, whereas in the adult forms patients can survive for 10 to 20 years. In the late onset forms of the disease psychiatric symptoms may precede the typical neurologic signs, which frequently leads to an initial misdiagnosis. The diagnosis of MLD is usually made by the determination of ASA activity in leucocytes or cultured skin fibroblasts. However, a deficiency of ASA is not a proof for MLD. One to two percent of the population have low residual enzyme activities (10%-15% of normal), but are healthy (Kolodny 1989). These individuals have been called pseudodeficient (PD). They are homozygous for the ASA PD allele (frequency 7-15%), which codes for only 5-10% of enzyme activity, when compared to the normal allele. Obviously these low enzyme activities are sufficient to prevent the outbreak of the disease. Whereas the allele is harmless for the carrier it causes problems in the diagnosis and genetic counselling of MLD, since based on enzyme activity determinations deficiencies associated with MLD or PD cannot be reliably distinguished. When low ASA activities are found in patients with neurologic symptoms of unknown origin these individuals are often diagnosed as suffering from an atypical form of MLD. It is very likely that they are pseudodeficient in ASA and that their symptoms are unrelated to MLD (Kihara 1980). In order to be able to reliably distinguish between PD and MLD so called cerebroside loading tests have been developed (Kappler 1991). In these type of assays cultured fibroblasts are exposed to radioactively labeled cerebroside sulfate and the in vivo degradation of the substrate is measured. Although this assay allows a distinction of PD and MLD it has considerable disadvantages: it depends on tissue culture facilities, the radioactive substrate is not commercially available and the results depend on tissue culture conditions. It takes some experience to perform the assay reliably. Frequently in genetic counselling individuals will be found (up to 15% of all probands) who have only 50 % of normal ASA activity. It cannot be determined wether they are carriers of a fatal MLD allele or a benign PD allele (Baldinger 1987). Precise genetic counselling is

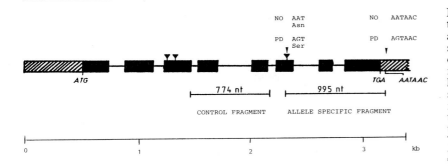

Figure 1: Fragments amplified in the PD allele specific PCR. The arylsulfatase A gene is shown schematically. Boxes indicate exons, lines introns. Black parts indicate coding sequences and hatched parts 5' and 3' untranslated sequences. ATG depicts the initiation codon, TGA the termination codon and AATAAC the polyadenylation signal. Triangles depict the positions of potential N-glycosylation sites. The mutations occuring in the PD allele are shown above, no: normal sequence, pd: sequences of the PD allele, arrows indicate the location of the mutations. Horizontal lines depict the fragments amplified in the PD allele specific PCR. The length is given in nucleotides (nt). A scale in kilobase is shown at the bottom.

impossible because even with the cerebroside loading test a distinction between heterozygosity for MLD and PD is impossible.

In order to improve the diagnostic procedures for a differentiation of PD and MLD we have analysed the mutations in the ASA PD allele and developed a rapid non radioactive assay for the direct detection of the PD allele.

Mutations in the ASA PD allele

Two A to G transitions have been found in the ASA PD allele (Gieselmann 1989) (see Fig 1). The first causes the loss of one of the two utilized potential N-glycosylation sites in the ASA polypeptide. The ASA in pseudodeficient individuals has lost one oligosaccharide side chain and is about 2.5 kd smaller than in normal individuals. This mutation however does not affect the stability or specific activity of ASA. It is a polymorphism and cannot explain the attenuated enzyme activity in pseudodeficient individuals. The second A to G transition causes the loss of the first polyadenylation signal downstream of the termination codon. This mutation causes the loss of about 90 % of ASA poly (A)+ mRNA. This causes a reduced synthesis of ASA polypeptides, which explains the attenuated enzyme activity in PD.

Allele specific amplification of the ASA PD allele

Based on our knowledge of the mutations characterizing the PD allele we have synthesized pairs of primers, which allow the allele specific amplification of the PD allele (Gieselmann 1991a). The primers are synthesized such that the 3' terminal base corresponds to the location of the mutation and either matches the normal or the PD allele sequence. When oligonucleotides which sequences correspond to the normal allele anneal to the PD allele, the 3' terminal base remains mismatched and does not allow the polymerase to extend the primer. Thus the DNA is only amplified when the sequence of the primers matches the genomic sequence. In this case the PCR yields an allele specific fragment of 995 bp (see fig. 1). To produce a control for the PCR we coamplified a fragment of 774 bp in the same reaction, amplification of which is independent of the PD mutations. With each DNA sample two PCRs have to be performed: one with a pair of primers specific for the PD allele and the other with a pair of primers specific for non PD alleles. The assay only detects the PD allele mutations and cannot show whether the non PD allele is a normal or MLD allele.

Genomic DNA of three healthy individuals (A, B, and C) with a known genotype was amplified as a control.

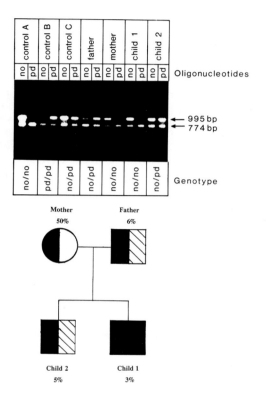

Figure 2: Determination of the ASA genotype by allele specific amplification. A) Top line gives the initials of the individuals from which the genomic DNA was isolated. Controls A,B,C are healthy individuals with a known genotype. The other individuals are from the family whose pedigree is shown below. Second line shows the combination of allele specific oligonucleotides used in the PCR, no: non PD allele specific primers, pd: PD allele specific primers. The 774 bp control fragment and the 995 bp allele specific fragment are indicated by arrows. The genotype is shown below no: non PD alleles, pd : pd alleles.
B) Pedigree of the family genotyped in figure 2 A. The filled area indicates the MLD allele, hatched area the PD allele and open parts the normal allele. Numbers give percentage of residual enzyme activity.

The 774 bp fragment was amplified in all reactions demonstrating that the PCR worked properly. The 995 bp fragment is only amplified when the corresponding allele is present in the genomic DNA. The individual A has no PD allele, B is heterozygous for a PD allele and C is homozygous for the PD allele.

Figure 2 B shows a pedigree of a family in which the first child was affected with MLD. The diagnosis was made at the age of two years when the brother was just born. The newborn child also had low ASA activities suggesting that both children suffered from MLD. When ASA activities were measured in the parents the healthy father had residual enzyme activities close to those of his children. This suggests that the father is a compound heterozygote of a MLD allele and a PD allele. Allele specific amplification of all family members (see fig. 2) revealed the presence of a PD allele in the father and the second child. Thus this child has inherited the PD allele from his father and is not affected with MLD.

Limitations of the allele specific amplification of the PD allele.

Allele specific amplification as well as allele specific oligonucleotide hybridization detect the two point mutations signifying the PD allele. These assays do not exclude the existence of mutations somewhere else in the gene. We have recently sequenced the ASA genes of a patient, who appeared to be honozygous for the PD allele mutations. However, there was no doubt that this patient suffered from MLD. Besides the two A to G transitions of the PD allele we found a third mutation in exon 2, which causes a serine 96 to glycine substitution (Gieselmann 1991b). Using in vitro mutagenesis we can show that this mutation leads to a complete loss of enzyme activity. The existence of MLD alleles derived from PD alleles calls for caution in the diagnosis of ASA PD using allele specific amplification. Based on theoretical considerations one can assume, that 1 in 200 alleles, which appear as PD alleles will carry additional mutations rendering them non functional (Gieselmann 1991b). Therefore the chances that an individual which appears to be homozygous for the PD allele will suffer from MLD is 1 in 40.000. Although this number is low, the existence of MLD alleles derived from PD alleles must be kept in mind and whenever such an allele is suspected a cerebroside loading test should be performed.

Mc Graw Hill, New York, 1721-1750

References

1. Baldinger S, Pierpont ME, Wenger DA. Pseudodeficiency of arylsulfatase A: a counselling dilemma. 1987, Clin Genet 31, 71-76

2. Gieselmann V, Fluharty AL, Tonnesen T, von Figura K. Mutations in the arylsulfatase A pseudodeficiency allele causing metachromatic leukodystrophy. 1991b, Am J Hum Genet 49, 407-413

3. Gieselmann V, Polten A, Kreysing J, von Figura K. Arylsulfatase A pseudodeficiency: loss of a N-glycosylation site and a polyadenylation signal. 1989, Proc Natl Acad Sci USA 86, 9436-9440

4. Gieselmann V. A rapid assay for the detection of the arylsulfatase A pseudodeficiency allele facilitates the genetic counselling and the diagnosis of metachromatic leukodystrophy. 1991a, Hum Genet 86, 251-255

5. Kappler J, Watts RWE, Conzelmann E, Gibbs DA, Propping P, Gieselmann V. Low arylsulfatase A activity and choreoathetotic syndrome in three siblings: Differentiation of pseudodeficiency from metachromatic leukodystrophy. 1991, Eur J Ped 150, 287-290

6. Kihara H, Chen King H, Fluharty AL, Tsay KK, Hartlage PL. Prenatal diagnosis of metachromatic leukodystrophy in a family with pseudoarylsulfatase A deficiency by the cerebroside loading test. 1980, Pediatric Research 14, 224-227

7. Kolodny E H. Metachromatic leukodystrophy and multiple sulfatase deficiency: sulfatide lipidosis. In: Scriver CR, Beaudet AL, Sly WS, Valle D (Eds.): Metabolic basis of inherited disease, Vol II 6th Ed, 1989,

Molecular Genetics of Neuromuscular Diseases - the Role of PCR in Diagnostics and Research

B Kadenbach, P Seibel

Until the discovery of deletions in mitochondrial DNA (mtDNA) in patients with mitochondrial myopathy by Holt et al. (1988), the characterization of neuromuscular diseases was restricted to the study of morphological, biochemical and immunological alterations and this mainly in skeletal muscle tissue (see reviews of Morgan-Hughes 1986, DiMauro 1987, Lombes 1989a). In the meantime multiple different deletions as well as point mutations of mtDNA were identified as being the molecular basis of various forms of neuromuscular diseases, as the possible cause of aging (Ikebe 1990, Cortopassi 1990) and of human death (Kadenbach 1990). In such studies the application of PCR is essential because the molecular analysis of these disorders can be acheived by using very small samples of tissue, these obtained by non-invasive methods. In fact a few hairs from patients with MERRF disease (Myoclonic Epilepsy with Ragged Red Fibers) were sufficient to determine quantitatively the amount of mutated mtDNA (Seibel 1990).

Mitochondrial diseases

Mitochondrial diseases, a subgroup of neuromuscular diseases, includes a heterogeneous group of disorders, based on insufficient or defective energy (ATP) synthesis in mitochondria. The defect can occur in one or in many tissues and can be fatal at infantile or juvenile age. Although mitochondrial diseases occur rather rarely, a number of as yet unknown diseases could be caused by defective mitochondrial energy synthesis. An impaired ATP synthesis in mitochondria does not necessarily lead to cell death because in all cells ATP can also be synthesized by glycolysis (about 5 % of total cellular ATP synthesis). The normal function of most cells and tissues, however, does require mitochondrial respiration and ATP synthesis.

Some forms of mitochondrial diseases might be based on defective nuclear coded enzymes involved in fatty acid oxidation or the citric acid cycle (Zeviani 1989b). Most mitochondrial diseases, however, are due to decreased activities of respiratory chain enzymes, in particular NADH dehydrogenase (complex I) and/or cytochrome c oxidase (complex IV), which are in part encoded in the mitochondrial genome.

The mitochondrial genome

Mitochondria contain a nucleus independent genome, occuring in 3-10 copies per mitochondrion and several hundred copies per cell. In contrast to nuclear DNA of nondividing cells, mtDNA is continuously synthesized and degraded (t1/2: 10-20 days) in all cells and tissues. The human double stranded circular mtDNA has a size of 16569 bp (Anderson 1981), and codes for only 13 protein subunits of energy transducing enzyme complexes of the respiratory chain and ATP synthase

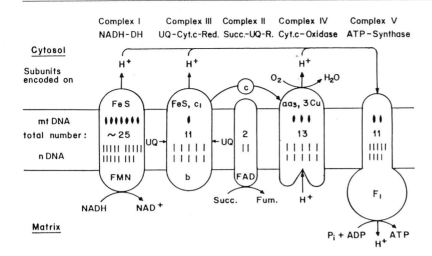

Figure 1: Scheme of respiratory chain enzyme complexes. The scheme indicates the number of mitochondrial coded and nuclear coded protein subunits of NADH dehydrogenase, ubiquinol-cytochrome c oxidoreductase, succinate-ubiquinone oxidoreductase, cytochrome c oxidase and ATP synthase. Only proton pumps (complex I, III and IV) and the proton dissipator ATP synthase contain mitochondrial coded proteins.

(see fig. 1). In addition mtDNA codes for two rRNAs and 22 tRNAs (fig. 2) which are all essential for the synthesis of the 13 mitochondrial coded proteins. While nuclear DNA is inherited by Mendel's rules, mtDNA is exclusively maternally inherited (Giles 1980, Case 1981). The recently described paternal inheritance of mtDNA in mice (Gyllensten 1991) appears to be a rare exception.

Deletions of mtDNA cause different mitochondrial diseases

Various deletions of up to more than 50 % of mtDNA have been found in skeletal muscle tissue of all patients with Kearns-Sayre syndrome (KSS) and of some patients with Chronic Progressive External Ophthalmoplegia (CPEO) (Holt 1988, Lestienne 1988, Ozawa 1988, Zeviani 1988, Saiffudin-Noer 1988, Schon 1989, Johns 1989, Shoffner 1989, Nelson 1989, Obermayer-Kusser 1990). The same deletion was also found in other tissues from patients, although to a smaller extent (Obermaier-Kusser 1990, Shanske 1990). The amount of deleted mtDNA is normally estimated from the intensity of deleted and wild-type mtDNA on Southern blots. We have applied PCR to determine more accurately the percentage of deleted mtDNA in different tissues of a patient with KSS by coamplification of deleted and normal mtDNA using two specific primer pairs and radioactive dATP. The deleted mtDNA was determined to 58 % in skeletal muscle, 37 % in heart, 26 % in kidney and 5 % in liver (Seibel 1991a). Since neither in KSS nor in CPEO a maternal inheritance could be proven (but

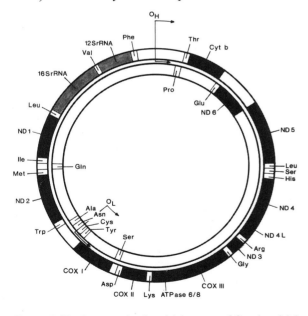

Figure 2: The human mitochondrial genome. Mitochondrial DNA codes for 13 proteins, 2 rRNAs and 22 tRNAs. The origins of replication of the heavy strand (OH) and light strand (OL) are indicated.

see Ozawa 1988), an acquired somatic mutation is assumed to be the cause of the deletion. The frequent occurrence of directly repeated sequences, up to 15 bp length, flanking the deleted region of mtDNA, suggests the involvement of a recombinational event (Schon 1989, Johns 1989) and/or a slip-replication mechanism (Shoffner 1989). In some patients multiple deletions were found to occur simultaneously, and it was suggested that a nuclear coded protein involved in replication of mtDNA might cause the deletions (Zeviani 1989a).

Because the amount of deletions is about 20-60 % of total mtDNA, and because the genes for tRNAs are distributed over the whole mitochondrial genome, interspersing the protein genes (see fig. 2), any deletion will result in the loss of one or more tRNA genes of which all are essential to the synthesis of protein. Therefore mitochondria with deleted mtDNA cannot synthesize functional enzyme complexes of oxidative phosphorylation.

Maternally inherited diseases are based on point mutations of mtDNA

From the pedigree of families with certain forms of mitochondrial diseases a maternal inheritance can be clearly established. By systematic sequencing of various PCR-amplified fragments of mtDNA from patients several point mutations have been identified as the cause of these diseases: LHON (Leber's Hereditary Optic Neuropathy) is related to a point mutation in the gene for subunit 4 of NADH dehydrogenase (nt 11778) (Wallace 1988).

The MERRF disease is related to two point mutations. One in the tRNALys gene (nt 8344) and another in the gene for 12S rRNA (nt 750) (Shoffner 1990). The second mutation at nt 750, however, could not be found in other patients with MERRF disease (Seibel 1991b). We have introduced "mispairing PCR" to determine quantitatively any point mutation at any site in the DNA

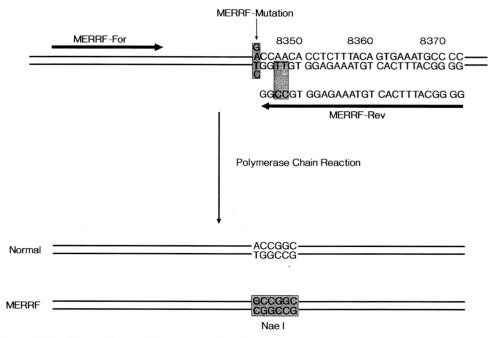

Figure 3: The "mispairing PCR" method to identify any point mutation as shown for the mitochondrial tRNALys gene in MERRF disease. The "mispairing primer" (MERRF-Rev) generates a new restriction site for Nae I endonuclease at its 3'end together with the adjacent mutated, but not wild-type, nucleotide. After amplification by PCR together with the primer MERRF-For, only the mutated mtDNA will be cleaved by Nae I, as visualized after agarose gel electrophoresis.

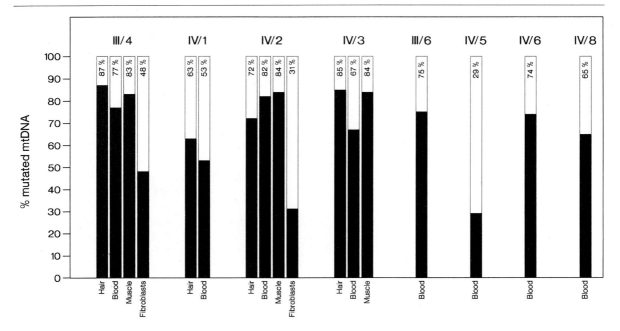

Figure 4: Percentage of mutated mtDNA in various tissues of eight members of a family presenting MERRF syndrome. The percentage mutated mtDNA was determined by "mispairing PCR" as described by Seibel et al., (1990). Roman numerals indicate the generation. III/4 and III/6 are sisters; IV/1, IV/2 and IV/3 are children of III/4; IV/5, IV/6 and IV/8 are children of III/6.

where no restriction site occurs and at restriction sites for which the endonuclease is not available. This method creates a new restriction site involving either the mutated or the wild-type nucleotide by using a mispairing primer (fig. 3). After amplification with labeled dATP, cleavage with the restriction enzyme and agarose gel electrophoresis, the amount of mutated DNA can be calculated from the radioactivity in the DNA bands (Seibel 1990). As shown in fig. 4 a varying percentages of mutated mtDNA was found in the various tissues of the same individual and in the same tissues of different individuals of a family presenting MERRF syndrome through the maternal lineage (Seibel 1991b). Since mutated mtDNA was also found in healthy individuals from the maternal lineage we suggest that a threshold of mutated mtDNA is required before the clinical symptoms become manifest.

A point mutation in the gene for subunit 6 of ATP synthase (nt 8993) was found to cause a new form of maternally inherited mitochondrial disease (Holt 1990).

MELAS (Mitochondrial Myopathy Lactic Acidosis and Stroke-like episodes) disease could be related to a point mutation in the tRNALeu (TTA) gene (nt 3243) (Goto 1990). Surprisingly another point mutation in the same tRNALeu(TTA) gene (nt 3260) was recently identified to cause a cardiomyopathy with quite different clinical symptoms (Zeviani 1991). Thus it appears that different point mutations in the same tRNA gene could result in different biochemical dysfunctions of the tRNA. The point mutation associated with MELAS is closely located to the 3' end of the 16S rRNA gene. Recently it has been shown by Hess et al. (1991) that this mutation results in severe impairment of 16S rRNA transcription termination. The further downstream mutation at nt 3260 in the tRNALeu(TTA) gene may directly effect the function of the tRNA. A changed specificity of mutated tRNAs may be caused by the modified kinetics of cytochrome c oxidase from MERRF patients (Lombes 1989b) and from the variable incorporation of labeled methionine into mitochondrial

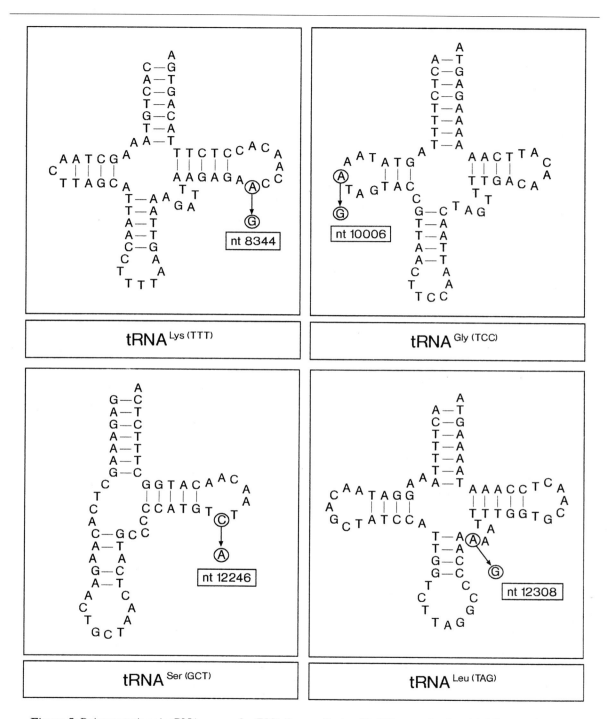

Figure 5: Point mutations in tRNA genes of mtDNA from patients with different mitochondrial diseases (see text).

proteins of skin fibroblasts of MERRF patients differing in their lysine content (Seibel 1991b).

Mitochondrial tRNA genes are hotspots for point mutations in mtDNA.

While some patients with CPEO display deletions of mtDNA others have normal length mtDNA (Moraes 1989). If a point mutation in a tRNA gene results in a defective tRNA any deletion of mtDNA associated with the loss of one or more tRNAs has the same consequence as any point mutation in a tRNA gene: the impaired synthesis of mitochondrial coded proteins and thus of mitochondrial ATP.

We sequenced all tRNA genes of mtDNA from the muscle tissue of a patient with CPEO without mtDNA deletion and of another patient with CIPO (Chronic Intestinal Pseudoobstruction with myopathy and ophthalmoplegia). From 19 PCR-amplified fragments encompassing all tRNA genes single strand DNA was synthesized by asymmetric PCR and sequenced by using internal primers (Lauber 1991). Three new point mutations were identified, tRNALeu(TAG) (nt 12308, A to G), tRNASer(GCT) (nt 12246, C to A), tRNAGly (nt 10006, A to G), as shown in fig. 5. All mutated nucleotides were shown to occur in conserved positions in the tRNA genes, i.e. none occured in the corresponding position of mitochondrial tRNA genes of various other species. Whilst in the mtDNA of the CIPO patient all 3 mutations occured and in the CPEO patient only the mutation in the tRNALeu (TAG) gene was found. This latter mutation (also identified by "mispairing PCR" (Seibel 1990)) was found to occur, at a lower percentage in two patients with myopathy and CPEO, respectively. Recently two further point mutations in the tRNAThr gene (nt 15924 and nt 15923) were identified in two unrelated infants with lethal respiratory chain defects (Yoon 1991). From all of these patients no maternal inheritance of the disease was proven. In contrast, the above described mutations in the genes for tRNALys and tRNALeu(TTA) (nt 3243 and 3260) are associated with maternally inherited diseases. It remains to be disclosed which factors determine the segregation during development and the rapid or slow amplification or even reduction of point mutated mtDNA in somatic cells (see fig. 4). Research on the biochemical consequences of point mutations in mitochondrial tRNA genes will help us to understand the multiple clinical symptoms of mitochondrial diseases.

References

1. Anderson S, Bankier AT, Barrell BG, de Bruijn MHL, Coulson AR, Drouin J, Eperon IC, Nierlich DP, Rose BA, Sanger F, Schreier PH, Smith AJH, Staden R, Young IG. Sequence and organization of the human mitochondrial genome. 1981, Nature 290, 457-465.

2. Case JT, Wallace DC. Maternal inheritance of mitochondrial DNA polymorphisms in cultured human fibroblasts. 1981, Som Cell Genet 7, 103-108.

3. Cortopassi GA, Arnheim N. Detection of a specific mitochondrial DNA deletion in tissues of older humans. 1990, Nucl Acids Res 18, 6927-6933.

4. DiMauro S, Bonilla E, Zeviani M, Servidei S, DeVivo DC, Schon E. Mitochondrial myopathies. 1987, J Inher Metab Dis 10 (Suppl. 1) 113-128.

5. Erlich HA, Gelfand D, Sninsky JJ. Recent advances in the polymerase chain rection. 1991, Science 256, 1643-1651.

6. Giles RE, Blanc H, Cann HM, Wallace, DC. Maternal inheritance of human mitochondrial DNA. 1980, Proc Natl Acad Sci USA 77, 6715-6719.

7. Goto YI, Nonaka I, Horai S. A mutation in the tRNALeu(UUR) gene associated with the MELAS subgroup of mitochondrial encephalomyopathies. 1990, Nature 348, 651-653.

8. Gyllensten U, Wharton D, Josefsson A, Wilson AC. Paternal inheritance of mitochondrial DNA in mice. 1991, Nature 352, 255-257.

9. Hess JF, Parisi MA, Bennett JL, Clayton DA. Impairment of mitochondrial transcription termination by a point mutation associated with the MELAS subgroup of mitochondrial encephalomyopathies. 1991, Nature 351, 236-239.

10. Holt IJ, Hardin AE, Morgan-Hughes. Mitochondrial DNA polymorphism in mitochondrial myopathy. 1988, Hum Genet 79, 53-57.

11. Holt IJ, Hardin AE, Petty RKH, Morgan-Hughes JA. A new mitochondrial disease associated with mitochondrial DNA heteroplasmy. 1990, Am J Hum Genet 46, 428-433.

12. Ikebe SI, Tanaka M, Ohno K, Sato W, Hattori K, Kondo T, Mizuno Y, Ozawa, T. Increase of deleted mitochondrial DNA in the striatum in Parkinson's disease and senescence. 1990, Biochem Biophys Res Comm 170, 1044-1048.

13. Johns DR, Rutledge SL, Stine OC, Hurko O. Directly repeated sequences associated with pathogenic mitochondrial DNA deletions. 1989, Proc Natl Acad Sci 86, 8059-8062.

14. Kadenbach B, Müller-Höcker J. Mutations of mitochondrial DNA and human death. 1990, Naturwissenschaften 77, 221-225.

15. Lauber J, Marsac C, Kadenbach B, Seibel P. Mutations in mitochondrial tRNA genes: a frequent cause of neuromuscular diseases. 1991, Nucl Acids Res 19, 1393-1397.

16. Lestienne P, Ponsot G. Kearns-Sayre syndrome with muscle mitochondrial DNA deletion. 1988, Lancet i, 885.

17. Lombes A, Bonilla E, DiMauro S. Mitochondrial encephalomyopathies. 1989a, Rev Neurol (Paris) 145 (10), 671-689.

18. Lombes A, Mendell JR, Nakase H, Barohn RJ, Bonilla E, Zeviani M, Yates AJ, Omerza J, Gales TL, Nakahara K, Rizzuto R, King Engel W, DiMauro S. Myoclonic epilepsy and ragged-red fibers with cytochrome oxidase deficiency: Neuropathology, Biochemistry and Molecular Genetics. 1989b, Ann Neurol 26, 20-33.

19. Moraes CT, DiMauro S, Zeviani M, Lombes A, Shanske S, Miranda AF, Nakase H, Bonilla E, Werneck L C, Servidei S, Nonaka I, Koga Y, Spiro AJ, Brownell KW, Schmidt B, Schotland DL, Zupanc M, DeVivo DC, Schon EA, Rowland LP. Mitochondrial DNA deletions in progressive external ophthalmoplegia and Kearns-Sayre syndrome. 1989, New Engl J Med 320, 1293-1299.

20. Morgan-Hughes JA. Mitochondrial diseases. 1986, Elsevier Science Publishers B.V.

21. Nelson I, Degoul F, Obermaier-Kusser B, Romero N, Borrone C, Marsac C, Vayssiere JL, Gerbitz K, Fardeau M, Ponsot G, Lestienne P. Mapping of heteroplasmic mitochondrial DNA deletions in Kearns-Sayre syndrome. 1989, Nucl Acids Res 17, 8117-8124.

22. Obermaier-Kusser B, Müller-Höcker J, Nelson I, Lestienne P, Enter C, Riedele TH, Gerbitz KD. Different copy numbers of apparently identically deleted mitochondrial DNA in tissues from a patient with Kearns-Sayre syndrome deleted by PCR. 1990, Biochem Biophys Res Commun 169, 1007-1015.

23. Ozawa T, Yoneda M, Tanaka M, Ohno K, Sato W, Suzuki H, Nishikimi M, Yamamoto M, Nonaka I, Horai S. Maternal inheritance of deleted mitochondrial DNA in a family with mitochondrial myopathy. 1988, Biochem Biophys Res Commun 154, 1240-1247.

24. Saiffuddin-Noer AN, Marzuki S, Trounce I, Byrne, E. Mitochondrial DNA deletion in encephalomyopathy. 1988, Lancet ii, 1253-1254.

25. Schon EA, Rizzuto R, Moraes CT, Nakase H, Zeviani M, DiMauro S. A direct repeat is a hotspot for large-scale deletion of human mitochondrial DNA. 1989, Science 244, 346-349.

26. Seibel P, Degoul F, Romero N, Marsac C, Kadenbach B. Identification of point mutations by mispairing PCR as exemplified in MERRF disease. 1990, Biochem Biophys Res Comm 173, 561-565.

27. Seibel P, Mell O, Hannemann A, Müller-Höcker J, Kadenbach B. A method for quantitatave analysis of deleted mitochondrial DNA by PCR in small tissue samples. 1991a, Meth. Cell. Mol. Biol. 2, 147-153.

28. Seibel P, Degoul F, Bonne G, Romero N, Francois D, Paturneau-Jouas M, Ziegler F, Eymard B, Fardeau M, Marsac C, Kadenbach B. Genetic, biochemical and pathophysiological characterization of a familial mitochondrial encephalomyopathy (MERRF). 1991b, J Neurol Sci, in press.

29. Shanske S, Moraes CT, Lombes A, Miranda AF, Bonilla E, Lewis P, Whelan MA, Ellsworth CA, DiMauro S. Widespread tissue distribution of mitochondrial DNA deletions in Kearns-Sayre syndrome. 1990, Neurology 40, 24-28.

30. Shoffner JM, Lott MT, Voljavec AS, Soueidan SA, Costigan DA, Wallace DC. Spontaneous Kearns-Sayre/chronic external ophthalmoplegia plus syndrome associated with a mtDNA deletion: a slip-replication model and metabolic therapy. 1989, Proc Natl Acad Sci USA 86, 7952-7956.

31. Shoffner JM, Lott MT, Lezza AMS, Seibel P, Ballinger SW, Wallace DC. Myoclonic epilepsy and ragged red fiber disease (MERRF) is associated with a mitochondrial DNA tRNALys mutation. 1990, Cell 61, 931-937.

32. Lezza AMS, Elsas LJ II, Nikoskelainen EK. Mitochondrial DNA mutation associated with Leber's hereditary optic neuropathy. 1988, Science 242, 1427-1430.

33. Yoon KL, Aprille JR, Ernst SG. Mitochondrial transfer RNAThr mutation in fatal infantile respiratory enzyme deficiency. Biochem. 1991, Biophys Res Commun 176, 1112-1115.

34. Zeviani M, Gellera C, Antozzi C, Rimoldi M, Morandi L, Villani F, Tiranti V, DiDonato S. Maternally inherited myopathy and cardiomyopathy: association with mutation in mitochondrial DNA tRNALeu(UUR). 1991, Lancet 338, 143-147.

35. Zeviani M, Moraes CT, DiMauro S, Nakase H, Bonilla E, Schon EA, Rowland LP. Deletions of mitochondrial DNA in Kearns-Sayre syndrome. 1988, Neurology 38, 1339-1346.

36. Zeviani M, Servidei S, Gelleva C, Bertini E, DiMauro S, DiDonato S. An autosomal dominant disorder with multiple deletions of mitochondrial DNA starting at the D-loop region. 1989a, Nature 339, 309-311.

37. Zeviani M, Bonilla E, DeVivo DC, DiMauro S. Mitochondrial diseases. 1989b, Neurologic Clinics 7, 123-156.

Acknowledgements

This work was supported by the Thyssen-Stiftung and Fonds der Chemischen Industrie. P. Seibel acknowledges a fellowship of the Boehringer Ingelheim Fonds für medizinische Grundlagenforschung.

The Application of Polymerase Chain Reaction for Studying the Phylogeny of Bacteria

G Köhler, W Ludwig, K H Schleifer

In contrast to animals or plants prokaryotes possess only a simple morphology and no fossil records are available. Therefore modern studies on the phylogeny of prokaryotes rely on comparative sequence analyses of homologous macromolecules that are ubiquitous among organisms, show functional constancy and are conserved enough to span a wide evolutionary spectrum. Suitable phylogenetic marker molecules are 16S and 23S rRNAs, elongation factors, ATP synthase subunits or RNA polymerases (Schleifer 1989, Woese 1987, Zillig 1989). The primary structures of these molecules are an alternating sequence of conserved and gradually less conserved regions reflecting the different phylogenetic levels, the different stages of evolution. The degree of sequence similarity of homologous molecules reflects the minimal number of base or amino acid changes

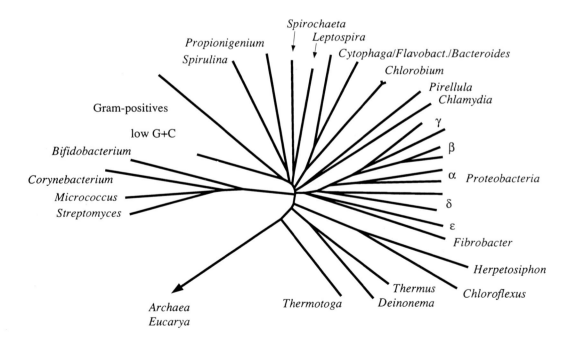

Figure 1.: Phylogenetic tree of the major lines of descent among eubacteria based upon 23S rRNA sequence comparisons (see text).

accumulated during evolution. Distance matrix or parsimony analyses of the aligned sequences allow the reconstruction of phylogenetic trees. The three kingdom as well as the phylum concept (Woese 1987) are supported by all phylogenetic marker molecules mentioned above.

The most comprehensive insight into phylogenetic relationships of bacteria, however, has been derived from the analysis of primary and secondary structures of ribosomal rRNAs, especially 16S rRNAs. An example is given in Figure 1. The phylogenetic tree based on 23S rRNA analyses shows the major lines of descent among the eubacteria.

The rRNAs and the corresponding genes are not only excellent phylogenetic markers but also suitable target molecules for specific hybridization probes. These probes are directed to primary structure regions which are unique for phylogenetically related organisms (Betzl 1990, Hertel 1991, Köhler in press). Probe techniques allow rapid and reliable detection and identification of organisms even in mixed populations. The introduction of polymerase chain reaction techniques has remarkably improved both, the comparative sequencing approach for phylogenetic analyses and the sensitivity of specific probe methodology.

The Impact of PCR Technology on Phylogenetic Studies

1. Comparative sequence analyses of rDNA

In the past the primary structures of bacterial rRNAs were determined by direct reverse transcriptase sequencing of the rRNAs or by DNA sequencing of cloned rRNA genes. Both techniques rely on the use of specific sequencing primers which are preferentially designed for well conserved target sites scattered along the primary structures. Using properly designed sets of primers any bacterial rRNA or rDNA can be sequenced applying the chain termination method. A major disadvantage of the reverse transcriptase approach is the susceptibility of the enzyme to pausing at modified bases or regions with strong secondary structures. Thus only partial sequences can be determined. Cloning of

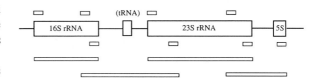

Figure 2: Schematic drawing of a typical eubacterial rRNA operon. Primer binding sites for PCR and the resulting amplified DNA fragments are indicated by white boxes (see text).

rRNA genes may be rather time consuming. Therefore, using the PCR technology *in vitro* amplification of rRNA gene fragments in combination with direct sequencing of the amplified DNA now allows more rapid and reliable sequence determination. With a limited number of primer pairs directed to well conserved regions of rDNA a set of partially overlapping fragments covering nearly complete eubacterial rRNA operons can be generated. Typically in bacterial rRNA operons the ribosomal RNA genes are arranged in the order 16S-, 23S-, 5S rRNA. Figure 2 schematically shows the target sites of primers commonly used for *in vitro* amplification of rDNA as well as the resulting rDNA fragments. Only at the 5' or 3' termini few bases of 16S and 5S rRNA genes, respectively, are not accessible following the approach outlined here.

2. Non culturable organisms

The PCR technique now allows for the first time in microbial history phylogenetic analyses of non culturable bacteria on the rDNA level, since small amounts of bacterial cells or DNA are sufficient for DNA amplification. After cloning of the rDNA fragments mixed populations can qualitatively be analysed. By using oligonucleotide primers directed to rRNA primary structure regions specific for phylogenetic groups it is even possible to selectively amplify rDNAs of distinct groups in mixed populations (Amann 1991).

3. Signature Analysis

Ribosomal RNAs contain signature elements (Woese 1987) which are unique for members of a phylogenetic

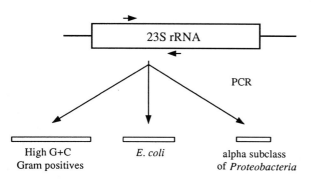

Figure 3: Detection of signature elements in bacterial 23S rRNA genes by PCR. High G+C Gram positives show insertions resulting in larger DNA amplificates in comparison to Escherichia coli. Smaller fragments found for members of the alpha subclass of Proteobacteria indicate a deletion (see text).

group of organisms. Single bases or sequence stretches, insertions or deletions can be used as signatures at the primary structure level. Also the presence or absence and characteristic lengths of higher order structure elements can be signatures. For example in comparison with the 23S rRNA of *Escherichia coli* Gram positive bacteria with high DNA G+C content contain a characteristic insertion of approximately 100 bp in domain III of 23S rRNA. A 80 bp deletion in domain III of the 23S rRNA sequence is suggested to be a signature for the alpha subclass of *Proteobacteria*. The presence of these insertions or deletions can simply be determined by a single PCR experiment using primers for conserved target sites flanking the region of interest. Differences in the length of the resulting rDNA amplificates can be analysed by using gel electrophoresis. For example with 23S rDNA of high G+C Gram positive bacteria a 380 bp fragment is generated. In comparision *E. coli* DNA delivers a "normal" fragment size of 272 bp without any deletion or insertion, whereas the homologous amplificated rDNA fragment of *Rhodobacter capsulatus*, a member of the alpha subclass of proteobacteria, has a size of approximately 190 bp. The approach is schematically shown in Figure 3. Applying this technique a rapid decision concerning the membership of a bacterial species to certain phylogenetic groups is possible.

4. Specific hybridization probes

Specific detection and identification of microorganisms by hybridization probes is an important spin-off of phylogenetic investigations. Ribosomal RNAs and their genes provide excellent target sequences for nucleic acid probes of different specifities. The PCR technique provides a rapid method for generation and labelling of polynucleotide probes. For example rRNA directed polynucleotide probes have been prepared by *in vitro* amplification of specific primary 23S rDNA structure regions and used for differentiation of waste water organisms [Dorn, Ludwig and Schleifer, unpublished studies]. The probes can be labeled during amplification by introduction of labeled nucleotides.

5. Probe target amplification

Probe target amplification by PCR increases the specifity of a detection system. With conserved primer pairs any bacterial target can be amplified. Subsequently the rDNA is analyzed for the presence of the target sequence by hybridization to specific probes. In an alternative approach one or both primers for PCR are designed as specific oligonucleotides. The corresponding rDNA is only amplified when primers match perfectly. Using a further specific probe for detection false positive results of the PCR detection experiment can be avoided (Fig.4).

Probe target amplification

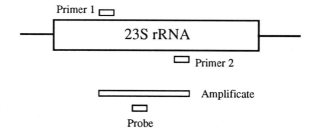

Figure 4: Schematic representation of the probe target amplification approach (see text).

References

1. Amann R, Springer N, Ludwig W, Görtz HD, Schleifer KH. Identification *in situ* and phylogeny of uncultured bacterial endosymbionts. 1991, Nature 351, 161-164.

2. Betzl D, Ludwig W, Schleifer KH. Identification of lactococci and enterococci by colony hybridization with 23S rRNA-targeted oligonucleotide probes. 1990, Environ Appl Microbiol 56, 2927-2929.

3. Hertel C, Ludwig W, Obst M, Vogel RF, Hammes WP, Schleifer KH. 23S rRNA-targeted oligonucleotide probes for the rapid identification of meat lactobacilli. 1991, System Appl Microbiol 14, 173-177.

4. Köhler G, Ludwig W, Schleifer KH. Differentiation of lactococci by rRNA gene restriction analysis. FEMS Microbiol Lett, in press.

5. Schleifer KH, Ludwig W. Phylogenetic relationships among bacteria. In: The Hierarchy of Life, Fernholm B, Bremer K, Jörnwall (Eds.), 1989, Elsevier Science Publishers BV, Amsterdam, 103-117.

6. Woese CR. Bacterial Evolution. 1987, Microbiol Rev 51, 221-271.

7. Zillig W, Klenk HP, Palm P, Pühler G, Gropp F, Garrett RA, Leffers H. The phylogenetic relations of DNA-dependent RNA polymerases of archaebacteria, eukaryotes and eubacteria. 1989, Can J Microbiol 35, 73-80.

Site-Directed Mutagenesis Facilitated by PCR

O Landt, U Hahn

Until recently site-directed mutagenesis necessitated subcloning of the target sequence and the preparation of single-stranded DNA as a template to allow annealing and extension of a mutagenesis primer. Sophisticated methods were required to select the mutated strand of the heteroduplexes created in this way (Carter 1985, Kunkel 1985, Nakamaye 1986, Stanssens 1989). The polymerase chain reaction (PCR) gives us the possibility of amplifying DNA fragments containing modified ends introduced by the 5'-ends of the oligonucleotides in use. If there are restriction sites suitable for recloning near the point of mutation it is possible to amplify the desired sequence and reclone it immediately (Kadowaki 1989). Yet usually the point of mutation is far from the next unique restriction site. In this case the standard PCR mutagenesis approach is to amplify the target sequence in two parts overlapping at the mutation site. The outer termini should overlap the appropriate restriction sites for recloning (Fig.1). Both fragments are generated individually. They are separated from the template DNA and fused in a PCR reaction using a pair of outer primers. This approach needs two complementary mutagenesis primers, two flanking primers, and three distinct PCR reactions (Higuchi 1988).

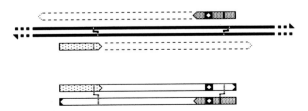

Figure 1: Principle of a two stage RNA amplification (for details see text).

Methods

We have developed a site-directed mutagenesis method which requires only one specific mutagenesis primer and a pair of flanking universal primers (Fig. 2) (Landt 1990). The idea is to use a double stranded DNA fragment obtained in a first PCR (spanned by one universal primer and the mutagenesis primer) as the mutagenesis primer for a second PCR, together with the

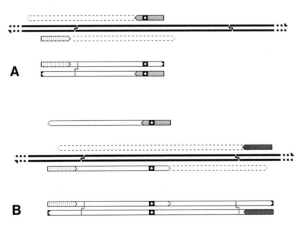

Figure 2: Two step PCR mutagenesis. 2a) The first PCR fragment is produced using a universal primer (on the left) and the mutagenesis primer. The upper strand of the reaction product (containing the mutation at the 3'-end) will be extended in the second PCR. 2b) Second PCR step. Using the purified fragment from the first PCR and a second universal primer (grey, on the right) the strand containing the mutation at its 3'end is extended. The product contains the mutation flanked by restriction sites suitable for cloning.

second universal primer. In the second PCR the strand extended from the first universal primer to the site of mutation will be elongated to the point where the second universal primer hybridizes. As any superfluous first universal primer would compete in the second PCR with the intermediate fragment and produce a non-mutated wild-type DNA fragment, this primer has to be removed after the first reaction. This mutagenesis approach has been of value for the construction of more than an hundred mutants in a protein engineering project in our laboratory. The complete amplified fragment should not be too long because of the risk of random mutations caused by the low fidelity of Taq polymerase. The proof reading activity of the thermostable Vent DNA polymerase (New England Biolabs) may reduce these problems. The first amplified fragment should be the shorter part of the whole sequence. The oligonucleotides used for PCR mutagenesis should

1. have roughly the same melting temperature (35-50°C are in the useful range; check with the programme OLIGO; Rychlik & Rhoads, 1989),
2. not be self complementary in order to avoid decreasing concentrations of free oligonucleotides,
3. be restricted from forming either homo- or hetero- "primer-dimers" (non-complementary 3'-ends; use again the OLIGO programme) - there is no need for C, G clusters at their 3'-ends to enhance hybridization because this runs the risk of unspecific hybridization elsewhere,
4. contain the desired mutation in the middle since the sequence has to be extended in both directions,
5. the 5'-end of the mutagenesis primer should be next to a T residue of the template (Landt & Hahn, submitted).

Oligonucleotides as short as 16 bases have been used successfully for single base changes in our laboratory. Standard lengths are about 20 bases.

1. First polymerase chain reaction

The hybridization temperature used has to be as high as possible to avoid mispriming and by-products. Unlike our first attempts, now we use up to 1 mg plasmid DNA as a template and we have reduced the number of thermocycles to keep the risk of random mutations low. Usually we run 15 cycles (94°C, 55°C, 72°C; 1 min. each) using 75 mmol/l of each of the four dNTPs, 1 mmol/l primers and 1 unit Taq Polymerase (Amersham Buchler). The product of the first reaction is purified by preparative agarose gel electrophoresis to eliminate superfluous primers and the template DNA. Alternatively we use 'PrimeErase Quik push columns' (Stratagene).

2. Second polymerase chain reaction

In reality the second PCR reaction is more of an extension reaction than an amplification. Therefore the amount of second PCR product is limited by the quantity of the fragment of the first reaction. To avoid too many single stranded wild-type copies being made, by extending the second universal primer, the concentration should be as low as 0.2-0.5 mmol/l and the hybridization temperature should be set relatively high. We usually use 25-40 cycles (94°C, 60°C, 72°C; 1 min. each) with 150 nmol/l of each dNTP, 100 ng plasmid DNA as template and 1 unit Taq polymerase. The product is isolated from a preparative agarose gel to remove the template DNA containing the wild-type sequence. The template DNA would contaminate the wild-type fragment after digestion. Instead of gel purification the second universal primer may be biotinylated, thus allowing the isolation of the product. Alternatively, and especially if a great number of mutants from the same wild-type source is needed, it is advantageous to destroy the restriction sites of the cloning template DNA and then to reintroduce it into the PCR fragment via the universal primers, prior to recloning.

3. Recloning

Due to contaminations from the PCR it is more difficult to cut the products with restriction endonucleases for recloning. Taq polymerase still seems to be responsible for PCR fragment contamination even after phenol extraction and agarose gel purification. Proteinase K digests have been known to destroy the polymerase and thereby to enhance recloning efficiency (Crowe 1991). Purification with glassmilk (Geneclean) was also successful in our laboratory. The PCR product is cut with the appropriate restriction enzymes and ligated with the cut vector.

4. Yields of the in-vitro mutagenesis procedure

With refined conditions and a careful purification of the products we found almost an 100 % yield in mutagenesis with respect to the wild-type as determined by DNA sequencing. Within a sequence of 300 base pairs we found up to 5 % clones containing a random mutation caused by the error rate of the Taq polymerase.

Conclusions

Investigations of the polymerase chain reaction have created new basic techniques and approaches. The site-directed introduction of a mutation into any cloned DNA fragment is now possible without the need to use mutagenesis plasmids, expensive nucleotide analoga or multiple enzymatic manipulations. The approach to site-directed mutagenesis as described above facilitates the mutagenesis and identification of any mutant within one week with little effort. In the field of protein engineering, this allows the rapid investigation of the structure function relationships of proteins.

References

1. Carter P, Bedouelle H, Winter G. Improved oligonucleotide site-directed mutagenesis using M13 vectors. 1988, Nucl Acids Res 13, 4431-4443.

2. Crowe JS, Cooper HJ, Smith MA, Sims MJ, Parker D, Gewert D. Improved cloning efficiency of polymerase chain reaction (PCR) products after proteinase K digestion. 1991, Nucl Acids Res 19, 184.

3. Higuchi R, Krummel B, Saiki RK. A general method of in vitro preparation and specific mutagenesis of DNA fragments: study of protein and DNA interactions. 1988, Nucl Acids Res 16, 7351-7367.

4. Kadowaki H, Kadowaki T, Wondisford FE, Taylor SI. Use of polymerase chain reaction catalyzed by Taq DNA polymerase for site-specific mutagenesis. 1989, Gene 76, 161-166.

5. Kunkel TA. Rapid and efficient site-specific mutagenesis without phenotypic selection. 1985, Proc Natl Acad Sci USA 82, 488-492.

6. Landt O, Grunert H-P, Hahn U. A general method for site-directed mutagenesis using the polymerase chain reaction. 1990, Gene 96, 125-128.

7. Nakamaye KL, Eckstein F. Inhibition of restriction endonuclease Nci I cleavage by phosphorothioate groups and its application to oligonucleotide-directed mutagenesis. 1986, Nucl Acids Res 14, 9679-9698.

8. Rychlik W, Rhoads RE. A computer program for choosing optimal oligonucleotides for filter hybridization, sequencing and in vitro amplification of DNA. 1989, Nucl Acids Res 17, 8543-8551.

9. Stanssens P, Opsomer C, McKeown Y, Kramer W, Zabeau M, Fritz H-J. Efficient oligonucleotide-directed construction of mutations in expression vectors by the gapped duplex DNA method using alternating selectable markers. 1989, Nucl Acids Res 17, 4441-4454.

Acknowledgements

We thank Udo Heinemann for his criticism of the manuscript and Sven Klages for his excellent technical assistance. The work was supported by the Deutsche Forschungsgemeinschaft (grant Ha 1366/2-1 and -2) and by the Studienstiftung des Deutschen Volkes.

Ectopic Transcription in the Analysis of Human Genetic Disease

J Reiss

The polymerase chain reaction (PCR) has drastically simplified the analysis of human genetic disease (reviewed in Reiss and Cooper, 1990). The complete analysis of complex genes such as CFTR, DMD/BMD or Factor 8 with 27, 26 and more than 75 individual exons, respectively, nevertheless remains a daunting task. Analysis of the mRNA concentrates on the functional parts of a given gene and enormously reduces the number of molecules needed for analysis. The need for biopsies to obtain expressing tissue can be circumvented by the exploitation of the recently described ectopic or illegitimate transcription. This phenomenon has been reported in a variety of genes (Chelly 1989, Sarkar 1989) and the detection of spermatid-specific transcripts in the lymphocytes of males and females indicated that this very low level of transcription might be a common property of all genes (Slomski 1991). Diagnostic applications have been described for Factor 8 (Berg 1990) and muscular dystrophies (Schlösser 1990). Furthermore, recent studies have shown that quantitative differences of ectopic transcripts in lymphocytes truely reflect RNA ratios in expressing tissues (R. Slomski, personal communication).

Materials and Methods

1. RNA preparation from peripheral blood lymphocytes

Lymphocytes are isolated from at least 10 ml of EDTA-anticoagulated blood either by pelleting or, better, by

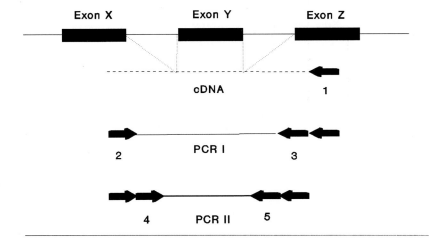

Figure 1: Principle of a two stage RNA amplification (for details see text).

centrifugation in a gradient (e.g. Ficoll-Paque, Pharmacia Sweden or Histopaque 1077, Sigma). In my laboratory yields are best when the blood is not older than two hours. Roberts et al. (1991), however, report the use of whole blood up to four days old. After washing twice with balanced salt solution (BSS) the cell pellet is dissolved in 100 µl BSS and transferred to a microcentrifuge tube. 400 µl 4 M guanidine isothiocyanate, 25 mM sodium citrate pH 7.0, 0.5 % sarcosyl, 0.1 M beta-mercaptoethanol (Chomszynski 1987) are added and the mixture is pipetted up and down approximately 10 times. 50 ml 2 M sodium acetate pH 4.0, 500 ml phenol (saturated with 10 mM Tris-HCl pH 7.5, 100 mM NaCL, 1 mM EDTA) and 100 ml chloroform isoamylalcohol (v/v 49:1) are added, the tubes vortexed for 10 s and placed on ice for 15 minutes. After centrifugation at 4° C for 15 min at 10000 g the aqueous phase is transferred to a fresh tube and mixed with 1 Vol isopropanol. Pellets are washed twice with 70 % ethanol and dissolved in H$_2$O (purest quality available). 10 ml EDTA blood yield approximately 25 µg RNA.

2. cDNA synthesis

For first strand cDNA synthesis 20 µg of total RNA are used. These are incubated with 200 ng of oligonucleotide 1 as primer and 200 units of reverse transcriptase (MMLV, preferably Superscript, BRL) with 40 units RNasin (Boehringer, FRG or Promega, USA) according to the manufacturer's recommendations.

3. cDNA amplification

Due to the extreme scarcity of ectopic transcripts a two-stage amplification is obligatory (Fig. 1). For the first round PCR the cDNA-primer (oligonucleotide 1) can be used together with an upstream primer (oligonucleotide 2) or a pair of primers both 5' to the cDNA primer (oligonucleotide 2 and 3). 1/25 of the first round PCR is subjected to a second round of amplification using 1 or 2 nested primers (internal to the primers of the first round). This primer "switch" serves to reduce non-specific coamplification of fragments with homologies with the oligonucleotides used before.

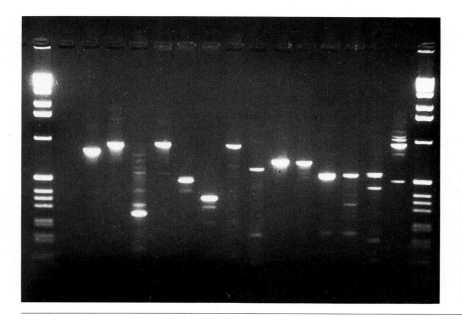

Figure 2: Ectopic transcripts of the DMD/BMD gene reverse-transcribed and amplified. The outside lanes are size standards (kb-ladder, BRL), the internal lanes are overlapping fragments covering the 5' part of the coding sequence over a length of 8 kb (courtesy of F. Rininsland).

Results

According to the strategy illustrated in Fig.1 the complete mRNA of the DMD/BMD gene can be reverse-transcribed and amplified using total RNA of peripheral blood lymphocytes. Fig.2 shows 14 overlapping fragments together covering the first 8 kb of the coding sequence. Approximately 60 % of DMD/BMD patients exhibit deletions, which can be identified in so-called "multiplex" amplifications. Due to the presence of a "normal" X-chromosome in female carriers, heterozygote detection using cDNA blots is difficult. Other possible techniques, e.g. pulsed field gel electrophoresis or CISS hybridization, are very complicated. Ectopic RNA analysis in these cases can be used to show pathological transcripts in the patients as well as in female carriers (Schlösser et al., 1990).

If no deletion is apparent after electrophoresis of the amplification products, mutations in the coding sequence can be identified by direct sequencing (Berg 1990). This step can be accelerated using one of the novel scanning techniques, e.g. chemical mismatch analysis, DGGE or SSCP analysis. A retrospective analysis of 72 sequenced CF alleles demonstrated an extremely high sensitivity and specificity of the rapid SSCP analysis (Plieth 1991).

Aberrant transcripts should be readily detectable and the regions in question could be analysed subsequently. Furthermore, if a mutation, responsible for aberrant transcripts, is not in the immediate vicinity of an exon (e.g. creation of a novel splice site within an intron) this mutation might go unnoticed in DNA analysis, since large introns are not normally sequenced. It remains to be seen, whether ectopic RNA analysis is also suitable for the detection of mutations within promotor regions. Since Chelly et al. (1991) reported that ectopic transcription proceeds through the usual promoters, such mutations might also influence the rate of ectopic transcription.

References

1. Berg LP, Wieland K, Millar DS, Schlösser M, Wagner M, Kakkar VV, Reiss J, Cooper DN. Detection of a novel point mutation causing haemophilia A by PCR/direct sequencing of ectopically transcribed factor VIII mRNA. 1990, Hum Genet 85, 655-658

2. Chelly J, Concordet JP, Kaplan JC, Kahn A. Illegitimate transcription: Transcription of any gene in any cell type. 1989, Proc Natl Acad Sci USA 86, 2617-2621

3. Chelly J, Hugnot JP, Concordet JP, Kaplan JC, Kahn A. Illegitmate (or ectopic) transcription proceeds through the usual promoters. 1991, Biochem Biophys Res Commun 178, 553-557

4. Chomczynski P, Sacchi N. Single-step method of RNA isolation by acid guanidinium thioisocyanate-phenol-chloroform extraction. 1987, Anal Biochem 162, 156-159

5. Plieth J, Rininsland F, Schlösser M, Cooper DN, Reiss J. Single strand conformation polymorphism (SSCP) analysis of exon 11 of the CFTR gene reliably detects more than one third of non ΔF508 mutations in German Cystic Fibrosis patients. Hum Genet, in press

6. Reiss J, Cooper DN. Application of the polymerase chain reaction to the diagnosis of human genetic disease. 1990, Hum Genet 85, 1-8

7. Roberts RG, Barby TFM, Manners E, Bobrow M, Bentley DR. Direct detection of dystrophin gene rearrangements by analysis of dystrophin mRNA in peripheral blood lymphocytes. 1991, Am J Hum Genet 49, 298-310

8. Sarkar G, Sommer SS. Access to a messenger RNA sequence or its protein product is not limited by tissue or species specificity. 1990, Science 244:331-334

9. Schloesser M, Slomski R, Wagner M, Reiss J, Berg LP, Kakkar VV, Cooper DN. Characterization of pathological dystrophin transcripts from the lymphocytes of a muscular dystrophy carrier. 1990, Mol Biol Med 7, 519-523

10. Slomski R, Schloesser M, Chlebowska H, Reiss J, Engel W. Detection of human spermatid-specific transcripts in peripheral blood lymphocytes of males and females. 1990, Hum Genet 87, 307-310

Acknowledgements

I thank my dear colleagues David N. Cooper (London) and Ryszard Slomski (Poznan) for their persistent cooperation and all the fun we had with it.

Suppliers of specialist items

Advanced Magnetics, Inc., 61 Mooney Street, Cambridge, MA 02138, USA

Ambion Inc., 2130 Woodward St. #200, Austin, Texas 78744-1832, USA

Amersham International PLC, Life Sciences Business, 1 Amersham Place, Little Chalfont, Bucks, HP7 9NA, UK; Amersham Buchler GmbH & Co.KG, Gieselweg 1, D-3300 Braunschweig, Germany

Amicon Div. W.R.Grace & Co.-Conn, 72 Cherry Hill Drive, Beverly, MA, 01915, USA

Applied Biosystems, Inc., 850 Lincoln Center Drive, Foster City, CA 94404, USA

Bachofer GmbH, P.O.Box 7058, D-7410 Reutlingen, Germany

Beckman Instruments, Inc., 2500 Harbor Blvd. Fullerton, CA 92634, USA; Frankfurter Ring 115, D-8000 München 40, Germany

Becton Dickinson, Immunocytometry Systems, 2350 Qume Dr., San Jose, CA 95131, USA; Tullastr. 8-12, D-6900 Heidelberg, Germany

Biochrom KG, Leonorenstr. 2-6, D-1000 Berlin 46, Germany

Bio-Med, Gesellschaft für Biotechnologie, Schloß Ditfurth, D-8729 Theres, Germany

Bio-Rad Laboratories/Chemical Div., 3300 Regatta Boulevard, Richmond, CA 94804, USA

Boehringer Mannheim Biochemicals, P.O.Box 50414, Indianapolis, IN 46250, USA; Sandhofer Str. 116, D-6800 Mannheim 31, Germany

Cangene Corporation, 3403 American Drive, Mississauga, Ontario L4V1T4, Canada

Clontech Laboratories, Inc., 4030 Fabian Way, Palo Alto, CA 94303, USA

Corbett Research, distributed in Europe by Labortechnik Fröbel, Hannoversche Straße 27a, D-1040 Berlin, Germany

Coy Coporation, 22 Metty Drive, Ann Arbor, Michigan 48103, USA

Diagen GmbH, Niederheiderstr. 3, D-4000 Düsseldorf; Qiagen Inc., 9259 Eton Ave, Chatsworth, CA 91311, USA

Drummond Scientific Company, 500 Parkway, Box 700, Broomall, PA 19008, USA

DuPont de Nemours GmbH, Du-Pont-Str. 1, D-6380 Bad Homburg, Germany

Dunn Labortechnik GmbH, Postfach 1104, D-5464 Asbach, Germany

Dynal AS, P.O.Box 158 Skoyen, N-0212 Oslo, Norway; 475 Northern Blvd., Great Neck, NY 11021, USA

Epicentre Technologies, 1202 Ann Street, Madison, Wi 53713, USA

Eppendorf-Netheler-Hinz GmbH, Barkhausenweg 1, D-2000 Hamburg 63, Germany; 45635 Northport Loop East, Fremont, CA 94538, USA

Ericomp, 6044 Cornerstone Court West, Suite E, San Diego, California 92121, USA

Fluka Chemical Corp., 980 S. Second Street, Ronkonkoma, NY 11779-7238, USA

FMC BioProducts, 5 Maple Street, Rockland, ME 04841, USA; FMC BioProducts Europe, Risingevej 1, DK-2665 Vallensbaek Strand, Denmark

Fröbel Labortechnik, Hannoversche Straße 27a, D-1040 Berlin, Germany

Gene-Trak Systems, Framingham, Massachusetts, USA

GIBCO BRL Life Technologies, Inc., Industrial Bioproducts, P.O.Box 6009, Gaithersburg, MD 20877, USA; Life Technologie Ltd., European Division, P.O.Box 35, Trident House, Renfrew Road, Paisley, PA3 4EF, Scotland

Glen Research Corporation, 44901 FalconPlace, Sterling, VA 22170, USA

Greiner GmbH, Postfach 1162, D-7743 Frickenhausen, Germany

Heraeus Instruments, Inc., 111-A Corporate Blvd., S. Plainfield, NJ 07080, USA

Hoefer Scientific Instruments, 654 Minnesota Street, Box 77387, San Francisco, California 94107-0387, USA

Hoffmann-La Roche AG, Diagnostica, Emil-Barell-Str. 1, D-7889 Grenzach-Wyhlen 1, Germany

Hybaid National Labnet, P.O. Box 841, Woodbridge, NJ 07095, USA

Idaho Technology, USA, phone: 001-208-5246354, USA

Invitrogen Corporation, 11588 Sorrento Valley Road #20, San Diego, CA 92121, USA

Knauer, Gerate GmbH & Co KG, Heuchelheimer Straße 9, D-6380 Bad Homburg v.d.H., Germany

Lark Sequencing Technologies Inc., 9545 Katy Freeway, Suite 200, Housten TX 77024-9870, USA

E. Merck, Reagents Division, Frankfurter Str. 250, P.O.Box 4119, D-6100 Darmstadt, Germany

MilliGen/Biosearch, Division of Millipore, 186 Middlesex Turnpike, Burlington, MA 01803, USA

Millipore Ltd., The Boulevard, Blackmoor Lane, Watford, Hertfordshire, WD1 2RA, UK; Hauptstr. 87, D-6236 Eschborn, Germany

MJ Research Inc., 24 Bridge Street, Watertown, Massachusetts 02172, USA

National Biosciences, 3650 Annapolis Lane, Plymouth, MN 55447, USA

Novagen, 565 Science Dr., Madison, Wi 53711, USA

A/S Nunc, P.O.Box 280, Kamstrup, DK-4000 Roskilde, Denmark; Hagenauer Str. 21a, D-6200 Wiesbaden, Germany

Organon Teknika, Boseind 15, 5281 RM Boxtel, The Netherlands

Peninsula Laboratories, Inc., 611 Taylor Way, Belmont, CA 94002, USA; Neckarstaden 10, D-6900 Heidelberg, Germany

Perkin-Elmer Cetus Instruments, 761 Main Avenue, Norwalk, CT 06859-0251, USA; P.O.Box 101164, D-7770 Überlingen, Germany

Pharmacia LKB Biotechnology AB, Bjorkgatan 30, Uppsala, Sweden; 800 Centennial Avenue, Piscataway, NJ 08855-1327, USA; Munzinger Str. 9, D-7800 Freiburg, Germany

Polaroid Corp., Technical Imaging Products, 575 Technology Square, Cambridge, MA 02139, USA; Ashley Road, St. Albans, Herts, AL1 5PR, UK

Polygen GmbH, Karlstr.10, D-6070 Langen, Germany

Promega Corp., 2800 Woods Hollow Road, Madison, WI 53711-5399, USA

Savant Instruments Inc., 110-103 Bi-County-Blvd., Farmingdale, NY 11735, USA

Schleicher & Schüll, Inc., 10 Optical Avenue, Keene, NH 03431, USA; P.O.Box 4, D-3354 Dassel, Germany

Serva Feinbiochemica GmbH & Co., Carl-Benz-Str. 7, D-6900 Heidelberg, Germany; 50 A & S Drive, Paramus, NJ 07652, USA

Sigma Chemical Co., P.O.Box 14508, St. Louis, MO 63178, USA; Fancy Road, Poole, Dorset BH17 7NH, UK

Stratagene, 11099 N. Torrey Pines Rd., La Jolla, CA 92037, USA; P.O.Box 105466, D-6900 Heidelberg, Germany

Synthetic Genetics, 3347 Industrial Court, San Diego, CA 92121, USA

Techne Incorporated, 3700 Brunswick Pike, Princeton, NJ 08540, USA

Tri-Continent Scientific Inc., 12555 Loma Rica Drive, Grass Valley, CA 95945, USA

Tropix Incorporated, 47 Wiggins Avenue, Bedford, Massachusetts 01730, USA

United States Biochemical Corp., P.O.Box 22400, Cleveland, OH 44122, USA; P.O.Box 2561, D-6380 Bad Homburg, Germany

Whatman BioSystems Inc., 22 Bridewell Place, Clifton, NJ 07014, USA; Springfield Mill, Maidstone, Kent, ME14 2LE, UK

List of Contributors

Bamborschke, Stephan
Department of Neurology, University of Köln, Joseph-Stelzmannstr. 9, 5000 Köln 41, FRG

Bartsch, Georg
Department of Urology, University of Innsbruck, Anichstr. 35, 6020 Innsbruck, Austria

Bauer-Hofmann, Richard
German Cancer Research Center, Project Group "Tumor Promotion in the Liver", 6900 Heidelberg, FRG

Bocklage, H.
Institute for Science of Health and Microbiology, University of Würzburg, Josef-Schneider-Str. 2, 8700 Würzburg, FRG

Bottner, Claudia
Private Institute of Immunology and Molecular Genetics, 7500 Karlsruhe, FRG

Buchmann, Albrecht
Institute of Toxicology, University of Tübingen, 7400 Tübingen, FRG

Eberle, Johannes
Department of Urology, University of Innsbruck, Anichstr. 35, 6020 Innsbruck, Austria

Ehninger, G.
Medical Clinics, Department II, Transplantation-Immunology and Immunohematology, University of Tübingen, Otfried-Müllerstr. 10, 7400 Tübingen, FRG

Einsele, H.
Medical Clinics, Department II, Transplantation-Immunology and Immunohematology, University of Tübingen, Otfried-Müllerstr. 10, 7400 Tübingen, FRG

Finckh, U.
Department of Neurology, Klinikum Steglitz, Free University of Berlin, Hindenburgdamm 30, 1000 Berlin 45, FRG

Flügel, Rolf M.
German Cancer Research Center, "Human Retrovirus Group", Im Neuenheimer Feld 280, 6900 Heidelberg, FRG

Gieselmann, V.
Institute for Biochemistry, Department II, Gosslerstr. 12d, 3400 Göttingen, FRG

Heesemann, J.
Institute for Science of Health and Microbiology, University of Würzburg, Josef-Schneider-Str. 2, 8700 Würzburg, FRG

Hahn, U.
Institute of Chemistry, Department of cristallography, Fabeckstr.4, 1000 Berlin 33, FRG

Henne, K.W.
Fred Hutchinson Cancer Research Center, Pathology Section, SC-111, 1124 Columbia Street, Seattle, USA

Huhn, Dieter
Klinikum Rudolf Virchow, Free University of Berlin, Department of Internal Medicine/Hematology, Spandauer Damm 130, 1000 Berlin 19, FRG

Kadenbach, B.
Institute for Biochemistry, Department of Chemistry, Philipps University, Hans-Meerwein-Str., 3550 Marburg, FRG

Karch, H.
Institute for Science of Health and Microbiology, University of Würzburg, Josef-Schneider-Str. 2, 8700 Würzburg, FRG

Kaspar, Felizia
Department of Urology, University of Innsbruck, Anichstr. 35, 6020 Innsbruck, Austria

Kaufhold, Achim
Institute for Medical Microbiology, Technical University of Aachen, Pauwelsstr. 30, 5100 Aachen, FRG

Klimek, Fritz
German Cancer Research Center, Project Group "Tumor Promotion in the Liver", 6900 Heidelberg, FRG

Klocker, Helmut
Department of Urology, University of Innsbruck, Anichstr. 35, 6020 Innsbruck, Austria

Köhler, Gerwald
Institute of Microbiology, Technical University Munich, Arcisstr. 21, 8000 Munich 2, FRG

Kölmel, H.W.
Klinikum Rudolf Virchow, Free University of Berlin, Department of Neurology, Cerebrospinal Laboratory, Spandauer Damm 130, 1000 Berlin 19, FRG

Landt, O.
Institute of Chemistry, Department of cristallography, Fabeckstr.4, 1000 Berlin 33, FRG

Lange, R.
Klinikum Rudolf Virchow, Free University of Berlin, Department of Neurology, Cerebrospinal Laboratory, Spandauer Damm 130, 1000 Berlin 19, FRG

Liu, Edison
Lineberger Cancer Research Center, University of North Carolina, Chapel Hill, NC, 27599-7295, USA

Lingenfelter, P.A.
Fred Hutchinson Cancer Research Center, Pathology Section, SC-111, 1124 Columbia Street, Seattle, USA

Ludwig, Wolfgang
Institute of Microbiology, Technical University Munich, Arcisstr. 21, 8000 Munich 2, FRG

Melzer, Beate
Institute for Medical Microbiology, Technical University of Aachen, Pauwelsstr. 30, 5100 Aachen, FRG

Müller, C.A.
Medical Clinics, Department II, Transplantation-Immunology and Immunohematology, University of Tübingen, Otfried-Müllerstr. 10, 7400 Tübingen, FRG

Müller, M.
Medical Clinics, Department II, Transplantation-Immunology and Immunohematology, University of Tübingen, Otfried-Müllerstr. 10, 7400 Tübingen, FRG

Muranyi, Walter
German Cancer Research Center, "Human Retrovirus Group", Im Neuenheimer Feld 280, 6900 Heidelberg, FRG

Myerson, David
Fred Hutchinson Cancer Research Center, Pathology Section, SC-111, 1124 Columbia Street, Seattle, USA

Neubauer, Andreas
Klinikum Rudolf Virchow, Free University of Berlin, Department of Internal Medicine/Hematology, Spandauer Damm 130, 1000 Berlin 19, FRG

Neubauer, Beatrix
Klinikum Rudolf Virchow, Free University of Berlin, Department of Internal Medicine/Hematology, Spandauer Damm 130, 1000 Berlin 19, FRG

Podbielski, Andreas
Institute for Medical Microbiology, Technical University of Aachen, Pauwelsstr. 30, 5100 Aachen, FRG

Porr, Angelika
Department of Neurology, University of Köln, Joseph-Stelzmannstr. 9, 5000 Köln 41, FRG

Rehse-Küpper, Brunhilde,
Department of Neurology, University of Köln, Joseph-Stelzmannstr. 9, 5000 Köln 41, FRG

Renz, M.
Private Institute of Immunology and Molecular Genetics, 7500 Karlsruhe, FRG

Reiss, Jochen
Institute for Human Genetics, University of Göttingen, Gosslerstr. 12d, 3400 Göttingen, FRG

Saal, J.G.
Medical Clinics, Department II, Transplantation-Immunology and Immunohematology, University of Tübingen, Otfried-Müllerstr. 10, 7400 Tübingen, FRG

Schleifer, Karl Heinz
Institute of Microbiology, Technical University Munich, Arcisstr. 21, 8000 Munich 2, FRG

Schmidt, Christian A.
Klinikum Rudolf Virchow, Free University of Berlin, Department of Internal Medicine/Hematology, Spandauer Damm 130, 1000 Berlin 19, FRG

Schwarz, Michael
German Cancer Research Center, Project Group "Tumor Promotion in the Liver", 6900 Heidelberg, FRG

Seelig, H.P.
Private Institute of Immunology and Molecular Genetics, 7500 Karlsruhe, FRG

Seelig, Renate
Private Institute of Immunology and Molecular Genetics, 7500 Karlsruhe, FRG

Seibel, P.
Institute for Biochemistry, Department of Chemistry, Philipps University, Hans-Meerwein-Str., 3550 Marburg, FRG

Siegert, Wolfgang
Klinikum Rudolf Virchow, Free University of Berlin, Department of Internal Medicine/Hematology, Spandauer Damm 130, 1000 Berlin 19, FRG

Steidle, M.
Medical Clinics, Department II, Transplantation-Immunology and Immunohematology, University of Tübingen, Otfried-Müllerstr. 10, 7400 Tübingen, FRG

Weisser, C.F.
Institute for Ecological Studies, 6729 Wörth/Rhein, FRG

Zentraf, H.W.,
German Cancer Research Center, 6900 Heidelberg, FRG

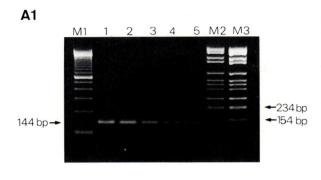

Figure A, chapter 14. A1: Agarose gel analysis of a 144bp PCR fragment (5SrRNA) from Legionella pneumophila (ATCC 43110 Oxford). 10µl, 7.5µl, 5µl, 2.5µl and 1.25µl (lane **1 to 5**) of a 100µl PCR sample were separated in a 3% agarose/Nusieve™ gel in 1xTBE buffer. Molecular weight markers: M1: 1µl 100bp-ladder (Gibco BRL), M2 and M3: 1µl and 2µl, respectively of the Boehringer VI marker (Boehringer Mannheim. PCR products and markers were visualized by ethidium bromide staining. Quantification of the 144bp fragments in lane 1-5 in correspondence to the 154bp fragment of Boehringer VI (M2: 8ng, M3: 16ng) lane **1** represents about 60ng product and lane 5 about 8ng. The eightfold amount (80-100ng) is sufficient to be sequenced in the assay described in the chapter. **A2-A4:** Demonstration of the sequencing results of the 144bp 5srRNA fragment of Legionella pneumophila using different amounts of DNA template for the sequencing reaction. In A2 250-300ng template has been used, in A3 60ng and in A4 30ng, respectively. It is clearly shown that there are no differences in quality whether the sequencing reaction was performed with 250-300ng or 60ng template. Below the cut-off from about 60ng we were not able to get sufficient sequencing signals (A4). For semiquantitative agarose gels see chapter 10.1.4

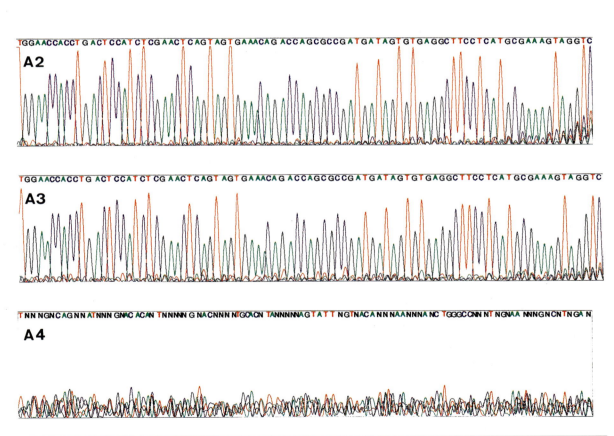

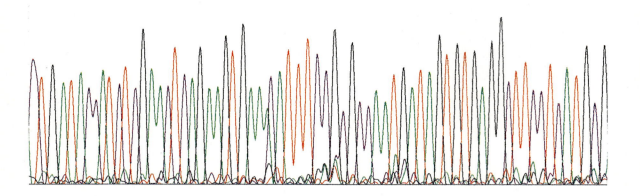

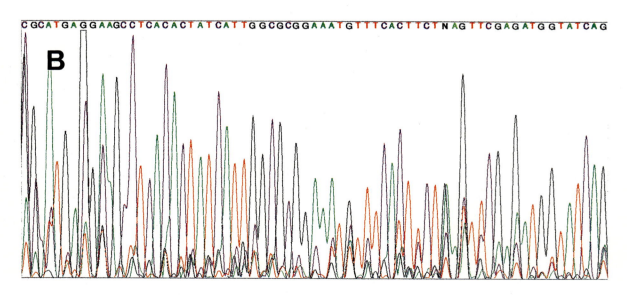

Figure B, chapter 14: Analyzed sequence data of a 144bp PCR fragment from the 5SrRNA gene of *Legionella bozemanae*. Immobilized strand (A) was sequenzed by Sequenase™, the eluted strand (B) by Taq polymerase. Note the even peak height of the four nucleotides using Sequenase™.

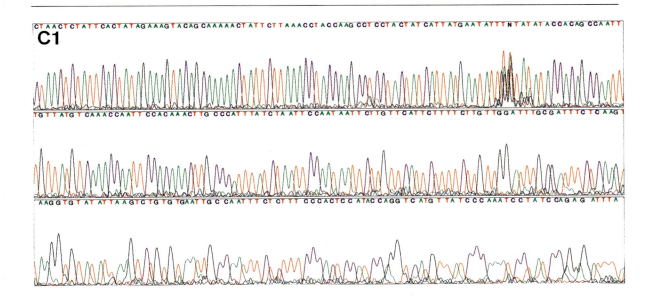

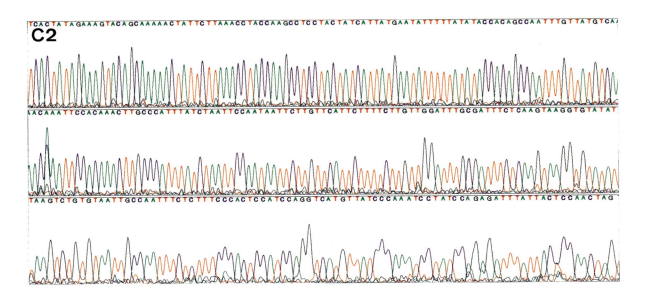

Figure C, chapter 14: Analyzed sequence data for a 501bp PCR fragment from the env-region of a HIV-1-DNA isolate performing solid-phase sequencing (Sequenase™). **C1:** Data obtained in manually performed sequencing. **C2:** Data obtained using the robotic workstation Biomek 1000 and PolySeq™. For further details see the procedures described in chapter 14, method 1 and 2..

ABC nuclease	155		249, 253
Acetone	52	Allele-specific primer	151
Acetonitril (HPLC grade)	230	Allelic mutation	136
Acid citrate dextrose	71	Allelity	151, 153
Acid guanidinium thiocyanate-phenol-chloroform extraction	92	Alpha-interferon gene	A11
		Alu family	39
Acridine orange	131	Alu PCR amplification	190
Acrylamide stock solution	127, 161, 176	Alu PCR assay	
		- efficiency	189
Actin, beta	102	- sensitivity	189
Aedes ägypti	A34, A35	- specificity	189
Aedes vexans	A34, A35	Alu repeat sequence	189
Agar plate	212	Alu repeats, polymorphism	164
Agarose gel	25, 27, 187	Alu-specific primer	189, 190
- casting	115	Alu-specific sequence	189
- electrophoresis	112	Amidite group	225
- electrophoresis buffers	112	Amidite monomer	225
- electrophoresis equipment	112	Amidite, acridine	233
- affinity	170	Amino acid, conserved	224
- ethidium bromide stained	109	Amino linker	240
Air, filter	64	Ammonium acetate	54, 95
- heat transfer	261	Ammonium bicarbonate	235
Air-conditioning	64	Ammonium chloride	54
Air-cycling	262	Ammonium hydroxide	226
Alkaline lysis	70, 75, 79, 88, A37	Ammonium persulfate (APS)	125, 161, 176
Allele	34, 39, 136, 137	Ampicillin	212
		Amplification	
Allele-specific amplification (ASA)	34, 35, 149, 150	- artifact	7
		- cycle	7
- 3'-end mismatch	149, 150	- efficiency	58, 202-206
- cycle number	151		
- dNTP concentration	150	- exponential	184, 198, 201
- double ASA	151		
- magnesium concentration	150	- grade	202
- one-tube nested PCR	152	- linear	184, 204
- optimization	150	- product	3, 4, 7, 8, 9, 11, 15
- primer concentration	150		
- specifity	150, 151	- biotinylated	170
Allele-specific hybridization	37	- size	14
Allele-specific oligonucleotide (ASO) hybridization	153, A1	- specifity	136, 141
		- structure	14
- optimization	154	- high-molecular-weight	220
Allele-specific oligonucleotide probe	137	- radioactive-labeled, detection	126
Allele-specific PCR (ASP)	34, 35, 149, 150,	Amplification refractory mutation system	34, 35, 149
		AmpliTaq™	7-9, 247

AmpliWave	262	Auto-immune reaction	A19
AmpliWax	16, 65, 132	Autoclave	64
AMPPD	122, A17	Automated DNA sequencing	180
Analytical PCR	4, 7, 12, 22	Bacillus stearothermophilus	245, 246, 252
Androgen receptor, cDNA	A5, A10		
Anion-exchange chromatography	227	Bacteria, lysing	89
Annealing	15, 56	- phylogenetic relationship	A57
- site	2, 4	- phylogenetic tree	A56
- temperature	4, 5, 6, 11, 23, 24, 26, 35, 40, 41, 51, 105, 223, 224	- DNA	137, 265
		- overgrowth	68
		- rRNA	A57
		Bacteriophage Qß replicase	268
		Balanced salt solution (BSS)	A64
- time	5, 6, 26, 41, 188	Bannwarth syndrome	A18
		Base monomer	224
- dissociation kinetics	6	BCIP	A39
Anopheles maculipennis	A34, A35	Bcr gene	A11
Anti-biotin alkaline-phosphatase conjugate	264	BCR-ABL	99
Antibody, calcium-dependent	209	Beads	173, 176
- DNA contamination	63	Bel-gene	A26, A27, A30
Arbo-virus	A36		
Argon ion laser	169	Benzoyl group	226
ARMS, see amplification refractory mutation system		Beta-A-globin genotypes	265
		BH10, HIV-clone	57
Arthropod vector	A32	Binary buffer system (HPLC)	227
Artifacts, amplification	7	Biopsy material	51, 76, 81
Arylsulfatase A polypeptide	A45	- prostate	A10
- activity	A44	Biotin	170, 226, 240
- deficiency	A44		
- pseudodeficiency	A44, A46	- phosphoramidite	233
- pseudodeficiency allele	A44, A46, A47	- p-dimethylamino cinnamaldehyde colorimetric test	239
- pseudodeficiency allele, mutation	A45, A46	- photoactive	236
- pseudodeficiency allele, specific amplification	A45, A46	- dUTP	28
		- XX-NHS ester	234, 239
- pseudodeficiency allele, specific primer	A46	Biotinylated PCR product, fully automatic sequencing procedure	180
ASA, see allele-specific amplification			
ASO, see allele-specific oligonucleotide hybridization		- manual sequencing procedure	172
ASP, see allele-specific PCR		- single-stranded PCR fragment	176
Asymmetric PCR	34, 169	Blood	52, 68
- sequencing	A10	- cell	69
Asymmetric reamplification	191	Blot membrane	117, 122, 154
ATP synthase	A48, A49, A51		
		Blotting procedures, see hybridization	
Auto extension	6	Blunt end restriction sites	138, 185,

		- synthesis	108, A4, A64
	187, 208, 248		
- staggered end	139	- amplification	A5, A64
- cloning procedure	208	Ceftriaxone	A17, A19
Bone marrow transplantation (BMT)	A22	Cell	68, 93, 95
Booster PCR	41	- lysis	53, 81
Borrelia burgdorferi	45, A15, A18	- lysis buffer	52
		- morphology	219
- flagellin gene	A17, A19	- smear	51, 219
- ospA gene	A17	- suspension	219
Bouin's fixative	52	- choroid plexus	219
Bovine serum albumin (BSA), DNA contamination	63	Central nervous system cells	220
		$(dT)_{17}$-primer, adaptor	197, 198
Bromphenol blue marker	129, 228	Cerebroside loading test	A44
Bronchoalveolar fluid	73	Cerebrospinal fluid	51, 76, A16, A21
Bst polymerase	252		
- DNA sequencing	252	Cetylpyridinium bromide	235
- fidelity	252	Chain termination	8, 169
- polymerization rate	252	Chaotropic agent	91
Buffered neutral formalin (BNF)	52	Chelating resin Chelex^R 100	79
Buffy coat	70, A37	Chemical cleavage of mismatches (CCM)	155, 156
Butanol	236	Chemical mismatch analysis	A65
C-abl gene	A11	Chemiluminescence-based detection	117, 122, 124
C-Ha-ras	A1		
C-Ha-ras codon 61	A1, A2	- background	122
C-Ha-ras mutations	A2	- film exposure	124
C-Ki-ras	A1	- sensitivity	122
C^7-dATP	169	Chemotherapeutic agent	99
C^7-dGTP	169, 175, 177	Chloroform	91, 187
		Chloroform/isoamyl alcohol	83
Cacodylate buffer	237	Chromogen	
Calf intestinal alkaline phosphatase	192	- BCIP	A38
Calf thymus DNA	246	- detection system	123
Candida albicans	45	- detection system, background	122
Capillary slab gel electrophoresis	168, 205	- NBT	A38, A39
Capillary thermal sequencer	261	Chromosome 9	A11
Carbodiimide binding	205	Chromosome 22	A11
Carboxyfluorescein [FAM]-labeled	164	Chromosome centromere	39
Carnoy's fixative	52	Circularization	184, 185, 187, 189
Carrier DNA	A37		
Carrier RNA	95	Citrate, acid citrate dextrose	71
Carryover	66	Clarke's fixative	52
- prevention	63, 66	Cleavage site	38, 185
cDNA	91, 99, 100, 193, 196, 197	Cloned rRNA, DNA sequencing	A57
		Cloning	136, 193, 208

- vector pKK233-2	211	Cytocentrifugation	219
CML, see leukemia, chronic myelogeneous		Cytochrome c oxidase	A48
CMV, see cytomegalovirus		Cytokines	A19
Coding DNA	39	Cytomegalovirus, see also human	
Codon	37, 38	cytomegalovirus	42, A22, A24
Complementary DNA, see also cDNA	99		
Contamination, see also cross-contamination	16, 18, 34, 52, 61-63, 65-66, 81-82, 190-191, 224, 246	- strain AD169	A23
		- active infection	201
		- culture	201
		- disease	A24
		- DNA	79, 201
		- infection	A22, A24
		- transcript	107
- risk	35, 79	Cytoplasmic DNA	69
- with DNA	94, 102, 104, 106, 107	Cytoplasmic RNA	69, 103
		D(T)$_{17}$-adapter	196
		D/ddATP termination mix	175, 177
- DNases	140	D/ddCTP termination mix	175, 177
- post-PCR	63	D/ddGTP termination mix	175, 178
- pre-PCR	63	D/ddTTP termination mix	175, 178
- prevention	64	DAF, see DNA amplification fingerprinting	
- ribonuclease	90	dATP tailing	194
- sources	63, 64	ddNTP	8
- sporadic	61, 62	Decontamination	65, 66
Control, DNA positive	62, 64, 141	Deep Vent DNA polymerase	249
Cosolvent	55, 57	- thermostability	249
Covalink NH plate	204, 205	Degradation	68
CPG carrier	225	Denaturing polyacrylamide gel	126, 169, 170
Cross-contamination	13, 16, 53, 63, 79, 81, 89, 93, 116, 170	- gradient gel electrophoresis (DGGE)	159, 160, 161
		Denaturation	2, 6, 41, 57
Cross-hybridization, see also hybridization	120	- of PCR fragments	109
Cross-link DNA	83	- temperature	6, 16, 35, 36, 255
Cross-link RNA	83		
Cryostat microtome	A1	- time	6
CsCl	91, 95, 104	Denaturing polyacrylamide gel	228
CSF, see cerebrospinal fluid		Denhardt's solution	154, A23
CSPD, see also AMPPD and chemiluminescence	122	Deoxynucleotide triphosphate	2, 4, 9, 244, 245
Culex p. pipiens	A34	DEPC treating	90, 91, 94, 96, 107
Cycle number	26, 255		
- sequencing	181	Dephosphorylation	193
- temperature profile	51	Deproteinization	91
- amplification	193	Detection of digoxigenin labeled hybrids	122
Cycling time reproducibility	262	- with AMPPD	122

- with BCIP	122	- dependent polymerase	100
- with NBT	122	- DNA hybrids	156
- chemoluminescent Dioxetane substrate for CSPD	122	- exon	99, 102, 105, 195
- nonradioactive	117	- extraction	65, 70, 71, 74
Detergent	53, 54	- automated	88, 89
DGGE analysis	159, 160, A65	- standardization	89
Dideoxy sequencing	248, 249	- fingerprint	39, 40
Dideoxy-mediated chain termination	A28	- fragment, branched	159
Diethyl pyrocarbonate, see also DEPC	90	- intron	99, 102, 104, 105
Diethylnitrosamine	A1		
Differential liquid phase hybridization	203, 205	- isolation	53, 68, 69, 79, 81, 85
DIG labelled DNA, see also digoxigenin	A42	- loss of DNA	79
DIG probe, see also digoxigenin	A37, A42	- needle biopsy, see also biopsy	79
Digestion using endonucleases	184, 186, 187, 189	- solid tissue	79
Digoxigenin labelling	A37	- library	185
Digoxigenin-11-dUTP (DIG)	29, A37	- ligase-encoding gene (ligT)	264
- in situ hybridization	A41	- loss	83
- incorporation	A40	- mapping	136
- labelled double-stranded probes	A41	- marker	140
Dimethoxytrityl (DMT)	225	- melting temperature (Tm)	3
Dimethyl sulfoxide (DMSO)	55, 57, 251, A5	- mutant	155
		- polymerase, see also polymerase	1, 3, 7, 37, 41
Direct sequencing of PCR fragments	168, A4		
Dissociation kinetics of hybrids	11	- polymerase II	244
Disulfide bond	93	- polymerase III	244
Dithiothreitol (DTT)	109, 196	- thermostable	245
DMD/BMD gene	A63, A65	- cycle number	255
DMSO, see dimethyl sulfoxide		- denaturation temperature	255
DMT-on synthesis, see also primer synthesis	232	- dNTP concentration	255
DNA		- enzyme concentration	255
- amplification fingerprinting (DAF)	38, 132	- error rate	254
- blot transfer, see also hybridization	117	- fidelity	253, 255
- capillary transfer, see also hybridization	117	- mismatches	253
- carry-over	89	- proofreading activity	253
- cleavage site	138	- terminal mismatch	253
- coding sequence	37	- infidelity	255
- concentration	203	- $MgCl_2$ concentration	255
- content	68	- mutation frequency	255
- damage	66	- proofreading activity	249, 255
- degradation	53, 66, 85	- polymorphisms	159
- enzymatic	66	- precipitation	83, 86
- denaturation	2, 55, 56, 159	- purification	65, 79, 193, 203

- sample	13, 18, 19, 84	Epidermal growth factor receptor	A5
- yield	79, 88	Epstein-Barr virus	42
- secondary structure	56	Escherichia coli (E. coli)	244, 247
- segments with overlapping cohesive termini	219	- ligase gene	264
		- pol I	246
- sequencing, automation	168	- pol I, fidelity	101
- chain termination method	A34, A50, A57	- rRNA	95
		- 23SrRNA	A58
		- RNase H	267
- electrophoretic separation	168	Ethanol	54, 83, 86, 87, 94, 95
- fluorescence detection	168		
- radio-active experiment	168	- precipitation	52-54, 79, 89, 187, 188, 247
- solid-phase sequencing	168		
- strand breakage	65		
- synthesis, see also primer synthesis	2, 6	Ethidium bromide	7, 113, 115, 131, 140, 141, 188
- synthesizer	225		
DNase treatment	102		
- RNase-free	103		
DNaseI	103	Ethyldimethylaminopropyl carbodiimide	204
DNTP	5, 7-9, 12, 17, 18, 26	Exogenous ribonuclease, contamination	90
		Exonuclease activity	14, 244, 245, 248
DNTP concentration	9, 13, 51, 255	- 3'-5'	35, 244, 245, 250
Dopamine D2 receptor	151	- digestion	170
Dot blot procedure, see also hybridization	99, 119, 120	Extension rate, see also polymerase, DNA polymerase	246
Duchenne muscular dystrophy (DMD)	38, 143		
Duralon UV	117	- step	188
dUTP	66	- time	188
Dye-labelled strands	176	False-negative result	16, 22, 36, 37, 38, 62, 91, 102, 107, 151, 246
Dynabeads, see also beads	174		
- binding capacity	172		
- preparation	172		
Ectopic RNA analysis	A65		
- transcript	A63, A64	FAM, see also dye primer	174, 177
EDTA	8, 13, 18, 52, 68, 71, 82, 84, 140	Fetal diagnosis	38
		FICOLL-PAQUE	71, 72
		- density gradient centrifugation	84
Efficiency factor F of PCR amplification	203	Fidelity, see also polymersases	4, 8, 22, 246, 248, 253-255
Elongation rate, see also polymerase, DNA polymerase	6, 247		
		Filter hybridization, see also hybridization	29
Eluted strand, see also sequencing	171		
Endogenous RNases, inhibition	90	Fingerprint band	39
Endonucleases, see also restriction enzymes	136, 208	FITC	204, 205
Endonucleolytic cleavage	193	- final extension	7
Enterokinase	213	- absorption maximum	239

- labelling of primer	241	- mapping	40
- amidite	233	Genomic DNA	102, 104
Fixative		Genotype	38
- alcohol formalin	52	GITC buffer, see also guanidinium	A8
- Bouin's	52	Glass	
- buffered neutral formalin (BNF)	52	- bead	193, A34
- Carnoy's	52	- capillary	261
- Clarke's	52	Glassware	64, 90
- formalin-alcohol-acetic acid	52	Glucose-6-phosphatase	A1
- paraformaldehyde	52, 219	Glyceraldehyde 3-phosphate dehydrogenase	
- Zamboni's	52	(GAPDH)	A5
- Zenker's	52	Glycerin	A5
Flagellin primer, see also Borrelia		Glycerol	55, 57
burgdorferi	A20, A21	Glycolipid cerebroside sulfate	A44
Flow cytometry	A14	Guanidinium	
Fluorescein, see also FITC	226	- chloride	91
Fluorescein-isothiocyanate, see also FITC	241	- rhodanid method	81
Fluorescence detection	A6	- thiocyanate	91, 92, 94,
- Fluorescence sequencing	180		95, A4,
- single-stranded sequencing	170		A64
- -detecting system	204		
- -labeled primer	40, 168,	- phenol-chloroform-isomylalcohol	
	205	extraction	105
Fluorescent dye	204, 226	- CsCl ultracentrifugation method	95
Foamy virus	A27	GuSCN, see guanidinium thiocyanate	
Formalin-alcohol-acetic acid	52	Hair, human	68
Formamide	15, 18, 55,	Hairpin	14
	57, 58,	Haplotypes	151
	245, A5	HCMV, see cytomegalovirus	
- loading buffer	128	Heat-stable DNA polymerases, see also	
Freeze-and-thaw procedure	74, 80, 213	polymerase	253
		Heating	
G-C clamp	35, 36, 159	- block	64
Gel analysis, see also agarose,		- magnet block	180
polyacrylamide	15	- agitation function	180
- loading buffer (GLB)	113	- cooling performance	181
- retardation	159	- heating performance	181
Gelatine	54	Heating rate	260
- DNA contamination	63	Heatstable bacteria	245
Gene walking	37, 190,	Heme	69
	191	Hemoglobin	
GeneAmp PCR System 9600	261	- C (β^C) sequence	153
Genetic		- β^A sequence	153
- disease	38, A63	Heparin	13, 52, 68,
- linkage	38		71
- study	149	Heparinase	52

Hepatitis virus		- LTR	45
- A virus	42	HTLV-2 (tax)	45
- B virus	42	Human cytomegalovirus (HCMV), see	
- C virus (HCV)	42, A32, A34, A36	also cytomegalovirus	106, A22, A24, A37, A39, A41
- C virus (HCV), RNA	A34, A35	- strain AD169	A22
- D virus	42	- PCR-analysis	A23
- E virus (HEV)	A32, A33	Human dopamine D2 receptor	
- F virus (HFV)	A32, A34, A36	- biallelic polymorphic site	151
- non-A, non-B (HNANB)	A32, A33, A36	- gene	151, 164
		Human genome	39, 189
HER-2/neu proto-oncogene	A12	- size	68
Herpes infection	201	Human herpes virus 6 (HHV-6)	43
- active	201	Human papilloma virus	265
- latent	201	- type 6	43
Herpes simplex virus 1+2	43	- type 16	43
Heteroduplex, see also hybrids	155, 159, 253	- type 18	43
		- types 6-11	43
High-melting domain, see also DGGE	159	Human spumaretrovirus (HSRV)	A26, A27
High-performance liquid chromatography		- bel gene	A26
(HPLC)	226	- cDNA	A27, A30
HIV-1	56, 58, 144, 201, 209, 251, A22, A27	Hybridization	13, 37, 61, 120, 121, 185
- env	5, 44, 56, 57, 186	- digoxigenin-11-dUTP-labeled DNA probe	120
- gag	44	- liquid-phase	267
- LTR	44	- nonradioactive	117
- nef	44	- nonspecific	120
- nucleocapsid gene, chemical cleavage	158	- probe	26, 27, 34
- provirus	5, 56	- synthesis	35
- RNA	268, 269	- solution	121
- tat	44	- temperature	120, 122
- zidovudine (AZT) resistance	268	- time	A42
HIV-2 (LTR)	44	- wash solution	121
HLA-DQ	55	Hydroxylamine reaction	157
Homopolymer tail	154	Hydroxyquinoline	83
Hot start	4, 16, 17, 41, 65, 132, 247	Hypervariable regions of the genome (HVR)	39
		Hypoxanthine-guanine phosphoribosyl- transferase gene	38
- in-situ PCR	220	Ice, source of contamination	64
HSRV, see human spumaretrovirus		Illegitimate transcription, see also	
HTLV-1		ectopic transcripts	A63
- gag	44	Imidazole, 1-methyl	204

Immediate early antigen transcript, see also cytomegalovirus	106	Kearns-Sayre syndrome (KSS)	A49
Immunochemical quantification techniques, see also PCR and quantification	204	Kieselguhr-polydimethylacrylamide support	230
		Klenow enzyme	187, 208, 209, 242, 254
In situ hybridization (ISH)	29, 99, 219, A39		
- non-isotopic DNA-DNA	A37	Label	
In-situ polymerase chain reaction	219	- nonradioactive	27
In-vitro mutagenesis, see also mutagensis	216, A62	- buffer	239
In-vitro translation	40, 90	- nucleotide	27, A58
Incorporation of labels	27	- probe	37
Incorporation rate, see also polymerase	16	- PCR	28
Infectious agent	41, 62, 76, 81	LacZ ribosome binding site	211
		Lambda DNA	139
Infidelity of DNA polymerases	255	Laminar air flow	64
Inhibition of PCR reaction	51, 53, 54	Latex spheres, antifluorescein antibody-coated	264
Inner fragment PCR, see also nested PCR	5		
Inorganic pyrophosphatase	169	Laureth	12, 53
Inosine	38, 224	LCR, see ligase chain reaction	
Insertion site	185	Leber's hereditary optic neuropathy (LHON)	A50
Interferon	A12, A13	Legionella	64
- beta-1	A11, A13	- bozemanae, analyzed sequence data	185
Internal amplification control	35-37, 62, 100, 151, 202-204, 206	- pneumophila	45, 171
		- pneumophila, sequencing result	184
		Length polymorphism	39
		Lesch-Nyhan syndrome	38
Internal PCR, see also nested PCR	35	Leucocyte	69, 84
Interphase	93, 94	Leukemia, acute lymphoblastic (ALL)	A11
Intestinal pseudoobstruction with myopathy and ophthalmoplegia (CIPO)	A53	Leukemia	
		- ALL	A11, A13
Intracellular bacteria	73	- ALL, myeloid-antigen expression	A11
Intracellular pathogen	74	- chronic myelogeneous (CML)	99, A11
Intronless gene	102	- chronic myelogeneous, blastic phase	A11
Iodoacetic acid	103	Ligase, see also DNA ligase	136, 139, 184, 185, 187, 188, 191, 193, 212, 244, 264
Ion-exchange resin	176		
IPTG (isopropyl-ß-D-thiogalacto-pyranoside)	213		
ISH, see in situ hybridization			
Isobutyryl group	226		
Isopropanol	88, 94	- buffer	187, 264
Isopsoralen	66	- DNA contamination	63
Ixodes	A18, A34, A45	- mismatches	265
		Ligase chain reaction (LCR)	263
		- cloning	265
JOE, dye 174, 177		- genomic sequencing	265
		- in-vivo footprinting	265

Ligated products, detection	264	Methylmercuric hydroxide, see also	
Linearization	184, 185, 188, 191	MeHgOH	96, 107
		MgCl$_2$, see magnesium	
Linker	226	MgSO$_4$	248
Liver tumors	A1	MicroAmp reaction tube	261
Loading buffer	141, 162	Microtiter plate	170, 172, 180
Loss of DNA material	190, 191		
Low-melting domain, see also DGGE	159	Microwave systems	262
Luminescence detection, see also detection	63	Mineral oil, see also oil overlay	13, 19, 65
Lyme disease, see also Borrelia burgdorferi	A18	Minimum medium	212
Lymphocyte	69, 71, 72	Minisatellite	39
- ectopic transcript	A63	Minisatellite variant repeat	39
Lysis buffer	69, 81, 82, 84, 87, 88	Misincorporation, see also polymerases	254
		- rate, see also polymerases	101
Lysozyme	89, 213	Mismatch	8, 35, 37, 105, 136, 137, 248
M13 primer, see primer	A10		
Magnesium, Mg^{2+}	8, 9, 18, 26, 51, 54, 56, 107, 138, 139, 245, 246, 247, 255	Mismatch, 3'	38, 204
		Mispairing PCR	A50, A51, A53
		Mitochondrial disease	A48, A53
		- ATP synthesis	A48
		- deletion	A48
		- point mutation	A48
Magnetic beads, see also beads	170, 180	- myopathy	A48
Magnetic cell sorting	A14	- lactic acidosis and stroke-like episodes (MELAS)	A51
Manganese, Mn^{2+}	101, 169		
Mastermix	16, 18, 65		
Maxam and Gilbert method, see also sequencing	A28	- tRNA, hotspot	A53
		Mobility retardation	159
Maximum temperature overshoot, see also thermocycler	262	Molar extinction coefficient (E$_m$)	221
		Molecular weight	244-247
MDV-1 RNA, see also Qß-replicase	269	- marker	62, 113
MeHgOH, see also RT-PCR	96, 107	- Boehringer V	114
Melting domain, see also DGGE	159	- Boehringer VI	114
Melting temperature (Tm)	4, 6, 10, 11, 15, 35, 54, 55, 56	- Clontech	114
		Molecule spacer, see also primer	233
		Mononuclear cell, isolation	71
Mercaptoethanol	54, 96, 91, 92, A64	Mouse major histocompatibility complex class-I gene	216
MERRF	A50, A51	Mouse mammary tumor virus	220
Metachromatic leukodystrophy	A44	mRNA	99, 100, 101, 193
Metal block PCR machine, see also thermocycler	260	- cDNA hybrid	100, 109
Methanobacterium thermoautotrophicum	245	- poly(A)-	91
Methyl green	131	- selective amplification	105
Methylase	137	- transcript	104

mtDNA	A51	dynabeads and sequencing	171, 181
- deletion	A50, A53	Nested PCR	5, 35, 56, 61, 171, 192, A18, A19
- point mutation	A50, A53		
Mucus-lysis	74		
Multidrug resistance gene (MDR)	99, 105		
Multiple sclerosis	A19	neu oncogene	A13
Mung bean nuclease	187	Neuroborreliosis, see also Borrelia burgdorferi	A15
Muscular dystrophies	A63		
Mutagenesis, see also site-directed mutagensis and in-vitro Mutagenesis	136	Neuromuscular disease, molecular genetics	A48
		NH_4Cl	69, 70, 71
- primer	A60, A61	Nitrogen	A9
- site-directed	216, A60	Non-biotinylated strand	170, 171, 173, 177
Mutagenicity	99		
Mutanolysin	73	Non-bound biotin	241
Mutated allele	38	Non-denaturing polyacrylamide gel	163
Mutation	137	Non-Hodgkin's lymphoma	A11, A13
- site	A60, A61	Nonidet P-40 (NP40)	53, 91
MVR, see minisatellite variant repeat		Northern blot	99
Mycobacteria		Nuclease	82
- culture	74	Nuclease activity	84, 92
- disruption	76	Nuclease protection assay	99
- DNA, preparation	74, 79	Nuclease-free bovine serum albumin	141
- genome	145	Nucleic acid isolation	68
- genome-multiplex PCR	145	Nucleic acid sequence based amplification (NASBA)	268
Mycobacterium (M.) tuberculosis	74, 143, 247, 265		
- primer	146	OD, see optical density	84
Mycoplasma pneumoniae	45	OD_{260}, see also optical density	12, 25, 221
Myoclonic epilepsy with ragged red fibers (MERRF) disease	A48	Oil overlay	4, 13, 51
		OLIGO program	221
Myosin heavy-chain gene	144	$Oligo(dT)_{12-18}$	101, 108
		$Oligo(dT)_{15}$	107, 108
N-Acetyl-L-Cystein (NALC), see also Mycobacteria	73	Oligodeoxynucleotide, antisense	A27
N-hydroxy-succimido biotin, see also biotin	240	Oligomer extension assay	191
N-lauryl sarcosine	121	Oligonucleotide	1, 9, 12, 221
N-octylglucoside	53		
Na-acetate	86	- 3'end biotin labelling	237
Na-citrate	68	- 3'end complementarity	223, 224
NADH dehydrogenase	A48, A49	- 3'modification	238
NAP5 column	241	- 5'-end biotin labelling	242
NASBA, see also self-sustained sequence replication (3SR)	268	- 5'-end labelling	240
		- chemical labelling	236
Nasopharyngeal carcinoma	A26, A27	- chemical modification	233
Negative control DNA	62	- concentration	221
NENSORB 20 column	241	- hybridization, TMACl buffer	154
Neodymium-iron-boron magnet, see also		- labelling	234

- length	224	PCR (Polymerase chain reaction)	
- melting temperature	221	- additives	26, 51, 55,
- purification	226		56, 57, 58,
- anion-exchange column	232		66
- gel electrphoresis	227	- Alu amplification	189, 190
- reverse-phase HPLC	229	- amplification of specific alleles	
- radio-labelled	236	(PASA)	34, 35, 149
- synthesis	224	- efficiency	57
OligoPak	231, 232	- artifact	10
Oncogene, expression	201	- booster	41
Ophthalmoplegia, chronic progressive		- by-product	34, 61, 259
external (CPEO)	A49	- cDNA fragment, direct sequencing	A6
Optical density (OD)	84, 221	- competitive	37, 202
Optimal annealing temperature (T_{opt})	221	- contamination	61
Organic phase	93	- diagnostic	63
Oropharyngeal mucosa	73	- differential	36
Osmium tetroxide reaction	157	- expression	40
Outer fragment PCR, see also nested PCR	5, 36, 56,	- fragment, cloning	A6
	A60	- generated site-directed mutant	217
Overlap extension	216	- grade	61, 63, 64,
Overnight culture of bacteria	212		82, 83
P53 gene	164	- inactivation	66
PAGE gel, see also polyacrylamide gel	39, 126,	- inhibition	13, 69
	226	- inverse (IPCR)	136, 139,
- autoradiography	126		184, 185,
- electrophoresis	129		186,
- formamide loading buffer	128	- jumping	64
- radioactive-labeled amplification		- mispriming	A61
products	126	- multiplex	36, 143,
- silver stain	131		144, 147
Pancreatic DNase I	103	- annealing time	145
Paraffin	52	- cosolvent	145
Paraffin embedded tissue	52, 53, 76,	- hot start set-up strategy	144
	85, 219,	- primer concentration	144
	A39, A41	- primer design	144
- and formaline fixed tissue	A39, A41	- sensitivity	144
Paraformaldehyde	52, 219	- single-copy gene	144
Paramagnetic beads, see also beads,		- mutagenesis	216, A60,
dynabeads	170		A61
- automated seperation	180	- oligonucleotide	216, A61
Paramagnetic particles	269	- nested one-tube	65
PASA, see PCR amplification of specific		- nested two-tube	65
alleles		- one-tube nested	35, 36
PBS buffer, see also phosphate buffered		- optimization	22, 185
saline	70, 81, 96	- panhandle	15, 37,
			191, 192

- post PCR contamination	18, 65	- RNA grade	93
- preparative	22, 26	- chloroform extraction	54, 79, 81, 85, 88
- plateau-phase	206		
- product	66	- chloroform/isoamyl alcohol	86
- biotinylated	173	Phenylketonuria	38
- quantification	25, 37, 40, 63, 201, 202, 219	Philadelphia chromosome	A12
		Phosphatase labeled antidigoxigenin Fab fragment	A38
- reaction		Phosphate buffered saline, see also PBS	96, 219
- buffer	7, 18	Phosphoramidite	
- sensitivity	62	- biotin	233
- specificity	62	- deoxyribonucleoside ß-cyanoethyl	225
- times	261	Photoactivable biotin reagent (PAB), see also biotin	236
- volume	4, 13		
- recombinant circle (RCPCR)	217	Phylogenetic marker molecules	
- reverse transcriptase (RT-PCR)	91, 99, 100, 105-110, A34	- 16SrRNA	A56
		- 23SrRNA	A56
		- ATP synthase subunit	A56
- SSCP	164	- RNA polymerase	A56
- set-up	16	Phylogenetic tree	A57
- single-strand conformation polymorphism (PCR-SSCP)	163	Picornavirus	44
		Piperidine	156, 157
- synthesis of double-stranded probe	30	Pipetting error	64, 90, 181
- synthesis of single-stranded probe	30	Pipetting robot	180
- touchdown	223	Plasma	76
PDH, see pyruvate dehydrogenase gene		- falciparum	45, 269
PEG	56, 57, 58	Plastic capillary	261
Peltier elements, see also thermocycler	260	Plasticware	90
Penicillin G	A17, A15	Plateau effect of PCR amplification	7
Peptide sequence	37, 38	Pneumocystis carinii	45
Peripheral blood cell	51, 68	Point mutation	37, 38, 149, 171
Peripheral blood lymphocyte, RNA preparation	A63	PolI	244
Pfu DNA polymerase	245, 250, 251, 252	PolIII	244
		Poly(A)-tail	101, 193, 198
- 3'-5'-exonuclease activity	250		
- 5'-3' DNA polymerase activity	250	- tract	104, 193
- annealing temperature	250	Poly-D-lysine	A39
- fidelity	250	Polyacrylamide gel	159
- salt concentration	250	- electrophoresis (PAGE)	39, 125, 164
Phast system	159		
Phenol	53, 54, 73, 83, 89, 91, 140, 187	- linear-gradient	159
		- slab gel format	168
		Polyethylene glycol	56
- extraction	91, 92, 94, 188	Polymerase	
		- activity	9, 244, 246

- Bst	252		210
- DNA sequencing	252	- dye-labeled	169, 174
- fidelity	252	- flanking	A60
- polymerization rate	252	- dimer	10, 24, 41, 223
- Deep Vent DNA	249	- dissociation	6
- Taq polymerase, see Taq polymerase		- elongation	2
Polymerization	244	- extension	6, 184, 185
- activity	101, 245	- specificity	101
- rate	246	- extension kinetics	203
Polymorphism	6	- gene-specific	108
Polymorphnuclear leucocyte	69	- adapter	197
Porphyrin compounds	52, 69	- hemi-specific	189
Positive control sample	25	- hexanucleotide	A6
Positive displacement pipet	63, 64, 82	- hybrid	195
Post-PCR		- junction	105, 106
- cross-contamination	62, 64	- junction and annealing	105
- sample handling	63	- M13	5, A6, A10
- sample loading	116	- M13 reverse	174
- sterilization	66	- M13 universal fluorescent sequencing	170
Pre-PCR	18, 65	- M13 universal sequencing	171
- equipment	64	- mismatched	37
- lab	64	- mispairing	A50, A51
Preamplification heating	41	- modification	35
Prehybridization	121	- mutant	216
Preparation, mini-prep DNA	212	- nested, see also nested PCR	26, 30, 35, 41, 56, 191
Primary aliphatic amine group	233, 238	- NNNNNN-adapter	195
Primer	1, 2, 9-13, 15-18, 26, 136, 137, 139, 170, 193, 196	- nonspecific	24, 191
		- oligo(dT)-adapter	108, 194, 195
- adaptor	193, 195, 196	- oligomerization	247
- annealing	1, 2, 9, 11, 15, 55, 105, 203	- overlapping	210
		- radioactively labelled	156
		- random	A5
		- secondary structure	55, 56
- site	2, 14	- self-annealing	41
- temperature	11	- sequence	37, 38, 42, 43, 44
- blocking-primer for PCR	170	- specificity	25
- carryover	26, 27	- target-hybrid	154
- competition	37	- internal mismatch	154
- concentration	12, 15, 24, 193, 221		
- consensus	40	- melting-temperature	154
- design	35, 104, 106, 203,	- template annealing	57
		- T_M-value	203

- universal	37, A60, A61	- buffer	A34, A61 86
- walking	190, 191	- method, PCR-adapted	84
- 21M13	177, 178, A6	- phenol-chloroform extraction	88
		Proteobacteria	A58
- 3'specific	196	Proto-oncogene	A1
Priming site	1	Pseudogene, processed	102, 103
Probe		Psoralene	66
- antisense	154	PT7-MDV-poly plasmid, see also Qß-replicase	269
- biotinylated	A42		
- capture	37	Pulsed field gel electrophoresis	A65
- double stranded	A37	Pyrimidine dimer	65, 66
- dsDNA	A38, A42	Pyrococcus furiosus	245, 246, 250
- in vitro amplification	A37		
- labelling, nonradioactive	8	Pyronine B	131
- purification	A39	Pyrophosphate	244
- quality	A39	Pyrophosphorolysis	169
- single stranded	A37	Pyruvate dehydrogenase gene (PDH)	57, 58, 88, 102, 105
- synthesis	26, 27		
- synthesis of dsDNA	A39		
- yield	A39	Q-beta replicase	
Processivity, see also polymerases	8, 246, 247	- double-stranded RNA	268
Product analysis	24, 25	- one-enzyme reaction	269
- nonspecific	58, 141, 190	- single stranded RNA	268
		Quantification of PCR-products (QPCR)	25, 37, 63, 201, 202, 203, 219
Promotor region	A65		
Proofreading activity, see also polymerase	8, 37, 41, 137, 149, 248, 254, 255	- 5'-end labeling	204
		- system	63
Prostate cell lines	A10	RACE, see rapid amplification of cDNA ends	
Prostate-specific antigen (PSA)	A5	Radiolabelling	8
Prostatic carcinoma	A4	Ramp time, see also thermoprofile	16, 23, 180
Protamine sulfate	52	Random	
Protease	54, 87, 147, 210, 213	- amplified polymorphic DNA	40
		- hexa-oligodeoxynucleotide	A27
		- hexamer sequence	195
Protein		- hexanucleotide	101, 109, A4, A9
- denaturation	53, 93		
- disulfide bond	91	- mutagenesis, see also mutagenesis	216, 217, A61, A62
- purification of recombinant	210		
Proteinase K	53, 54, 74, 76, 77, 82, 85, 87, 88, 220, A16, A21, A23,	- nicking	185
		RAPD	40
		RAPD marker	40
		Rapid amplification of cDNA ends (RACE)	37, 108, 193, 194,

			195, 196, 197
ras		- XhoI	139
- mutations	A1	- XhoII	138
- oncogen	A1	- digested vector DNA	217
- proto-oncogene	153, 164	- endonucleolytic cleavage	136
rDNA	99, A1	- enzyme	
- amplification	A58	- activity	140, 141, 189
- cloning	A57	- analysis	A28
Reamplification	A57	- buffer	186
Recloning	26, 27, 29	- recognition sequence	193
Recognition	A60, A61	- DNA contamination	63
- sequence	137, 139, 185	- fragment	139, 191, 192, 193
- site	136-139	- analysis	136, A21
Recombinant RNA	269	- length polymorphism (RFLP)	38
Red blood cell	69	- map	185
Red blood cell lysis buffer	69	- modification system	137, 138
Repetitive DNA sequence	39, 253, 255	- site	39, 66, 136, 137, 139, A60
Replication factor	201	- sites, flanking sequences	208
Reproducibility of results	22, 62	Retroviral RNase H	267
Respiratory chain enzyme complex	A49	Reverse	
Restriction		- M13 fluorescent sequencing primer	170
- analysis, see also endonucleases	137, 140, A19	- M13 sequencing primer	171
- digestion	139, 140, 188	- transcriptase	91, 100, 109, A64
- reaction buffer	140, 188	- activity	101, 246
- endonuclease, see also endonucleases	136, 137, 139, 206, A61	- AMV	101, 267, A4, A6, A9
		- buffer	107, 196, 197
- cleavage site	139	- DNA contamination	63
- Bam HI	138, 216	- endogenous RNase H activity	267, 268
- BclI	138	- MoMLV	101, 107, 196-197
- BglII	138		
- BstEII	242	- optimal conditions	100-101
- EcoRI	138, 139, 216	Reverse transcription	91, 96, 100-102, 106-108, 193, 195, A27
- HindIII	139, 209		
- NaeI	A50		
- NcoI	211	- amount	108
- SacI	139, 209	- components	196, 197
- SalI	139, 209	- efficiency	100
- SauIIIa	138, A19	- oligo dT	101, 109
- XbaI	139, 209		

- priming	101	- template	101
- random hexanucleotides	101, 109	- template, secondary structure	107
- specific	101, 109	- transcript	91, 105
Reverse-phase chromatography	227	- yield	100
RFLP, see restriction fragment length polymorphism		RNase	90, 103
		RNase activity	90
Rhipicephalus sanguineus	A34, A35	- inhibitor, see RNasin	
Rhodamine, see also primer, dye	204, 205, 226	- free DNase I	103
		- free DNase I treatment	102, 103
Rhodamine-amidite	233	- H activity	100
Rhodobacter capsulatus	A58	RNasin	91, 108, 109, 196, 197, A34
Ribonuclease	90, 155		
- endogenous activity	93		
Ribosomal RNA		Robotic workstation	63, 180
- 16SrRNA	A57	Rotavirus	45
- 23SrRNA	A57	ROX, see also sequencing primer	174, 177
- 5SrRNA	A57	RT buffer, see also reverse transcriptase	107, 196, 197
RNA			
- 12Sr	A50	RT-PCR, selective	102
- 16Sr	A51, A57	RTth reverse transcriptase	250
- aggregation, non-specific	93		
- degradation	91, 100, 107	S-adenosylmethionine	138
		S_1 nuclease	187
- dependent DNA polymerase	100, 268	Saline buffer	52
- DNA hybrids	156	Salmon sperm DNA	119, 264, A37
- extraction	69, 71, 81		
- genome	99	Salt solution, balanced	72
- hydrolysis	90, 93	Sample	
- isolation	90, A4, A8	- DNA content	14
- isolation, quick	96	- degradation, see also degradation	68
- leakage	201	- homogeneity	14, 23
- maximum solubility	93	- preparation	68
- pellet	91, 94, 95	- storage	68, 84
- poly(A)$^+$	105, 108, 196, 197	Sanger's enzymatic sequencing method, see also sequencing	169
- polymerase	244	Sarcosyl	53, 92
- preparation	94, 100, 102, 104	Satellite repetitive DNA	39
		Scanning autoradiographs	27
- procedures	90	Scintillation counting	27
- quantification	102	SDS, see sodium dodecyl sulfate	
- quantity, in vivo	201	Selective mRNA, amplification	106
- sample	103, 106	Selective transcript amplification	106
- sample, DNA contamination	102, 105	Self sustained 3SR RNA transcription	267
- secondary structure	96, 100, 101	Selfpriming	24
		Semiquantitative	
- SSCP	164	- fluorescence analysis	25

- gel analysis	113	- fragment, generation	169
Sense probe	154	- template	169
Sep-Pak C18 column	235	Site-directed mutagenesis, restriction enzymes	216
Sephadex column (G-50)	235		
Sephadex G-25 spin column	238	Site-directed mutagenesis, see also mutagenesis	216, A60, A62
Sequenase			
- DNA polymerase	171, 174, 181	Slot blot procedure, see also hybridization	99, 119
- dye-primer sequencing kit	174	Soaking process	119
- 3'-5'exonuclease activity	169	Sodium acetate	83, 93, 103, 104
- polymerization	169		
- processivity	169	Sodium chloride	54, 83
Sequence		Sodium citrate	92
- dependent mobility	159	Sodium desoxycholate	53
- polymorphism	38, 39	Sodium diatrizoate	71
Sequencer	171	Sodium dodecyl sulfate (SDS)	53, 54, 56, 82, 91, 94, 140
Sequencing	36, 191		
- androgen-receptor,	A7		
- automated DNA	176, 180	Sodium hypochlorite	66
- binding buffer	172, 176	Solid phase-bound capture probe	40
- gel	176, 205	Solid-phase	170
- primer	5	Solid tissue, see also biopsy	76, 88
- reaction, see also primer	8, 34	- hybridization system	204
Serum	62, 76, 81, 87	- sequencing	171, 174, 176
Sheep antidigoxigenin Fab-alkaline phosphatase	A39	- synthesis of oligonucleotides	224
		Sonication	77
Sickle ßS-globin genotypes	265	Southern blot	15, 24, 26, 117
Sickle-cell (β^S) sequence	153		
Sickle-cell disease	38	- hybridization, see also hybridization	185
Silane	88, 89	- denaturing buffer	117
Silicate-based controlled pore glass (CPG)	224	- neutralization buffer	118
Siliconization	228	SP6 polymerase promotor sequence	164, 265
Silver stain	39, 131, 159	Specific hybridization probe	A58
		Specific primer	101, 189, 193, 195
- of denaturing PAGE	133		
Single base change	149	Specific product	190
- detection	149	Specific transcript	99
Single copy		Sputum	51, 73, 74
- DNA	39	SSCP analysis, see also single-strand conformation polymorphism	164, A65
- gene	102, 202		
- PCR amplification	36	SSCP, PCR single-strand conformation polymorphism (PCR-SSCP)	163
- base point mutation	265, 268		
Single-stranded conformation polymorphism (SSCP)	165	ssDNA	
		- DIG probe	A42
Single-stranded DNA	34, 36	- probe	A42

A 93

- probe, synthesis	A39	- concentration	7, 51
SSPE	155, 173	- degradation	75
Staggered end of oligonucleotides	185, 187	- DNA contamination	63
Stained gel		- error rate	245, A6, A62
- photography	113		
- UV illumination	113	- exonuclease activity	16
Sticky-end cloning procedure	208, 242	- fidelity	9, 245, 248, A61
Stoffel buffer	9, 19, 247		
Stoffel fragment	14, 247	- half life	4, 8, 55
Strand-displacement activity, see also		- inhibition	53
polymerases	248	- primer-target mismatch	151
Strand-separation	203	- polymerization	9
Stratalinker, see also UV-irradiation	118	- recombinant	246
Streptavidin bridges, see also biotin	173	- recombinant	55
- magnetic bead	168	Taq dye primer cycle sequencing kit	177
Structural-protein-coding gene	39	Target	
Subcloning, ligase-free	209	- amplification	203
Substrate competition	37	- DNA	202, 203, 204
Succinate-ubiquinone oxidoreductase	A49		
Sulfolobus acidocaldarius	245	- gene	36
Sulfolobus solfataricus	245	- primer	190, 191
Sulfolobus species	245	TAS, reverse transcriptase	265
Supernatant of sequencing procedure	173, 176	TBE buffer	187
Synthesis rate of Taq polymerase	8	TE buffer	84, 86, 87, 188
Synthetase	244		
		Telomere	39
T4 DNA ligase, see also ligase	187, 208, 212, 265	TEMED	125, 161, 176
T4 DNA polymerase	244, 254	Temperature	
T4 polynucleotide kinase	234	- accuracy	262
T7 polymerase promotor sequence	164	- controlling	262
T7 RNA polymerase	208, 267	- optimum (T_{opt})	246
T7-RNA polymerase binding sequence	265	- uniformity	262
Tailing	198	Template secondary structure	55
TAMRA, see also primer and sequencing	174, 177	Terminal deoxynucleotidyl transferase (TdT)	237
Tandem repeat region	39, 253	Termination reaction	175
Taq DNA polymerase	4-7, 14, 16, 19, 26, 54, 91, 109, 137, 169, 171, 245, 247	Tetramethyl ammonium chloride, see TMACl-solution	
		Tetrazol	225
		Thermal	
		- conductivity	262
		- cycling	3, 4, 16, 23
Taq DNA polymerase, activity	53-57, 69, 247	- mass	262
- bound to the DNA	208		
- buffer	247		

Thermocycler	2, 13, 18, 19, 64
- air	259, 261
- cooling rate	260
- metal blocks	259
- microwaves	259
- temperature homogeneity	259
- water	259
- well-comparability	259
- well-to-well uniformity	259
Thermoplasma acidophilum	245
Thermoprofile	5
- irridation distance	66
- irridation time	66
- light	64
- sensitivity	65
- transillumination	139, 140
Thermococcus litoralis	208, 245, 247, 248
Thermostability	
Thermus	
- aquaticus, see Taq polymerase	
- flavus	208, 245, 246, 254
- ruber	245
- thermophilus	101, 245, 264
- thermophilus DNA polymerase	250
- 5'-3' exonuclease activity	250
- extension rate	250
- half-life	250
- RT activity	250
Thesit	54
Thermus thermophilus DNA polymerase,	
Thin-walled reaction tube	261
Thiol group	226, 233
Tissue	
- adherence	219
- biopsies, RNA-Isolation, see also biopsy	A4
- DNA	
- homogenizer	64
Tm, see melting temperature	
TMACl solution	154
Toluidine blue	131
Toxoplasma gondii	45

Transcription	201
- activitiy	201
- buffer	267
Transcription-based amplification system see TAS	
Translocation	99
Trc promotor	211
Tricine	54
Triethyl ammonium acetate solution (TEAA)	230
Trifluoroacetic acid (TFA)	233
Tris-HCl	54, 107
Tris-saturated phenol	83
Triton-X-100	53, 69, 172
Trityl cartridge minicolumn	226
Trityl-off synthesis, see also primer synthesis	238
Truncation product	25
Tth pol, see also Taq polymerase	101, 250
Ubiquinol-cytochrome c oxidoreductase	A49
Ultrafree-MC unit	241
Ultrasonication	76
Universal promoter sequence	40
Uracil N-glycosylase (UNG)	8, 66
Urea	127, 176
Urine	51, 76
UV	
- crosslink	118
- damage	65, 66
- inactivity	65
	246, 248
- DNA polymerase	249
Vacuum centrifuge	64
Vanadyl-ribonucleoside complex (VCR)	91
Varizella zoster	43
Vector	136, 208, A61
Vent DNA polymerase	208, 248, 249, 254
- proof-reading activity	A61
Vent-(exo-)DNA polymerase	248, 249
Viral	
- disease	99
- DNA	79, 87, 265
- gene	201
- replication	201

Visna virus	219	Wobble base	224
Water bath, contamination, see also		Wobble primer	224
thermocycler	260	X-chromosome	A65
- temperature transfer	261	Xylene	77, 85, 86
Well-to-well		Xylene cyanol	129
- comparability	262		
- uniformity	262	Y chromosome	A37-A39, A42
Western blot (WB)	214, A18, A20		
Wild-type		Zamboni's fixative	52
- DNA	155, 162	Zenker's fixative	52
- probe	162		
- sequence	A61		

Printing: Mercedesdruck, Berlin
Binding: Buchbinderei Lüderitz & Bauer, Berlin